# HERNIA SURGERY
# Simplified

**System requirement:**

- Operating System: Windows XP or above
- Web Browser: Internet Explorer 8 or above, Google Chrome, Mozilla Firefox and Safari
- Essential plugins: Java and Flash player
  - Facing problems in viewing content—it may be your system does not have Java enabled.
  - If videos do not show up—it may be the system requires Flash player or need to manage Flash setting.
  - You can test Java and Flash by using the links from the troubleshoot section of the CD/DVD.
  - Learn more about Flash setting from the link in the troubleshoot section.

**Accompanying DVD-ROM is playable only in Computer and not in DVD player.**

CD/DVD has Autorun function—it may take few seconds to load on your computer. If it does not work for you, then follow the steps below to access the contents manually:

- Click on my computer
- Select the CD/DVD drive and click open/explore—this will show list of files in the CD/DVD
- Find and double click file—"launch.html".

# DVD CONTENT

**Hernia Repair with Prolene Mesh Implant**

(This video does not have voice over)

# HERNIA SURGERY
# Simplified

**Sachin Kuber** MS (General Surgeon)
Director (Panel Surgeon)
Oyster and Pearl Hospital, Pune, Maharashtra, India
Rajiv Gandhi Medical University, Karnataka, India
Sanjeevan Hospital, Pune, Maharashtra, India
Yashada Hospital, Pune, Maharashtra, India

JAYPEE BROTHERS MEDICAL PUBLISHERS (P) LTD
New Delhi • London • Philadelphia • Panama

**Jaypee Brothers Medical Publishers (P) Ltd.**

**Headquarters**
Jaypee Brothers Medical Publishers (P) Ltd.
4838/24, Ansari Road, Daryaganj
New Delhi 110 002, India
Phone: +91-11-43574357
Fax: +91-11-43574314
**Email: jaypee@jaypeebrothers.com**

**Overseas Offices**

J.P. Medical Ltd.
83, Victoria Street, London
SW1H 0HW (UK)
Phone: +44-2031708910
Fax: +02-03-0086180
**Email: info@jpmedpub.com**

Jaypee-Highlights Medical Publishers Inc.
City of Knowledge, Bld. 237, Clayton
Panama City, Panama
Phone: + 507-301-0496
Fax: + 507- 301-0499
**Email: cservice@jphmedical.com**

Jaypee Brothers Medical Publishers Ltd.
The Bourse
111 South Independence Mall East
Suite 835, Philadelphia, PA 19106, USA
Phone: + 267-519-9789
**Email: joe.rusko@jaypeebrothers.com**

Jaypee Brothers Medical Publishers (P) Ltd.
17/1-B, Babar Road, Block-B, Shaymali
Mohammadpur, Dhaka-1207
Bangladesh
Mobile: +08801912003485
**Email: jaypeedhaka@gmail.com**

Jaypee Brothers Medical Publishers (P) Ltd.
Shorakhute, Kathmandu
Nepal
Phone: +00977-9841528578
**Email: jaypee.nepal@gmail.com**

Website: www.jaypeebrothers.com
Website: www.jaypeedigital.com



**Inquiries for bulk sales may be solicited at:** jaypee@jaypeebrothers.com



***Hernia Surgery Simplified***

*First Edition:* **2013**

ISBN: 978-93-5025-949-8

*Printed at Ajanta Offset & Packagings Ltd., New Delhi*

**Dedicated to**

*My mother*
*Late Mrs Anjali Bhaskar Kuber*

*My father*
*Mr Bhaskar D Kuber*

*My better half*
*Dr (Mrs) Mugdha Sachin Kuber*

*My teacher*
*Dr Laxmikant Shah*

# PREFACE

It is my great pleasure to introduce to you, all readers another marvel from M/s Jaypee Brothers Medical Publishers (P) Ltd, New Delhi, India, and me. The book *Hernia Surgery Simplified* is a totally new concept of book writing. This is very vast and complicated subject and any book written on this subject can never be perfect. As medical field is changing and evolving so fast, that to accomplish this information in a single book is too difficult to comply.

Here, we have come up with a short book explaining about the facts of hernia repair. The aim of the book is to present the latest techniques of hernia surgery prevalent today. We have tried to cover this huge subject in short but adequate manner. All the chapters contain new and relevant, useful techniques of various types of hernia repair. All the obsolete techniques are eliminated from the book. Our book also lets readers to know about the latest mesh products available in the market, to make them familiar.

Our outlook in writing the book is to make hernia surgery easy for learners, surgeons in a way that they will get the ready and useful information on this subject. To prepare a book in a handy manner is difficult than writing a huge book. We have compiled the latest techniques on hernia repair in the book. This will surely help the undergraduate and postgraduate students to understand what is happening in the medical and surgical field today.

It is our sincere attempt to put this valuable information on hernia surgery for your approval. We hope that this detailed book dedicated to hernia repair will be useful in updating the knowledge of the learners.

Sincerely, I thank M/s Jaypee Brothers Medical Publishers (P) Ltd, New Delhi, India, for giving me an opportunity to write the book.

**Sachin Kuber**

# CONTENTS

# Chapter 1

# Milestones in Hernia Surgery

## Introduction

Hernia is defined as an abnormal protrusion of viscus through normal openings in the body. Hernia is a quite common problem of today's civilization. It was very commonly known condition in ancient times too. Before going to the vast intricate details of the hernia and its surgery we will take a brief look at the milestones of hernia surgery. How near perfect surgery has evolved in these recent years and the creditors of this surgery is worth noticing.

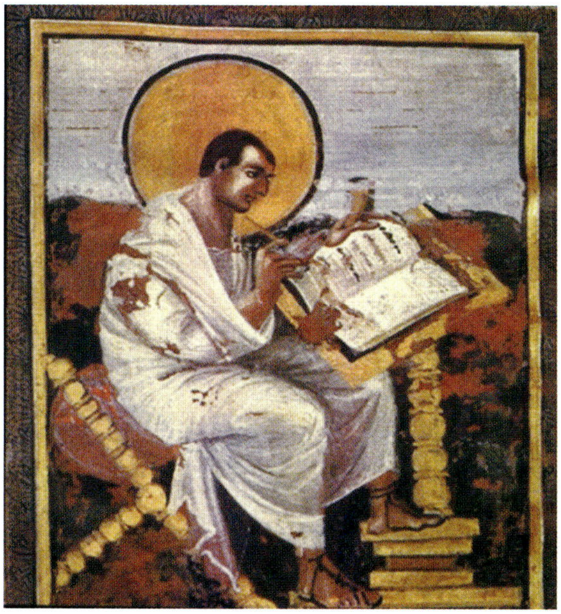

**Fig. 1.1:** Paul of Aegina in 700 AD—complete ligature of sac

1. First record of hernia condition: 1500 BC By Greeks.
2. First surgery of inguinal hernia: First century AD by Celsus involved excision of sac, testis, chord.
3. Paul of Aegina in 700 AD: Complete ligature of sac and cord at external ring (Fig. 1.1).
4. Guy de Chauliac in 1363 differentiated inguinal and femoral hernia.
5. Franco in 1556 described technique to repair the strangulated hernia to avoid injury to bowel (Fig. 1.2).
6. Casper Stromayr 1559 distinguished between direct and indirect hernia.
7. Early 19th century correct description of inguinal anatomy.
8. Dawn of modern surgery by Joseph Lister 1865 in relation with antiseptic use in surgery (Fig. 1.3).

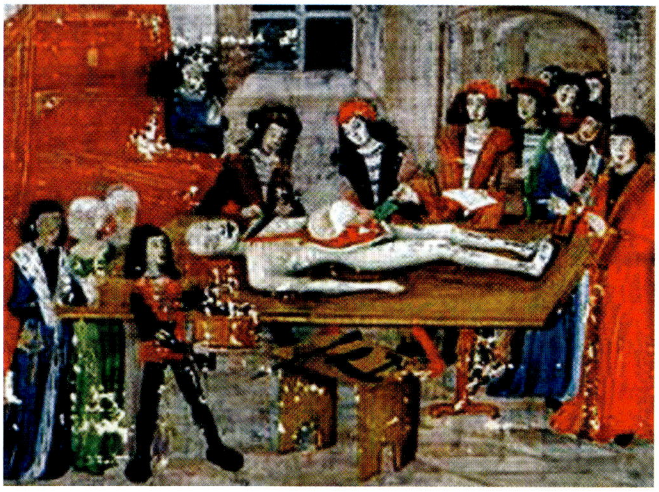

**Fig. 1.2:** Franco (1556) described technique to repair the strangulated hernia to avoid injury to bowel

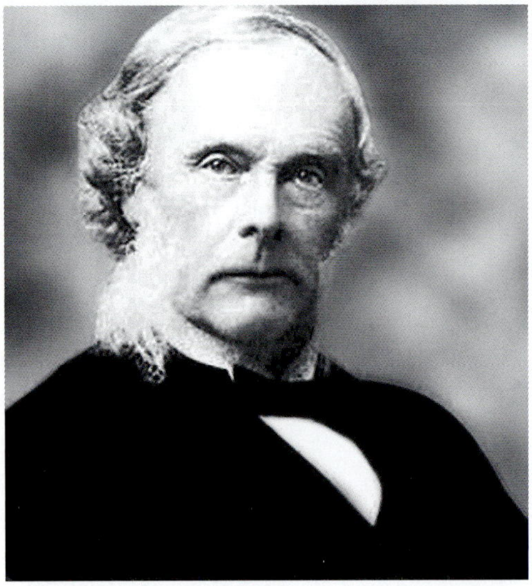

**Fig. 1.3:** Dawn of modern surgery by Joseph Lister 1865 in relation with antiseptic use in surgery

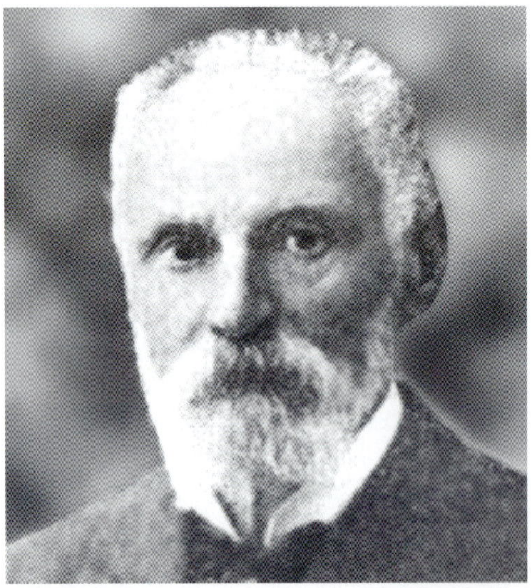

**Fig. 1.4:** Edoardo Bassini (1884) implemented repair of transversalis fascia and reinforcing the posterior wall of inguinal canal with interrupted silk sutures.He is called father of modern hernia surgery.It was a herniorrhaphy surgery

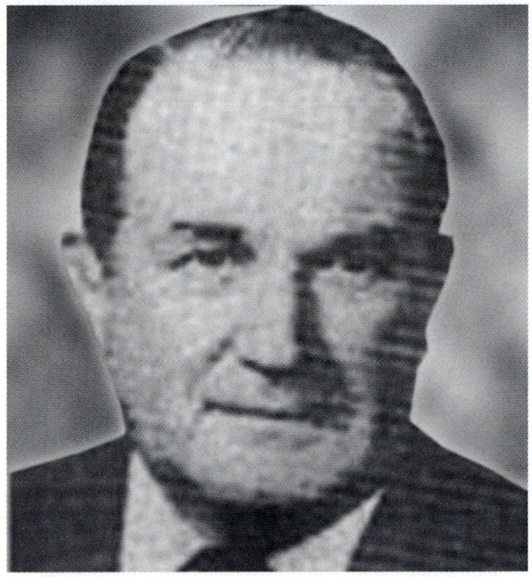

**Fig. 1.5:** Maingot (1941)—advocated floss silk for darning

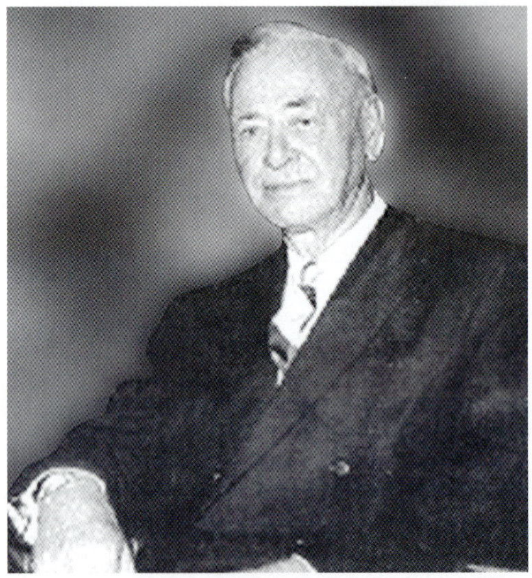

**Fig. 1.6:** Shouldice (1953)—multilayered repair by pure tissue repair

9. Marcy 1871 introduced antiseptic use in hernia surgery.
10. Lucas in 1881 opened external oblique aponeurosis and dissected sac.
11. Edoardo Bassini 1884 implemented repair of transversalis fascia and reinforcing the posterior wall of inguinal canal with interrupted silk sutures. He is called father of modern hernia surgery. It was a herniorrhaphy surgery (Fig. 1.4).
12. George Lotheissen 1898 restructured the inguinal hernia surgery by repairing the femoral ring and inguinal defects.
13. McArthur 1901 used pedicle strips of external oblique aponeurosis interlinked between conjoint tendon and inguinal ligament.
14. Kirschner 1910 used fascial grafts from thigh.
15. Handley 1918 invented "Darn and Staylace" procedure.

16. Ogilvie 1937 nonabsorbable silk lattice repair.
17. Maingot 1941 advocated Floss silk for darning (Fig. 1.5).
18. Melick 1942 used first time Braided, multifilament nylon for inguinal hernia.
19. Tanner 1942 Coined the SLIDE operation.
20. Shouldice 1953 multilayered repair by Pure tissue repair (Fig. 1.6).
21. Usher 1958 first used knitted polypropylene mesh in hernia repair.
22. In 1979 first attempt of laparoscopic hernia repair in inguinal region.
23. Gilbert 1984 described umbrella plug for inguinal hernia repair.
24. Read 1985 described relation between smoking and herniation.
25. Lichtenstein 1986 described the tension free repair of inguinal hernias.
26. Robbins and Rutkow 1990 coined the concept of introducing preformed mesh plug in hernia defect.
27. Schultz 1990 first used a synthetic prosthetic biomaterial in laparoscopic repair of an inguinal hernia.
28. LeBlanc 1991 describes the attempt of laparoscopic incisional hernia repair.
29. Popp 1991 described a method to dissect the peritoneum away from abdominal wall prior to the incision of the peritoneum in TAPP repair.

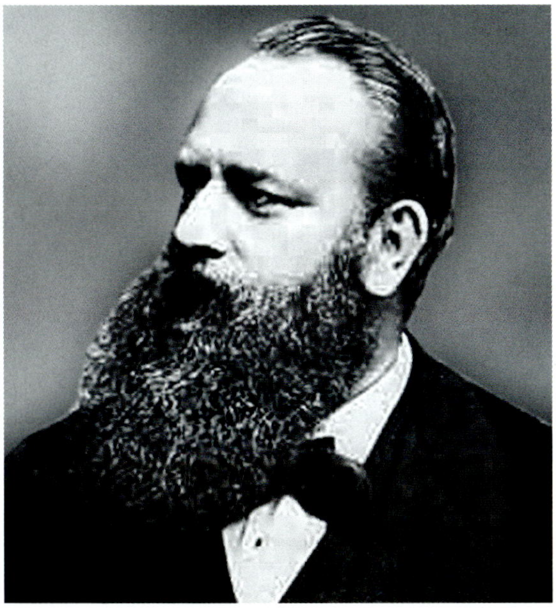

**Fig. 1.7:** Theodor Billroth (1878)—envisaged prostheses before Bassini's sutured cure (1887)

## At a Glance

Theodor Billroth (1878) envisaged prostheses before Bassini's sutured cure (1887) (Fig. 1.7). Phelps (1894) reinforced with silver coils. Metals were replaced by plastic (Aquaviva 1944). Polypropylene (Usher 1962), resisting infection, became popular. Usher instituted tensionless, overlapping preperitoneal repair. Spermatic cord was parietalized, to obviate keyholing. Stoppa (1969) championed the sutureless Cheatle-Henry approach encasing the peritoneum. His technique, "La grande prosthese de renforcement du sac visceral" (GPRVS), was adopted by laparoscopists. Newman (1980) and Lichtenstein (1986) pioneered subaponeurotic positioning. Kelly (1898) inserted a plug into the femoral canal; Lichtenstein and Shore (1974) followed. Gilbert (1987) plugged the internal ring, and Robbins and Rutkow (1993) treated all groin herniae thus. Incisional herniation has been controlled by prefascial, retrorectus prosthetic placement (Rives-Flament 1973). ePTFE (Sher et al. 1980) is useful intraperitoneally, since it evokes few adhesions. Here, laparoscopy (Ger 1982) is competitive. Beginning in 1964 (Wirtschafter and Bentley) experimental and clinical studies have shown herniation may be associated with aging and genetic or acquired (smoking, etc.) systemic disease of connective tissue. These data, with prospective trials, all but mandate tensionless prosthetic repair.

## History of the Procedure

Hippocrates used the Greek *hernios* for bud or bulge to describe abdominal hernias. Statues of the era portray this condition. The Ebers papyrus, from approximately 1550 BCE, detailed the use of a truss. Celsius used transillumination to differentiate a hernia from a hydrocele and advocated gradual pressure (taxis) in the management of incarcerated hernia. The earliest recorded surgical efforts were to reduce the hernia through a scrotal incision, to remove the sac and the testis, and to close the area with sutures that spontaneously extruded.

As the church forbade physicians from surgical procedures, nonphysicians (barbers) began developing therapy for surgical problems. De Chauliac advocated escharotics with gradual cicatrization accompanied by prolonged bed rest as the solution for inguinal hernias. Parë followed the operation of Gerald of Metz using a cerclage wire of gold to retard further intestinal protrusion into the scrotum.

In 1700, Littre reported an omphalomesenteric duct trapped in a hernia. Richter described an incarcerated but nonobstructing hernia in 1785. Hunter, in 1756, detailed the embryological origin of the indirect inguinal hernia. De Gimbernat advocated cutting the ligament that is eponymically associated with him in management of incarcerated femoral hernia. Teale reported the first prevascular femoral hernia in 1846.

Other eponyms associated with inguinal hernias relate to anatomical descriptions by Camper (fascia) (1801), Cooper (ligament) (1804), Cloquet (hernia) (1817), Grynfeltt (hernia) (1866), Hesselbach (triangle) (1814), Laugier (hernia) (1833), Nuck (canal) (1650-1692), Petit (hernia) (1783), and Scarpa (fascia) (1814). Scarpa also previously described a sliding hernia and a Spiegelian hernia in 1645.

The advent of antisepsis by Lister in 1865 paved the way for a more precise surgical approach to hernia. Finally, physicians could expect success of an operation not being disrupted by infection. In 1871, Marcy felt that closure of the fascia adjacent to the internal ring would provide a reliable repair of the inguinal hernia. Over a decade later, Bassini (1884) formulated an approach to hernia repair that remains the foundation of the modern hernia repair, namely, reconstruction of the floor of the inguinal canal. In the last century, Cheatle used a properitoneal approach in 1920, while McVay (1948) made popular the use of Cooper's iliopectineal ligament in repair.

Chapter 2

# Surgical Anatomy of Hernia Sites

## Surgical Anatomy of Hernia Sites

*"The anatomy of the inguinal region is misunderstood by surgeons of all levels of seniority." Robert E Condon, MD.*

Success of hernia repair is measured primarily by the permanence of the operation, fewest complications, minimal costs, and earliest return to normal activities. This success depends largely on the surgeon's understanding of the anatomy and physiology of the surgical area as well as a knowledge of how to use most effectively the currently available techniques and materials.

The surgeon who seeks to make a success of hernia repairs should fully understand the anatomical variations in the hernia site. Today it is mandatory for the surgeon to individualize the surgery according to the anatomy encountered.

### Anatomy of the Abdomen and Groin

Much of what we know about the anatomy of the abdomen and groin comes from the work of the early anatomists and surgeons. A thorough understanding of these and later anatomical "discoveries" is essential to successful hernia repair (Table 2.1).

*Original drawing:* Hesselbach's original (1814) drawing detailing the triangular area bordered by the deep

**Table 2.1**

| Anatomical discoveries | |
|---|---|
| Vesalius (Flemish) and Fallopius (Italy) Poupart (France) | Described the inguinal ligament |
| Heister | First to describe direct hernias (1724) |
| Pott (England) | Anatomy of congenital hernias; methods of incarceration |
| Camper (Holland) | Described the superficial subcutaneous fascia |
| Scarpa (Italy) | Described deep subcutaneous fascia; anatomic and surgical importance of sliding hernias (En Glissade) (1814) |
| Sir Ashley Cooper (England) | Described anatomy and surgical treatment of crural and umbilical hernias; anatomy of the groin including the superior pubic (Cooper) ligament; cremasteric fascia and the transversalis fascia |
| Hunter | Emphasized the role of the processus vaginalis |
| Morton | Described the conjoined tendon |
| Cloquet | Noted postnatal closure of the processus vaginalis; made observations of the iliopubic tract |
| Hesselbach (Germany) | Defined iliopubic tract; described importance of the medial triangle of the groin (included the femoral canal).; described the "corona mortis" (arterial circle formed by the deep epigastric and obturator arteries) |
| De Gimbernat | Described medial ligament of the femoral canal (lacunar ligament), and division of that ligament in the treatment of strangulated femoral hernias |
| Richter (Germany) | Described partial obstruction and incarceration of a wall of the bowel in a hernia defect |

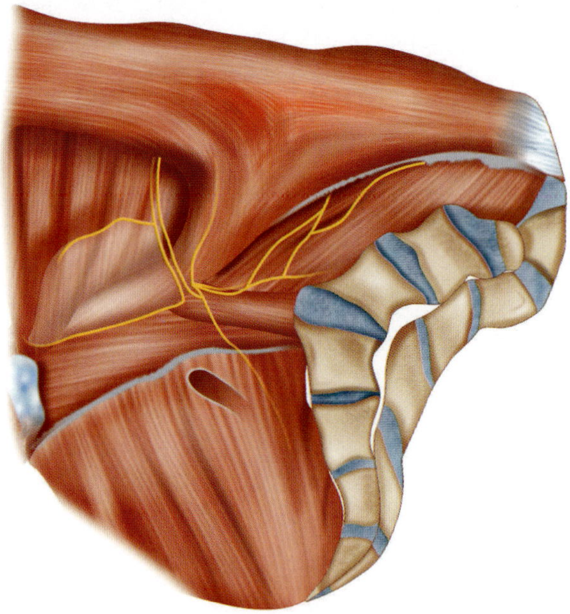

Fig. 2.1: Original drawing–Hesselbach's original (1814) drawing detailing the triangular area bordered by the deep epigastric vessels, the lateral border of the rectus muscle, and the superior pubic ligament (Cooper)

epigastric vessels, the lateral border of the rectus muscle, and the superior pubic ligament (Cooper) (Fig. 2.1).

*Current interpretation:* Current version of the Hesselbach's triangle substitutes the inguinal ligament for the superior pubic ligament (Fig. 2.2).

# External Anatomy of Abdominal Wall—The Surface Markings

## Anterior Abdominal Wall Anatomy

The anatomical layers of the abdominal wall include skin, subcutaneous tissue, superficial fascia, deep fascia, muscle, extraperitoneal fascia, and peritoneum. This anatomy may vary with respect to the different topographic regions of the abdomen. The major source of structural integrity and strength of the abdominal wall is provided by the musculofascial layer. The main paired abdominal muscles include the external oblique muscles, internal oblique muscles, transversus abdominis muscles, and rectus abdominis muscles and their respective aponeuroses, which are interdigitated with each other, and provide core strength and protection to the abdominal wall viscera. The integrity of the abdominal wall is essential not only to protect the visceral structures but also to stabilize the trunk and to aid trunk movement and posture.

### *Surface Anatomy*

The abdomen can be divided into quadrants or nine abdominal regions (Fig. 2.3). The midline in the sagittal plane is the linea alba. The lateral edge of the rectus sheath is the linea semilunaris. The lower costal margin, the iliac crest and pubic tubercle can be palpated.

*Surface lines:* For convenience of description of the viscera and of reference to morbid conditions of the

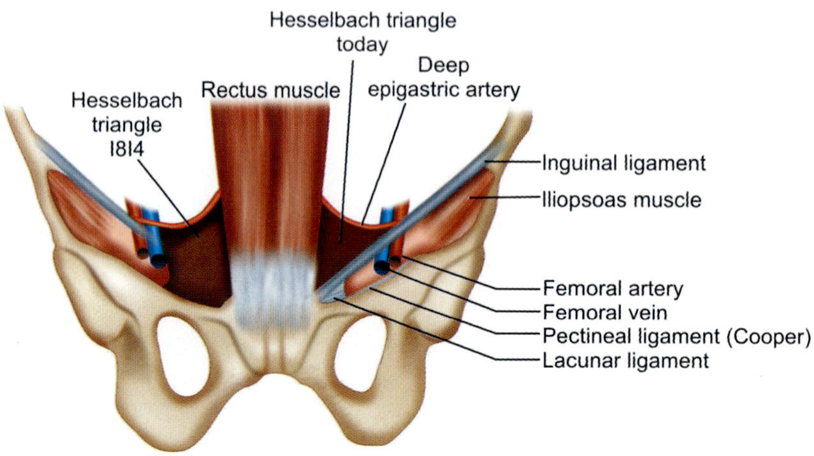


Fig. 2.2: Current interpretation–current version of the Hesselbach's triangle substitutes the inguinal ligament for the superior pubic ligament

contained parts, the abdomen is divided into nine regions, by imaginary planes, two horizontal and two sagittal, the edges of the planes being indicated by lines drawn on the surface of the body. In the older method the upper, or subcostal, horizontal line encircles the body at the level of the lowest points of the tenth costal cartilages; the lower, or intertubercular, is a line carried through the highest points of the iliac crests seen from the front, i. e. through the tubercles on the iliac crests about 5 cm behind the anterosuperior spines. An alternative method is that of Addison, who adopts the following lines:

(1) An upper transverse, the transpyloric, halfway between the jugular notch and the upper border of the symphysis pubis; this indicates the margin of the transpyloric plane, which in most cases cuts through the pylorus, the tips of the ninth costal cartilages and the lower border of the first lumbar vertebra; (2) a lower transverse line midway between the upper transverse and the upper border of the symphysis pubis; this is termed the transtubercular, since it practically corresponds to that passing through the iliac tubercles; behind, its plane cuts the body of the fifth lumbar vertebra.

By means of these horizontal planes the abdomen is divided into three zones named from above, the subcostal, umbilical, and hypogastric zones. Each of these is further subdivided into three regions by the two sagittal planes, which are indicated on the surface by a right and a left lateral line drawn vertically through points halfway between the anterosuperior iliac spines and the middle line. The middle region of the upper zone is called the epigastric, and the two lateral regions the right and left hypochondriac. The central region of the middle zone is the umbilical, and the two lateral regions the right and left lumbar. The middle region of the lower zone is the hypogastric or pubic, and the lateral are the right and left iliac or inguinal. The middle regions, viz., epigastric, umbilical, and pubic, can each be divided into right and left portions by the middle line. In the following description of the viscera the regions marked out by Addison's lines are those referred to.

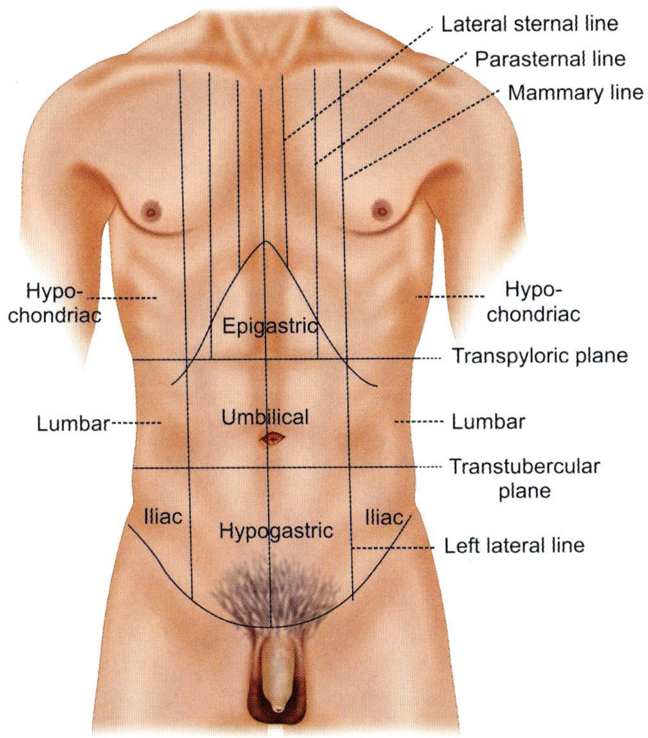


**Fig. 2.3:** Abdomen can be divided into quadrants or nine abdominal regions

## The Fascia

Below the skin the superficial fascia is divided into a superficial fatty layer, Camper's fascia, and a deeper fibrous layer, Scarpa's fascia. The deep fascia lies on the abdominal muscles. Inferiorly Scarpa's fascia blends with the deep fascia of the thigh. This arrangement forms a plane between Scarpa's fascia and the deep abdominal fascia extending from the top of the thigh to the upper abdomen (Figs 2.4A and B). Below the innermost layer of muscle, the transversus abdominis muscle, lies the transversalis fascia. The transversalis fascia is separated from the parietal peritoneum by a variable layer of fat, subcutaneous tissue.

### Superficial Fascia

The superficial fascia of the abdominal wall is divided into a superficial and a deep layer. It may be as thin as half an inch or less or as thick as 6 inches or more. Above the umbilicus, the superficial fascia consists of a single layer. Below the umbilicus, the fascia divides into two layers: the Camper fascia (a superficial fatty layer) and the Scarpa fascia (a deep membranous layer). The superficial epigastric neurovascular bundle is located between these two layers. The abdominal subcutaneous fat, which is separated by the Scarpa fascia, is highly variable in thickness.

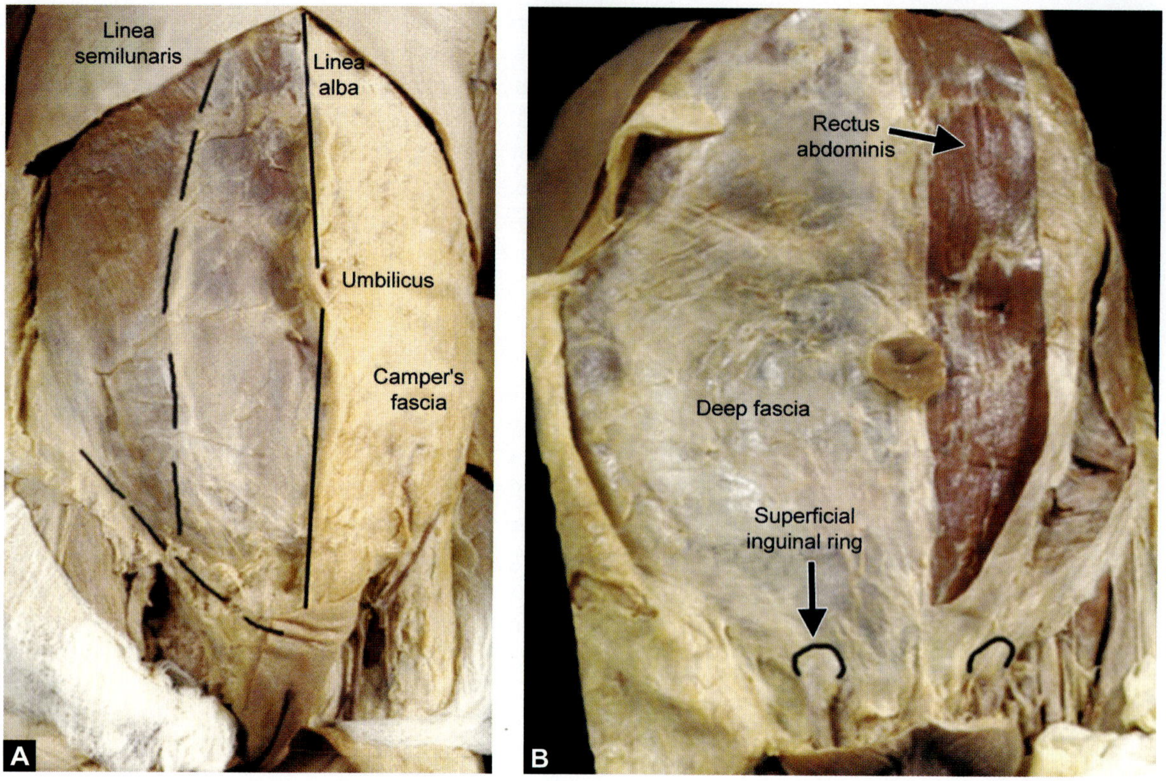


**Figs 2.4 and B:** Anterior abdominal wall in cadaveric dissection

### *Deep Fascia*

The deep fascia is a thin, tough layer that surrounds and is adherent to the underlying abdominal muscles. Each abdominal muscle has an aponeurotic component that contributes to the deep fascia. The individual abdominal muscles are described below:

### *Subserous and Peritoneal Fascia*

The subserous fascia is also known as extraperitoneal fascia and serves to bond the peritoneum to the deep fascia of the abdominal wall or to the outer lining of the gastrointestinal tract. It may receive different names depending on its location (i.e. transversalis fascia when it is deep to that muscle, psoas fascia when it is next to that muscle, iliac fascia, and so on). The peritoneum is a thin (one cell thick) membrane that lines the abdominal cavity. It is useful in reconstructive efforts because it provides a layer between the bowel and mesh.

## Rectus Abdominis and Rectus Sheath

The rectus muscle extends from the xiphoid process of the sternum and 5, 6, 7th costal cartilages to the pubic symphysis and pubic crest. The muscle is enclosed within the rectus sheath formed by the aponeuroses of the lateral abdominal muscles (Fig. 2.5). Along the length of this strap muscle there are three fibrous intersections separating the muscle into four segments. The fibrous intersections are attached to the anterior surface of the rectus sheath, but not to the posterior surface. This allows the superior and inferior epigastric vessels to pass along the posterior surface of the muscle without encountering a barrier.

The most important feature from the surgical perspective is that the fibers of the rectus sheath run from side-to-side. Vertical incisions divide fibers while horizontal incisions down closure with sutures encircling fibers rather that between fibers (Fig. 2.6).

The posterior rectus sheath has a similar trilaminar criss-cross pattern above the umbilicus, where it is composed of the posterior lamina of the internal oblique and the aponeurosis of the transverses abdominis muscle from either side.

## Lateral Muscles

The lateral muscles arise from the lower part of the rib cage, the lumbar fascia and the iliac crest.

The external oblique muscle arises from the lower eight ribs. The fibers run downwards and forwards to form an aponeurosis anteriorly. The aponeurosis passes anteriorly to the rectus muscle to insert into the aponeurosis from the other side at the linea alba. Inferiorly the aponeurosis inserts into the anterosuperior iliac spine and stretches over to the pubic tubercle, forming the inguinal ligament.

The internal oblique muscle arises from the lumbar fascia, the iliac crest and the lateral two-thirds of the inguinal ligament and runs upwards and forwards to form an aponeurosis. Above the arcuate line the aponeurosis splits to enclose the rectus muscle. Below the arcuate line the aponeurosis passes anterior to the rectus muscle. The inferior part of the aponeurosis inserts into the symphysis pubis. At this insertion the aponeurosis is fused with the aponeurosis of the transversus abdominis muscle to form the conjoint tendon.

The transversus abdominis muscle arises from the lower six costal cartilages, the lumbar fascia and the iliac crest. The fibers run forwards to form an aponeurosis. Superiorly the aponeurosis passes behind the rectus muscle. Below the arcuate line the aponeurosis passes anterior to the muscle. The inferior fibers of the aponeurosis are fused with those of the internal oblique to form the conjoint tendon.

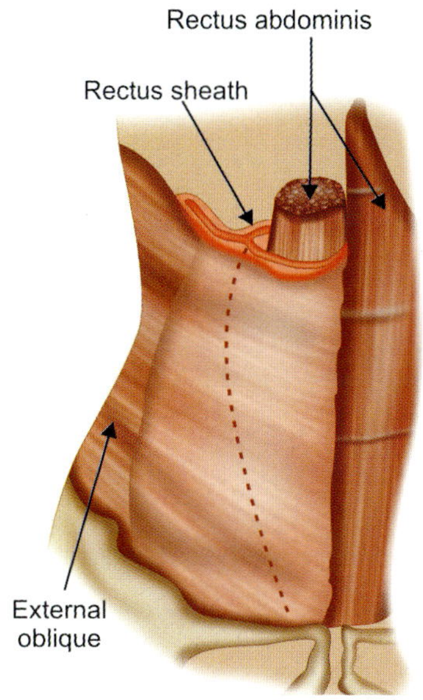


**Fig. 2.5:** Lateral abdominal wall muscles

## Musculofascial Layer

The abdominal wall includes 5 paired muscles (3 flat muscles, 2 vertical muscles). The 3 flat muscles are the external oblique, internal oblique, and transversus abdominis. The 3-layered structure, combined with extensive aponeuroses, works in a synkinetic fashion not only to protect the abdominal viscera but also to increase abdominal pressure, which facilitates defecation, micturition, and parturition. The 2 vertical muscles are the rectus abdominis and pyramidalis. Fusion of the fascial layers of these muscles forms 3 distinct fascial lines: the linea alba and 2 semilunar lines. The linea alba is formed by the fusion of both rectus sheaths at the midline, while the semilunar lines are formed by the union of the external oblique, internal oblique, and transversus abdominis aponeuroses at the lateral border of the rectus abdominis muscle (Figs 2.8A to C).

## External Oblique (Fig. 2.9)

The external oblique muscle is the largest and thickest of the flat abdominal wall muscles. It originates from the lower 8 ribs, interlocks with slips of latissimus dorsi and serratus anterior, and courses inferior-medially, attaching via its aponeurosis centrally at the linea alba. Inferiorly, the external oblique aponeurosis folds back upon itself and forms the inguinal ligament between the anterior superior iliac spine and the pubic tubercle. Medial to the pubic tubercle, the external oblique aponeurosis is attached to the pubic crest. Traveling superior to the medial part of the inguinal ligament, an opening in the aponeurosis forms the superficial inguinal ring. The innervation to the external oblique is derived from the lower 6 thoracic anterior primary rami and the first and second lumbar anterior primary rami.

## Internal Oblique (Figs 2.6 and 2.10)

The internal oblique muscle originates from the anterior portion of the iliac crest, lateral half to two-thirds of the inguinal ligament, and posterior aponeurosis of the

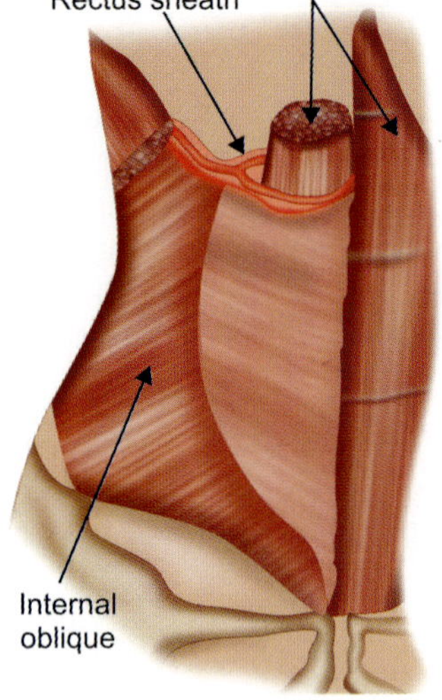


**Fig. 2.6:** Internal oblique muscles

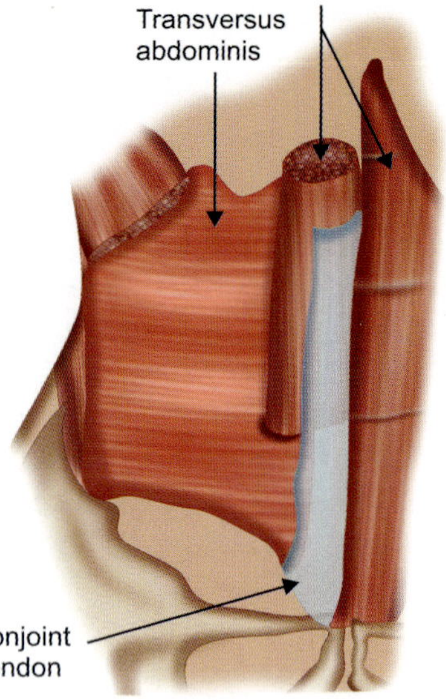


**Fig. 2.7:** Transversus abdominis muscle

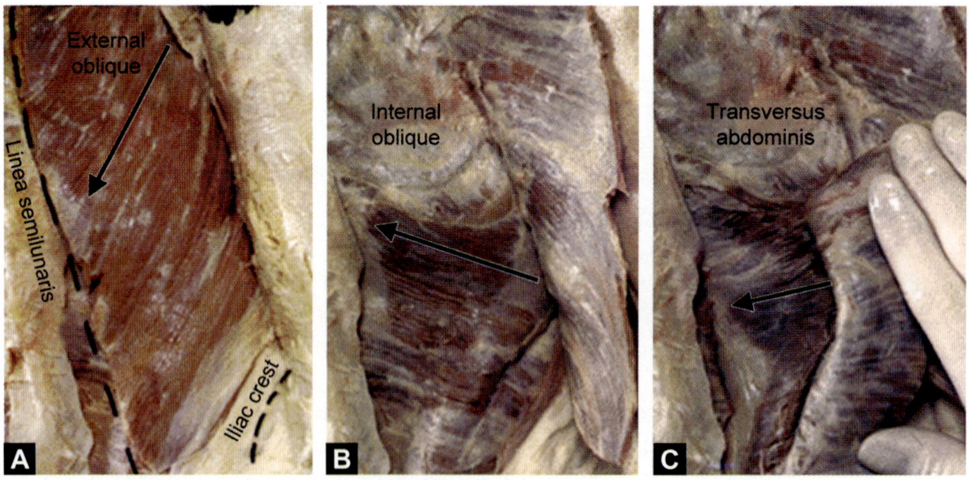


**Figs 2.8A to C:** (A) Cadaveric dissection view of external oblique muscle; (B) Cadaveric dissection view of internal oblique muscle; (C) Cadaveric dissection view of transversus abdominis muscle

transversus abdominis muscle. The internal oblique fibers run superior-anteriorly at right angles to the external oblique and insert on the cartilages of the lower 4 ribs. The anterior fibers become aponeurotic at around the ninth costal cartilage. At the lateral border of the rectus abdominis muscle and above the arcuate line, the aponeurosis splits anteriorly and posteriorly to enclose the rectus muscle to help form the rectus sheaths. However, beneath the arcuate line, the internal oblique aponeurosis does not split, resulting in an absent posterior rectus sheath. The inferior aponeurotic fibers arch over the spermatic cord, pass through the inguinal canal and then descend posterior to the superficial ring to attach to the pubic crest. The most inferior medial tendinous fibers fuse with the aponeurotic fibers of the transversus abdominis muscle to form the conjoint

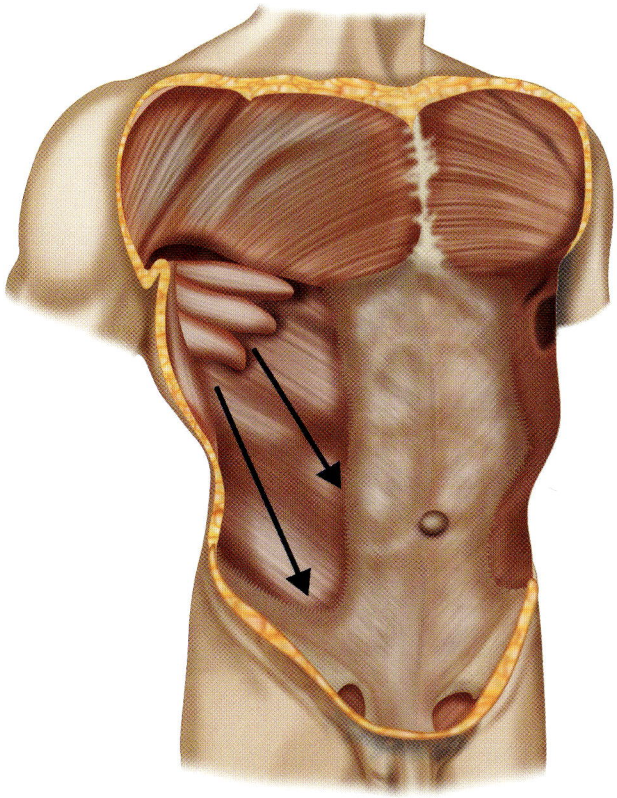

Fig. 2.9: External oblique

tendon, which also inserts on the pubic crest. The internal oblique is not invariable in its anatomy in the inguinal region. Its origin may commence at the internal ring or at a variable distance lateral to the ring. The muscle may then insert either into the pubic crest and tubercle or into the lateral margin of the rectus sheath a variable distance above the pubis. There are thus four combinations of origin and insertion of the internal oblique in the groin. The contribution of the internal oblique too groin anatomy and in particular to the defenses of inguinal canal is very variable.

The internal oblique muscle in its lateral fleshy part is not uniform in its structure; it is segmented or banded. The muscular bands terminate just lateral to the border the rectus muscle and are most marked in the inguinal and lower abdominal region. The bands are generally arranged like the "blades of a fan" with the interspaces increasing as the medial extremities are reached. Spigelian hernias occur through these defects of the semilunar line, which are more pronounced in the lower abdomen.

## Transversus Abdominis

The transversus abdominis muscle is the innermost of the 3 flat abdominal muscles. The fibers of the transversus abdominis course predominately in a horizontal orientation. It has 2 fleshy origins and 1 aponeurotic origin. The first fleshy origin is from the anterior three-fourths of the iliac crest and lateral third of the inguinal ligament, while the second origin is from the inner surface of the lower 6 costal cartilages where they interdigitate with fibers of the diaphragm. Between the 2 fleshy origins is the aponeurotic origin from the transverse processes of the lumbar vertebrae. These fibers course medially to the lateral border of the rectus muscle. From about 6.6 cm inferior to the xiphoid process to the arcuate line, the insertion is aponeurotic and contributes to the formation of the posterior rectus sheath (Figs 2.7 and 2.11).

## Fascia Transversalis

The transversalis fascia (or transverse fascia) is a thin aponeurotic membrane which lies between the inner surface of the transversus abdominis and the extraperitoneal fascia (Fig. 2.12).

It forms part of the general layer of fascia lining the abdominal parietes, and is directly continuous with the iliac and pelvic fasciae.

In the inguinal region, the transversalis fascia is thick and dense in structure and is joined by fibers from the aponeurosis of the transversus, but it becomes thin as it ascends to the diaphragm, and blends with the fascia covering the under surface of this muscle.

### *Borders*

Behind, it is lost in the fat which covers the posterior surfaces of the kidneys.

Below, it has the following attachments: posteriorly, to the whole length of the iliac crest, between the attachments of the transversus and iliacus; between the anterosuperior iliac spine and the femoral vessels it is connected to the posterior margin of the inguinal ligament, and is there continuous with the iliac fascia.

Medial to the femoral vessels it is thin and attached to the pubis and pectineal line, behind the inguinal falx, with which it is united; it descends in front of the femoral vessels to form the anterior wall of the femoral sheath (Fig. 2.13).

Beneath the inguinal ligament it is strengthened by a band of fibrous tissue, which is only loosely connected to the ligament, and is specialized as the iliopubic tract.

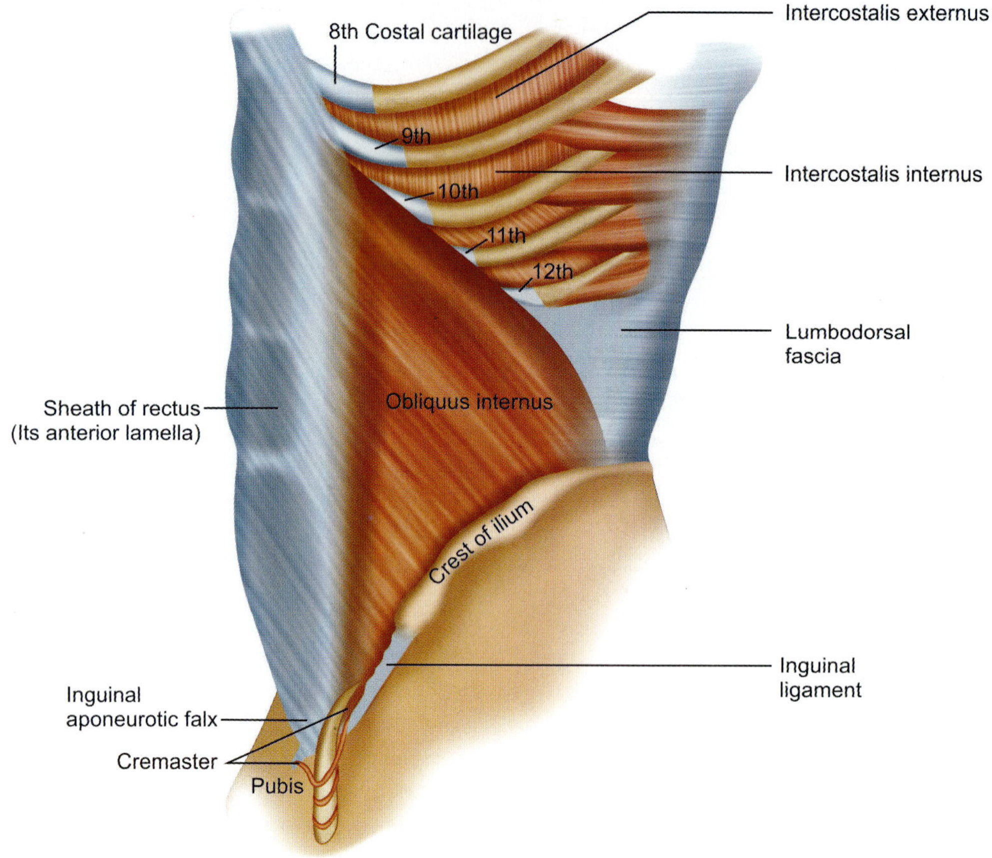


**Fig. 2.10:** Internal oblique

### *Opening*

The spermatic cord in the male and the round ligament of the uterus in the female pass through the transversalis fascia at a spot called the deep inguinal ring.

This opening is not visible externally, since the transversalis fascia is prolonged on these structures as the internal spermatic fascia.

### *Transversalis Fascia*

The most important, and at the same time, most puzzling entity in the infraumbilical space is the transversalis fascia. This fascia has been described as being bilaminal: a superficial sheet and a deep, translucent, usually tough sheet. The transversalis fascia covers the deep aspect of the musculus transversus abdominis. Medially, it lies deep to the posterior sheath of the musculus rectus abdominis. This sheath however ends abruptly distally, at a distance from the pubis constituting the semilunar line of Douglas.

At that level, both layers of transversalis fascia separate on their way to the midline. The most superficial one passes anterior to the rectus muscle and blends with other fascial layers constituting the linea alba1. The deepest layer of transversalis fascia remains deep to the rectus muscle, thus constituting the only posterior fascial reinforcement of the muscle at that level. The rectus muscle inserts on the pubic bone. The posterior layer of the transversalis fascia blends with the periosteum of the pubis and forms Cooper's ligament laterally to the insertion of the rectus muscle. Even more laterally, just where superficial and deep layer of transversalis fascia separate, the deep layer is pierced from posterior to anterior by the epigastric vessels, immediately cephalad to their origin from the iliac vessels. The epigastric vessels therefore run between the 2 sheets of transversalis fascia,

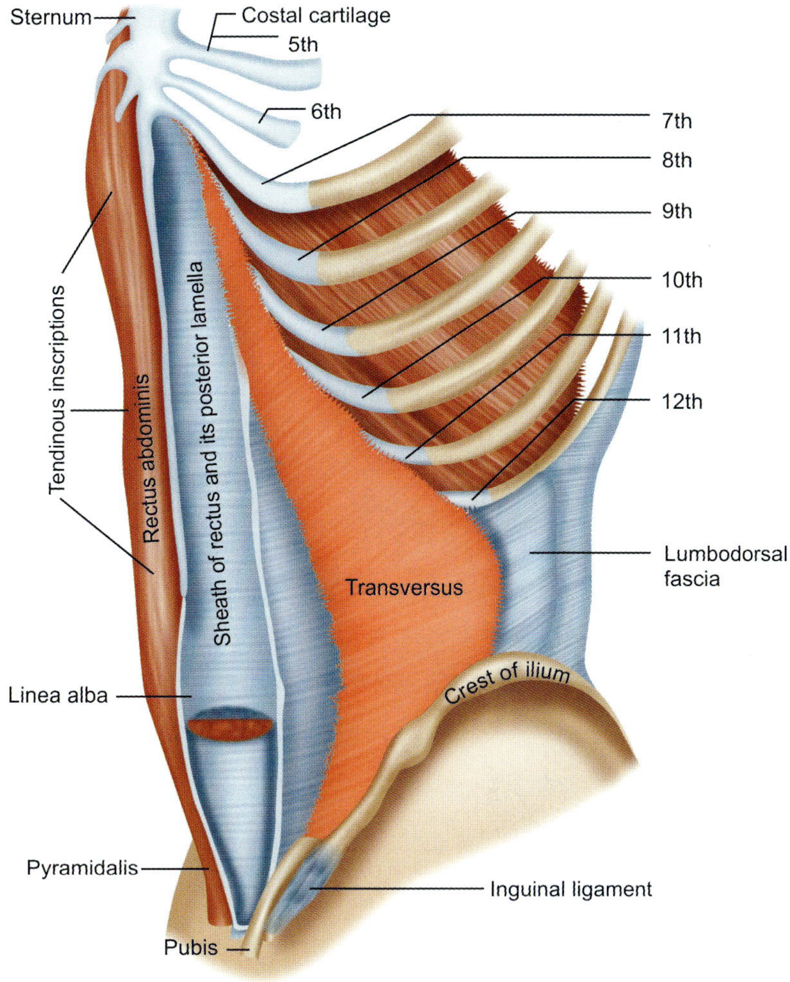


**Fig. 2.11:** Transversus abdominis muscle

but as they run more cranially and medially in close contact with the lateral end of the rectus muscle, they remain adherent to the posterior layer of transversalis fascia.

### *Bogros' Space (Fig. 2.14)*

Bogros' space is situated laterally and cranially to Retzius' space. It represents the retroinguinal preperitoneum, limited anteriorly by the deep layer of transversalis fascia, enveloping the epigastric vessels, medially by the adherent zone of umbilicovesical fascia, transversalis fascia and peritoneum situated just behind the epigastrics, laterally by the pelvis wall and iliacus muscle and inferiorly by the psoas muscle, with medially to it the external iliac vessels and femoral nerve. Cranially, Bogros' space is in free continuity with the lumbar retroperitoneum. This continuity explains the inferior expansion of perirenal abcesses appearing in the groin.

If one insufflates Retzius' space and Bogros' space separately, the adherence of fascia behind the epigastric vessels will give to this part of the retroperitoneum the aspect of an hour glass with long axis running cranially and laterally.

The rectus abdominis muscles (Fig. 2.16) are paired, long, straplike muscles that are the principal vertical muscles of the anterior abdominal wall. The rectus abdominis is interrupted throughout its length by 3 to 4 tendinous inscriptions, all of which are adherent to the anterior rectus sheath and separated by the linea alba. These inscriptions can be visualized externally in a

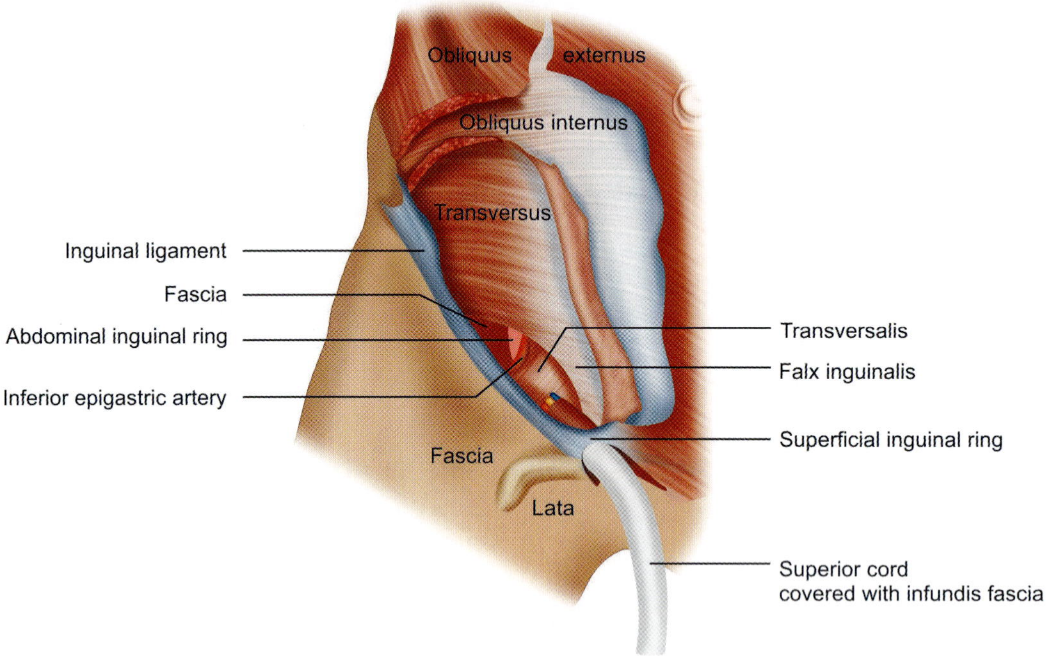


**Fig. 2.12:** Transversalis fascia (or transverse fascia)

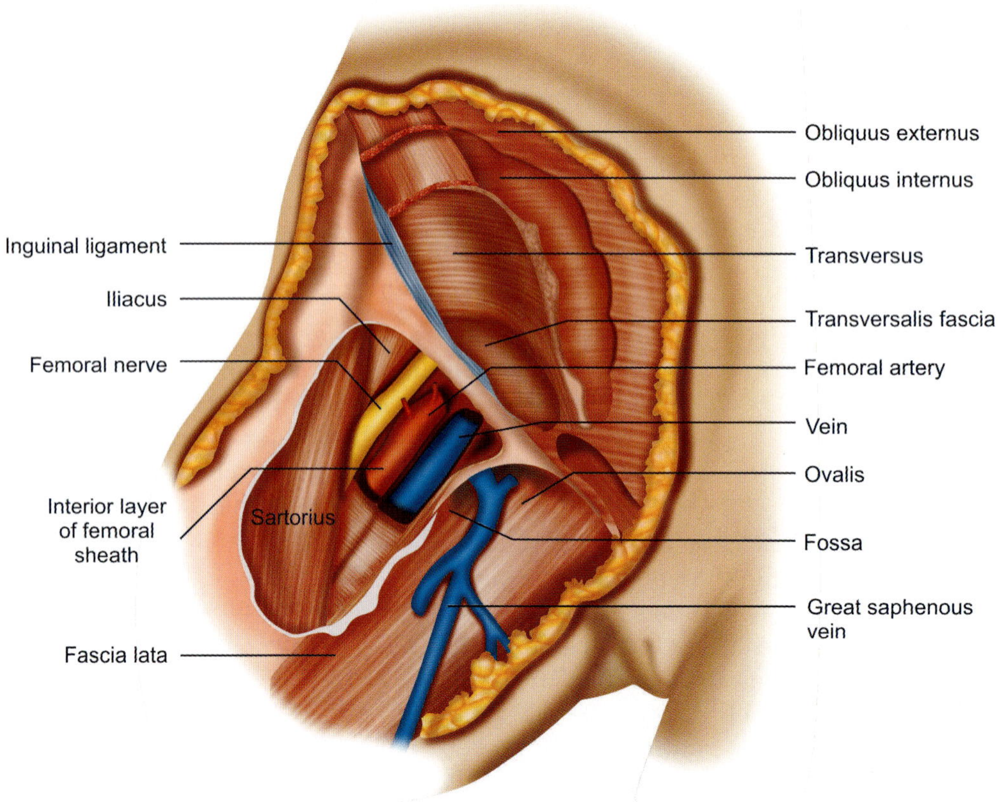


**Fig. 2.13:** Femoral vessels

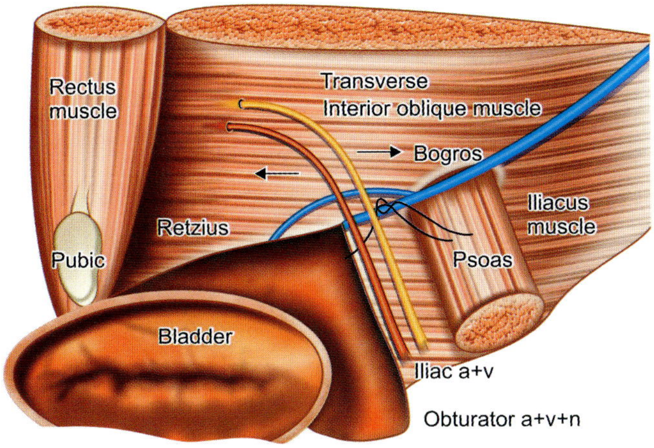


**Fig. 2.14:** Bogros' space

well-developed individual secondary to fasciocutaneous ligaments. The medial tendon of the rectus abdominis originates from the pubic symphysis and the lateral tendon of the rectus abdominis originates from the pubic crest (Fig. 2.15). It inserts to the anterior surfaces of the fifth, sixth, and seventh costal cartilages and xiphoid process. The lateral border of each rectus muscle and its sheath merge with the aponeurosis of the external oblique to form the linea semilunaris. The rectus abdominis (*See* Fig. 2.4B) muscle functions as a tensor of the abdominal wall and flexor of the vertebrae. Additionally, this muscle helps to stabilize the pelvis during walking, protects the abdominal viscera, and aids in forced expiration.

The rectus sheath is a strong, semifibrous compartment that houses the rectus muscles, the superior and inferior epigastric vessels, and the inferior 5 intercostal and subcostal nerves. It is formed by interlacing aponeurotic

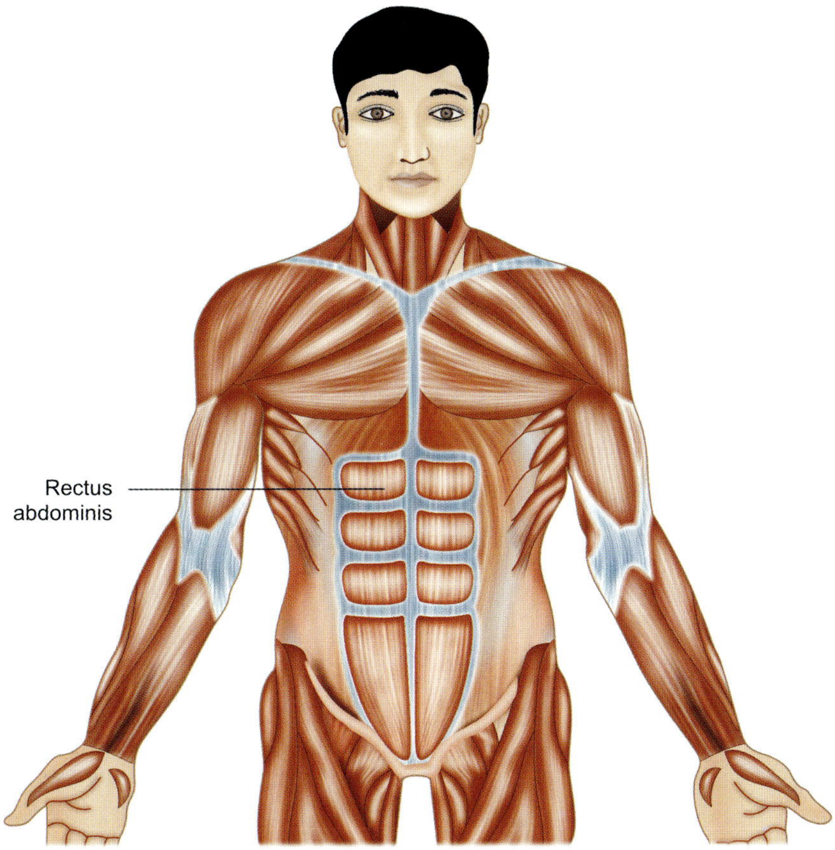


**Fig. 2.15:** Rectus abdominis

fibers from the 3 flat abdominal muscles. The anterior rectus sheath is the union of the external oblique aponeurosis and the anterior layer of the internal oblique. The posterior rectus sheath is composed of the posterior layer of the internal oblique aponeurosis, the transversus abdominis aponeurosis, and the transversalis fascia. Superior to the costal margin, the posterior rectus sheath is absent because the internal oblique muscle is attached to the costal margin and the transversus abdominis courses internal to the costal cartilages.

### Pyramidalis (Fig. 2.16)

The pyramidalis is a small triangular muscle located anterior to the inferior aspect of the rectus abdominis; the pyramidalis is absent in about 20% of the population. The pyramidalis originates from the body of the pubis directly inferior to the insertion of the rectus abdominis and inserts into the linea alba inferior to the umbilicus to assist in stabilization of the lower midline.

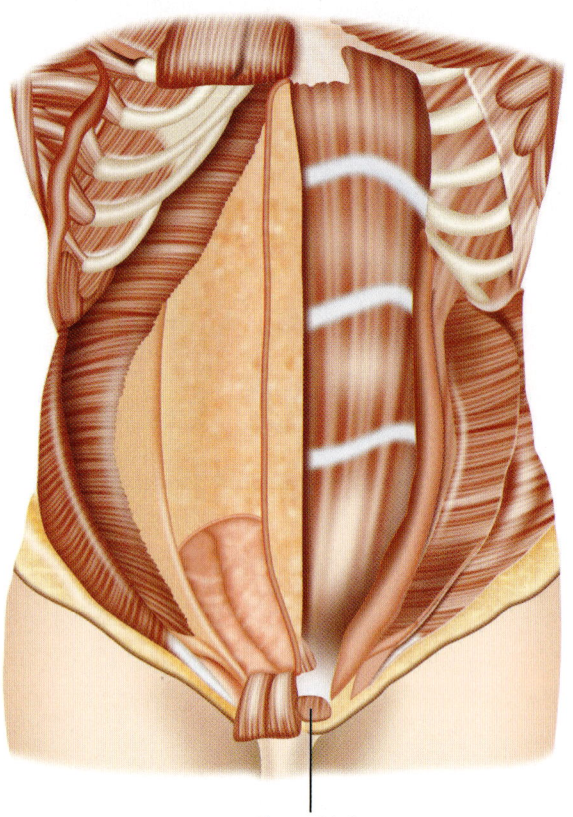


**Fig. 2.16:** Pyramidalis

### Arcuate Line (Fig. 2.17)

Above the arcuate line, the anterior rectus fascia exists anterior to the rectus muscle, and the posterior rectus fascia is posterior to the rectus muscle. Below the arcuate line, the 3 aponeuroses merge together to form exclusively the anterior rectus sheath, with little or no posterior sheath. The arcuate line is generally located 2 fingerbreadths from the umbilicus to midway between the umbilicus and pubis. However, some reports in the literature state that the arcuate line is closer to 75% of the distance between the pubic crest and the umbilicus or 1.8 cm superior to the anterior superior iliac spine (ASIS).

### Linea Alba

The linea alba is the fusion of the anterior and posterior rectus fascia; it is located in the abdominal midline, between the rectus muscles, from the xiphoid to the pubis. The linea alba is a 3-dimensional composition of tendon fibers from abdominal wall muscles. Midline insertions of these fibers play a significant role in stabilizing the abdominal wall. The cranial aspect is attached to the xiphoid process, while, caudally, it inserts at the pubic symphysis.

### Linea Semilunaris

The linea semilunaris can be seen as a pair of linear impressions in the skin that correspond with the most lateral edges of the rectus abdominis. These lines are visible in a person who is physically fit but obscured in a person who is obese. They are formed by the band of aponeuroses of the external oblique, the internal oblique, and the transversus abdominis muscles.

## Importance of Langer's Lines in Hernia Surgery

### History

These lines correspond to the alignment of collagen fibers within the dermis. They were first given detailed attention in 1861 by Austrian anatomist Karl Langer (1819-1887), though he cited the surgeon Baron Dupuytren as being the first to recognize the phenomenon. Langer punctured numerous holes at short distances from each other into

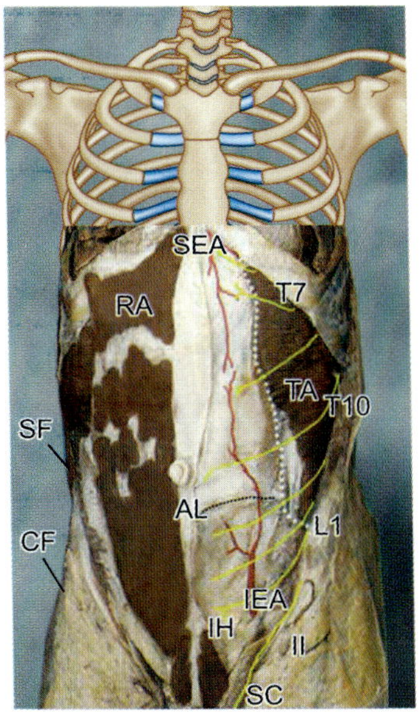


Fig. 2.17: Arcuate line

the skin of a cadaver with a tool that had a circular-shaped tip, and noticed that the resultant punctures in the skin had ellipsoidal shapes. From this testing he observed patterns and was able to determine "line directions" by the longer axes of the ellipsoidal holes.

### Uses

Knowing the direction of Langer's lines within a specific area of the skin is important for surgical operations, particularly cosmetic surgery. Usually, a surgical cut is carried out in the direction of Langer's lines, and incisions made parallel to Langer's lines generally heal better and produce less scarring. Sometimes the exact direction of these lines are unknown, because in some regions of the body there are differences between different individuals. Directional changes of Langer's lines have been known to occur within the course of a person's lifetime.

The orientation of stab wounds relative to Langer's lines can have a considerable impact upon the presentation of the wound.

Langer's lines (Figs 2.18A and B) are lines of tension or cleavage within the skin that are characteristic for each part of the body. In microscopic sections cut parallel with these lines, most of the collagenous bundles of the reticular layer are cut longitudinally, while in sections cut across the lines, the bundles are in cross-section. The cleavage lines correspond closely with the crease lines on the surface of the skin in most parts of the body. These cleavage lines are of particular interest to the surgeon because an incision made parallel to the lines heals with a fine linear scar, while an incision across the lines may set up irregular tensions that result in an unsightly scar. In other areas of the body, Langer's lines are visible or can easily be seen by compressing the skin. On the scalp Langer's lines are not obvious due to the presence of hair and thickness of the skin.

## Vascular Supply of Abdomen

### Vascular Supply and Innervation

The plane between the internal oblique muscle and transversus abdominis muscle contains the neurovascular structures that supply the abdominal muscles. The superior and inferior deep epigastric vessels enter the rectus muscle superiorly and inferiorly. Transperitoneal vessels enter the rectus in the periumbilical region. The abdominal wall receives its blood supply from direct cutaneous vessels and musculocutaneous perforating vessels. The two subdivisions of perforators course medially and laterally. The lateral branch is usually the dominant branch and contains most of the perforator vessels. The lateral fasciocutaneous perforators pierce the aponeuroses of the internal and external oblique muscles. They may pass through the linea alba and emerge on the lateral aspect of the rectus abdominis.

El-Mrakby et al performed microdissections to analyze the vascular anatomy of the anterior abdominal wall. They concluded that the musculocutaneous perforators are the main providers of blood supply to the anterior abdominal wall. Also, the vessels were further categorized into large (direct) or small (indirect) perforators. The indirect perforators generally have diameters less than 0.5 mm and terminate in the deep layer of the subcutaneous fat. Conversely, the direct perforators have diameters greater than 0.5 mm and course into the subdermal plexus to supply the superficial subcutaneous fat and skin. In addition, El-Mrakby et al described the area lateral and inferior to the umbilicus as the area with the richest concentration of perforator vessels. This vascular network allows multiple flap designs that may incorporate one or several perforator vessels.

***Study by Huger et al Classified the Vascular Blood Supply of the Abdominal Wall into Three Simple Zones***

Zone I is defined by the midabdomen and is supplied primarily by the deep epigastric arcade. As the internal thoracic artery passes behind the costal cartilages to enter the abdominal wall, it gives rise to the superior epigastric artery. This vessel then enters the abdomen and travels underneath the surface of the posterior rectus sheath. The superior epigastric artery joins the deep inferior epigastric artery through a series of choke vessels within the rectus above the umbilicus.

Zone II is defined by the lower abdomen and is supplied by branches of the epigastric arcade and the external iliac artery. Blood supply superficial to the fascia is provided by the superficial epigastric and superficial pudendal arteries. Both of these arteries originate from the femoral artery. The deep iliac circumflex artery originates from the external iliac and runs deep to all abdominal muscles to provide blood supply to the area

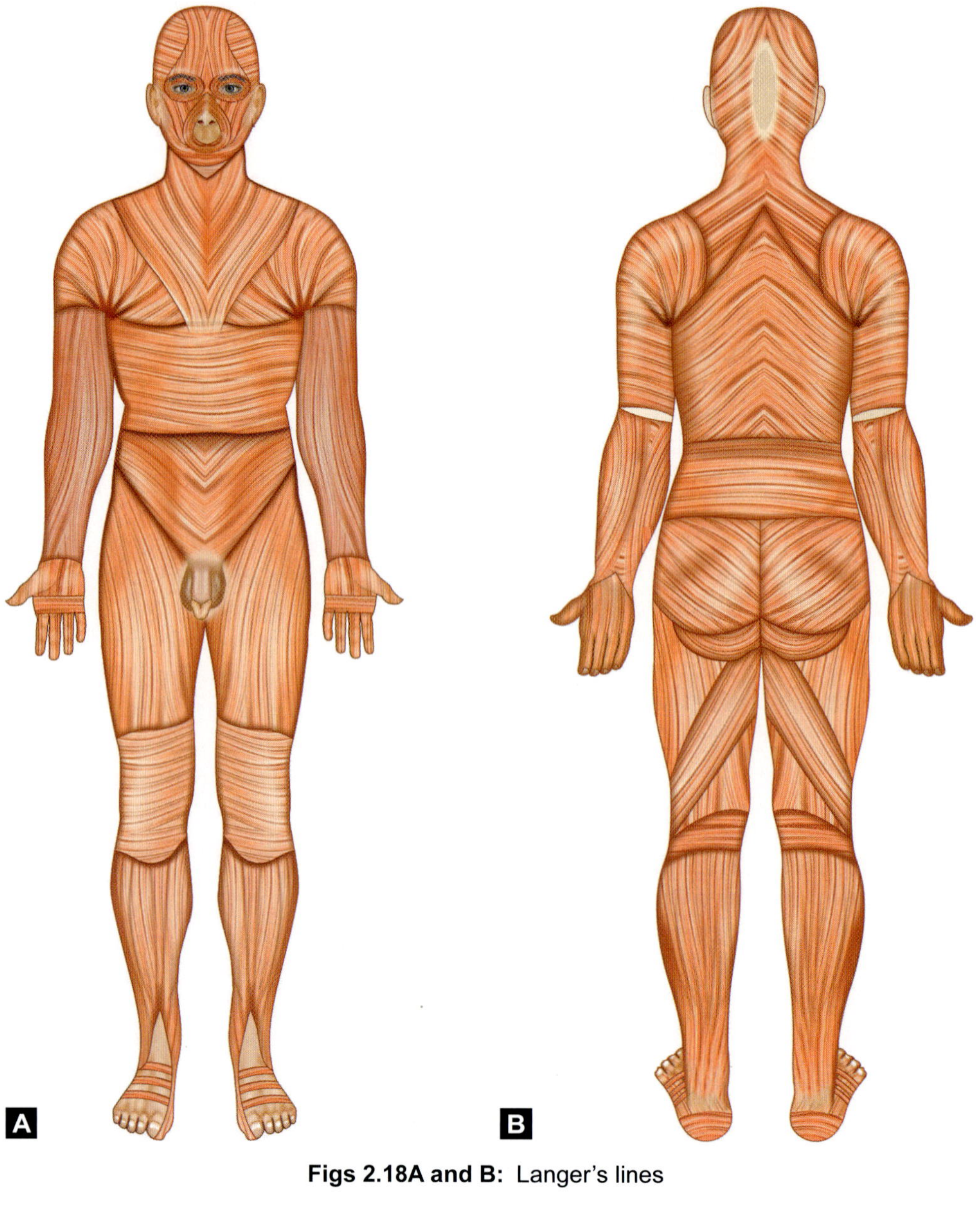


**Figs 2.18A and B:** Langer's lines

of the anterior iliac spine; it also pierces all 3 muscles of the lateral abdominal wall and provides a sizable musculocutaneous perforator.

Zone III comprises the flanks and lateral abdomen. Blood supply to this area comes from the intercostal, subcostal, and lumbar arteries. The intercostal vessels leave the rib cage and enter the abdominal wall between the transversus abdominis and internal oblique muscles, where they anastomose with the lateral branches of the superior epigastric artery and deep inferior epigastric artery.

Sensory innervation to the abdomen is derived from the roots of the nerves T7 to L4. These nerves travel in the plane between the internal oblique and transversus abdominis muscles. Motor innervation is provided by the intercostal, subcostal, iliohypogastric, and ilioinguinal nerves. These nerves must be preserved during abdominal wall reconstruction in order to maintain abdominal wall sensation and muscular function.

## Blood Supply (Table 2.2)

- *Superior epigastric arteries:* Continuation of the internal thoracic arteries. They run inferiorly in the rectus sheath, deep to the rectus abdominis muscle. The superior epigastric arteries anastomose with the inferior epigastric arteries within the rectus sheath.
- *Inferior epigastric arteries:* Branches of the external iliac arteries. They run superiorly in the rectus sheath, deep to the rectus abdominis. The inferior epigastric arteries anastomose with the superior epigastric artery within the rectus sheath.
- *Deep circumflex iliac arteries:* Branches of the external iliac arteries. They run deep in the abdominal wall, parallel to the inguinal ligament.
- *Superficial circumflex iliac arteries:* Branches of the femoral arteries. They run superficially in the abdominal wall, parallel to the inguinal ligament.
- *Superficial epigastric arteries:* Branches of the femoral arteries. They run superficially, superiorly toward the umbilicus.

### Innervation

- *Thoracoabdominal nerves (branches of the VPR of T7-T11):* Travel anteroinferiorly between the internal oblique and transverse abdominal muscles (remember the analogous situation in the thorax). Supplies motor (to the muscles) and sensory (cutaneous) fibers. Distribution is as follows:
  - T7-T9—superior to umbilicus
  - T10—at level of umbilicus
  - T11 (along with subcostal, iliohypogastric, and ilioinguinal nerves)—inferior to umbilicus.

**Table 2.2**

| Blood supply of inguinal canal | | | | |
|---|---|---|---|---|
| *Artery* | *Source* | *Branches* | *Supply to* | *Notes* |
| Epigastric, inferior | External iliac artery | Cremasteric artery | Lower rectus abdominis muscle, pyramidalis muscle, lower abdominal wall | Inferior epigastric artery anastomoses with the superior epigastric artery within the rectus abdominis muscle |
| Epigastric, superficial | Femoral artery | Cutaneous branches | Superficial fascia and skin of the lower abdominal wall | Superficial epigastric artery is one of three superficial arteries that arise from the femoral artery (see also: superficial circumflex iliac artery and superficial external pudendal artery) |
| Epigastric, superior | Internal thoracic artery | No named branches | Upper rectus abdominis muscle, upper abdominal wall | Superior epigastric artery is the direct continuation of the internal thoracic artery; it anastomoses with the inferior epigastric artery within the rectus abdominis muscle |
| Intercostal, posterior | Highest intercostal (upper 2 intercostal spaces), descending thoracic aorta (3rd-11th intercostal spaces) | Posterior branch, spinal branch, anterior branch, collateral branch, lateral cutaneous branch | Intercostal muscles, spinal cord and vertebral column, deep back muscles, skin and superficial fascia overlying the intercostal spaces | Posterior intercostal arteries supply the lateral and posterior portions of the intercostal space; anterior intercostal arteries supply the anterior portions of the intercostal spaces |
| Subcostal | Descending thoracic aorta | Spinal branch, collateral branch, lateral cutaneous branch | Vertebrae, spinal cord; muscles, skin and fascia of the upper abdominal wall | Subcostal artery is equivalent to a posterior intercostal artery, but is named subcostal because it courses inferior to the 12th rib |

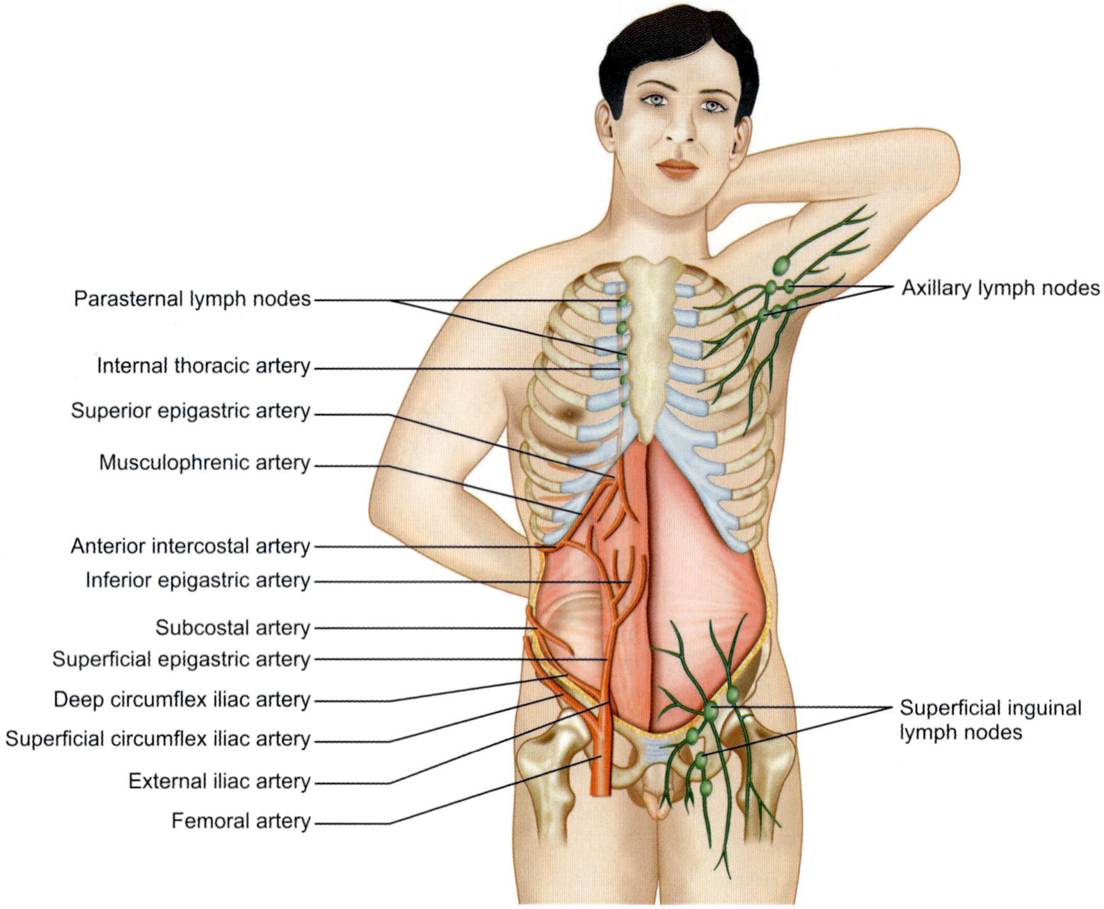


**Fig. 2.19:** Blood supply of inguinal canal

- *Subcostal nerves (T12):* Travel anteroinferiorly between the internal oblique and transverse abdominal muscles (remember the analogous situation in the thorax) to innervate the wall inferior to the umbilicus. Supplies motor (to the muscles) and sensory (cutaneous) fibers.
- *Iliohypogastric nerves (L1):* Path is somewhat similar to thoracoabdominal nerves and subcostal nerves, that is, anteroinferiorly between the internal oblique and transverse abdominal muscles for part of the way. However, the iliohypogastric nerves and ilioinguinal nerves are different in that they pierce the internal abdominal oblique at the anterosuperior iliac spine to travel superficial to it and deep to the external abdominal oblique. Supplies motor (to the muscles) and sensory (cutaneous) fibers to the wall inferior to the umbilicus.
- *Ilioinguinal nerves (L1):* Supplies motor (to the muscles) and sensory (cutaneous) fibers to the wall inferior to the umbilicus. Sometimes considered separate from the iliohypogastric nerves because ilioinguinal nerves also innervate the scrotum or labia by sending branches through the inguinal canal. The iliohypogastric nerves and ilioinguinal nerves are different in that they pierce the internal abdominal oblique at the anterosuperior iliac spine to travel superficial to it and deep to the external abdominal oblique.

## Lymphatic Drainage

- *Superficial lymphatic vessels:* Accompany superficial arteries. Most of them above the umbilicus ultimately drain into the axillary lymph nodes. Below the umbilicus, the vessels drain into the superficial inguinal lymph nodes.

- *Deep lymphatic vessels:* Drain to the external iliac, common iliac, and lumbar lymph nodes, eventually reaching the cisterna chyli and thoracic duct.
  *Note:* The deep inguinal lymph nodes receive most of the drainage from the lower extremity. Efferent vessels from them drain into the external iliac, common iliac, and lumbar lymph nodes, eventually reaching the cisterna chyli and thoracic duct.

## Posterior Abdominal Wall

The posterior abdominal wall extends from the twelfth rib to the pelvic brim. Vertebrae T12 to L5 are located in the midline posteriorly and the iliolumbar and sacroiliac ligaments anchor the ilium of the hip bone to the 5th lumbar vertebra and sacrum. Muscles located in the posterior abdominal wall include diaphragm, psoas major and minor (if present), quadratus lumborum, iliacus, and transverses abdominis.

The kidneys, ureters and suprarenal glands are deeply embedded in and supported by subserous fat and fascia on the posterior wall between peritoneum and the transversalis fascia lining the abdominal cavity. The aorta, inferior vena cava and other vessels supplying gonads, kidneys, adrenal glands and body wall lie in subserous fascia on the posterior wall. The inferior vena cava lies to the right of the aorta. Both vessels bifurcate to form common iliac vessels. These again bifurcate into external and internal iliac vessels before leaving the posterior abdominal wall. The bed of the posterior abdominal wall is made up of three bony and four muscular structures; the bones are the bodies of the lumbar vertebrae, the sacrum, and the wings of the ileum. The muscles are the diaphragm—posterior portion, the quadratus lumborum, the psoas major, and the iliacus (Table 2.3).

### Major Muscles of the Posterior Abdominal Wall

The muscles of the posterior abdominal wall are the psoas, quadratus lumborum and the iliacus (Fig. 2.20).

The psoas muscle arises from the sides of the upper lumbar vertebrae and the intervertebral disks. The muscle runs downwards into the pelvis and out again under the inguinal ligament. It inserts into the lesser trochanter of the femur in common with the iliacus muscle. The psoas is innervated by the L2,3,4 lumbar nerves. The psoas is enclosed within the psoas fascia, a compartment which may limit the spread of a psoas abscess. The psoas muscle flexes the hip, or flexes the lumbar spine. Several structures such as the kidney and ureter, gonadal vessels, appendix and lumbar nerves have a close relationship to the muscle. Patients attempt to immobilize the psoas muscle when there is pain

**Table 2.3**

| Major nerves of the posterior abdominal wall | | | |
|---|---|---|---|
| *Source* | *Branches* | *Motor* | *Sensory* |
| Iliohypogastric and ilioinguinal nerves (*L1*)<br>Lumbar plexus (ventral primary ramus of spinal ?) | Lateral and anterior cutaneous branches | Muscles of the lower abdominal wall | Skin of the lower abdominal wall, upper hip and ? |
| Subcostal (*T12*)<br>Ventral primary ramus of *T12* | Lateral cutaneous branch, anterior cutaneous branch | Muscles of the abdominal wall | Skin of the anterolateral abdominal wall |
| Femoral (*L2,3,4*)<br>Lumbar plexus (ventral primary) | Anterior femoral cutaneous branches to sartorius muscle, rectus femoris muscle, vastus lateralis muscle, vastus intermedius muscle, vastus medialis muscle, pectineus muscle | Sartorius, rectus femoris, vastus lateralis, vastus intermedius, vastus medialis, pectineus | Skin of anterior thigh |
| Obturator (*L2,3,4*)<br>Emerging in the pelvis from the medial side of the psoas muscle | | | |
| Genitofemoral (*L1,2*)<br>emerging through the psoas muscle onto its anterior surface | | | |

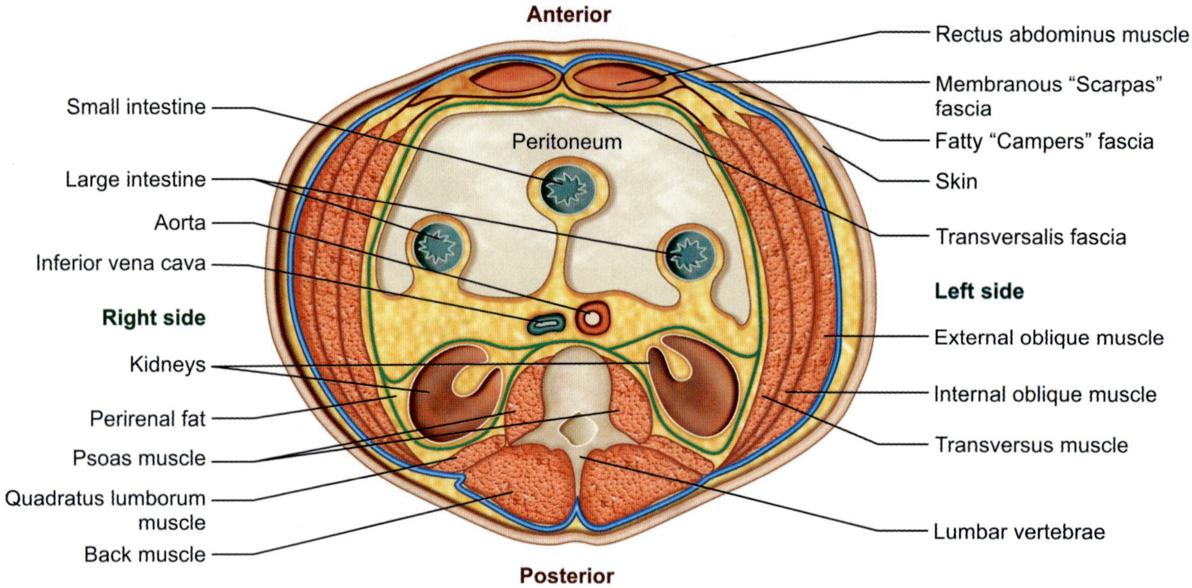


**Fig. 2.20:** Coronal section of abdomen showing posterior abdominal wall

from many of these structures. This is accomplished by drawing the knees upward passively.

The quadratus lumborum muscle arises from the medial half of the twelfth rib and inserts into the iliac crest. It forms a bed for the kidney. It is innervated by the T12 and lumbar nerves. Its action is to fix the twelfth rib during inspiration. The iliacus muscle arises from the iliac fossa in the pelvis. It runs below the inguinal ligament to insert together with psoas into the lesser trochanter. It is innervated by the femoral nerve.

### Blood Supply to the Posterior Abdominal Wall

The aorta passes into the abdomen from the thorax in the midline lying on the vertebral bodies. The crura of the diaphragm form an opening so that the aorta passes behind the diaphragm under the median arcuate ligament. The aorta gives off four pairs of lumbar arteries that supply the abdominal wall (similar to the intercostals arteries of the thorax). Four other pairs are also given off: the inferior phrenic arteries supplying the diaphragm; the middle suprarenal arteries; the renal arteries; the gonadal arteries. There are three unpaired arteries which arise from the anterior aorta: the celiac trunk; the superior mesenteric artery; the inferior mesenteric artery. At the lower border of the L4 lumbar vertebra the aorta bifurcates into the common iliac arteries.

## Blood Supply of Posterior Abdominal Wall (Figs 2.21A and B)

### Crura of Superficial Inguinal Ring

The superficial inguinal ring is bounded below by the crest of the pubis; on either side by the margins of the opening in the aponeurosis, which are called the crura of the ring; and above, by a series of curved intercrural fibers.

- The inferior crus (or lateral, or external pillar) is the stronger and is formed by that portion of the inguinal ligament which is inserted into the pubic tubercle; it is curved so as to form a kind of groove, upon which, in the male, the spermatic cord rests.
- The superior crus (or medial, or internal pillar) is a broad, thin, flat band, attached to the front of the symphysis pubis and interlacing with its fellow of the opposite side.

#### *Superficial Inguinal Ring (Fig. 2.22)*

In the aponeurosis of the external oblique, immediately above the crest of the pubis, is a triangular opening, the subcutaneous inguinal ring (superficial inguinal ring, external inguinal ring), formed by a separation of the fibers of the aponeurosis.

The subcutaneous inguinal ring is situated 1 centimeter above and lateral to the pubic tubercle. It has medial and lateral crura. It is at the layer of the aponeurosis of the obliquus externus abdominis.

The superficial inguinal ring forms the exit of the inguinal canal, through which the ilioinguinal nerve, the genital branch of the genitofemoral nerve, and the spermatic cord (in males) or the round ligament (in females) pass. The deep inguinal ring is the entrance to the inguinal canal (Fig. 2.23).

## Deep Inguinal Ring (Fig. 2.19)

### Inguinal Ligament (Fig. 2.24)

The inguinal ligament is formed by the aponeurotic fibers of the external oblique muscle. The ligament stretches from the anterior superior iliac spine (ASIS) to the pubic tubercle. At the medial end of the inguinal ligament, fibers are reflected backwards to insert into the superior ramus of the pubis, forming the lacunar ligament. The iliopsoas muscles, the femoral vein artery and nerve, all pass below the inguinal ligament. The inguinal canal passes obliquely through the abdominal wall above the ligament. The inguinal canal transmits the vas deferens in the male and the round ligament in the female. The deep ring is the entrance to the inguinal canal on the inside of the abdominal wall. The deep ring is formed in the transversalis fascia. As the canal passes through the abdominal wall it receives a layer of muscle from the internal oblique, the cremaster muscle. At the superficial ring the inguinal canal passes through the external oblique aponeurosis and receives a layer from the aponeurosis, the external spermatic fascia in the male. The deep inguinal ring lies lateral to the inferior epigastric vessels. The superficial ring lies above and medial to the pubic tubercle.

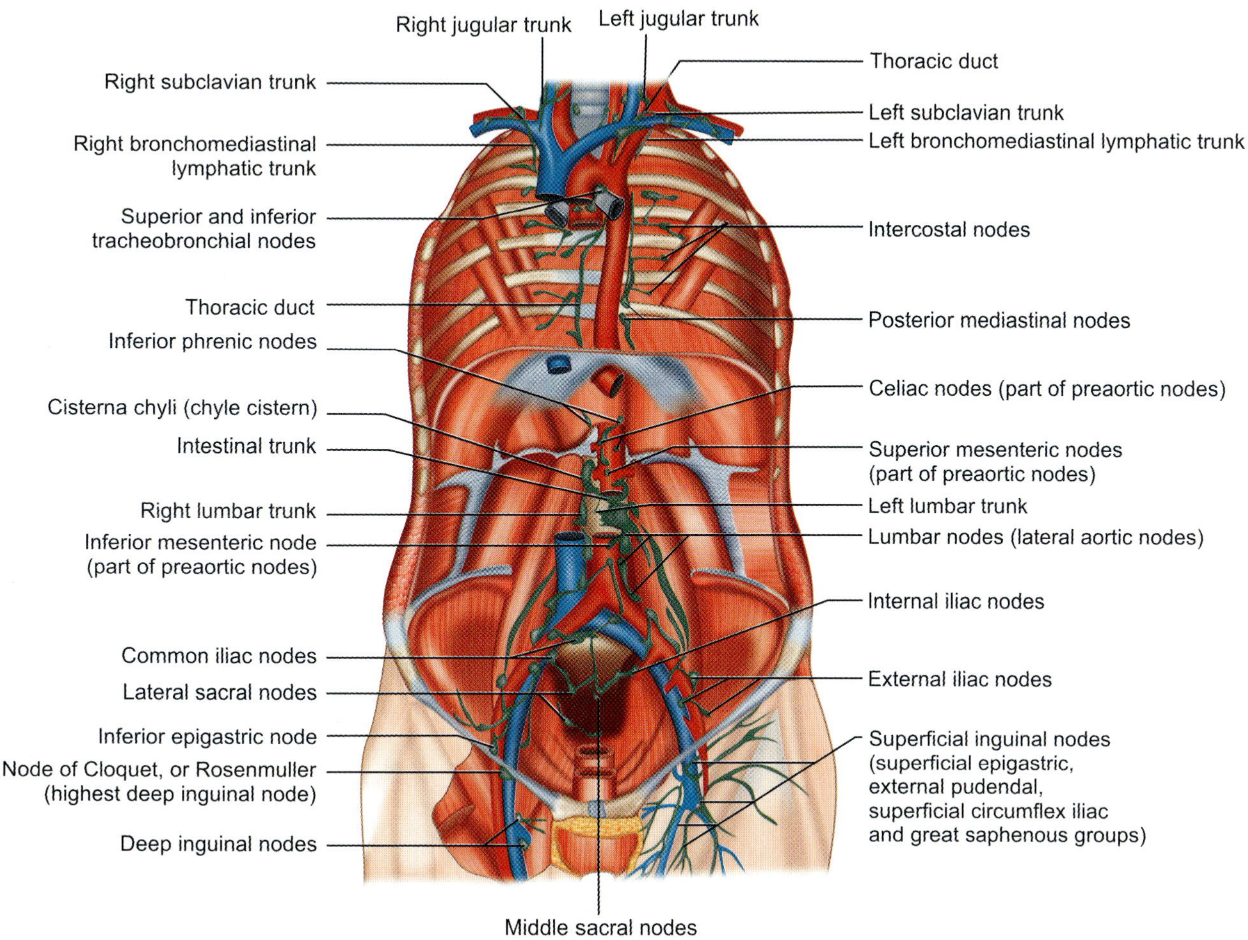


**Fig. 2.21A**

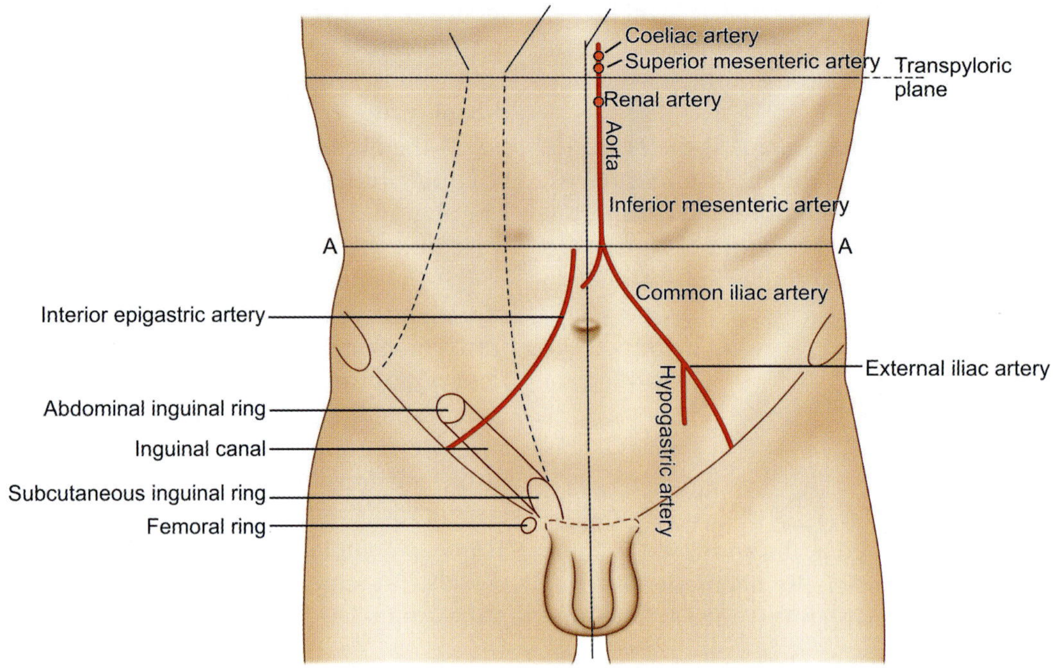


**Fig. 2.21B**

**Figs 2.21A and B:** Blood supply of posterior abdominal wall

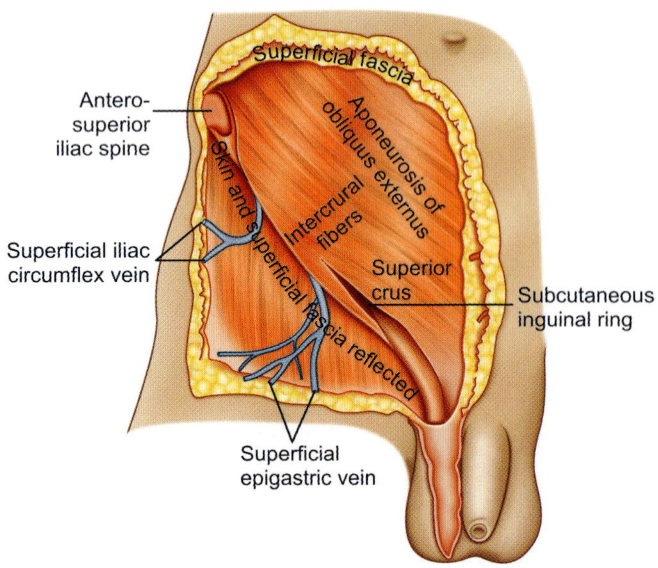


**Fig. 2.22:** Superficial inguinal ring

## Eponym

It is incorrectly referred to as Poupart's ligament (Fig. 2.26), because Poupart gave it its relevance to hernial repair (he called it *"le suspenseur de l'abdomen"*, the suspender of the abdomen). It is also incorrectly termed the Fallopian ligament.

A direct inguinal hernia (Fig. 2.25) occurs when a loop of gut pushes peritoneum and conjoint tendon through the superficial ring. An indirect hernia occurs when a loop of gut pushes peritoneum through the deep ring into the inguinal canal.

## Spermatic Cord

The spermatic cord passes through the inguinal canal to the testis. The vas deferens, testicular artery and veins, lymph vessels, autonomic nerves, cremasteric artery, artery of the vas and the genital branch of the femoral nerve are covered by three layers of fascia derived from the abdominal wall. The fascial covering of the spermatic cord is formed by the external spermatic fascia derived from the aponeurosis of the external oblique, the cremasteric fascia derived from the internal oblique and the internal spermatic fascia derived from the transversalis fascia.

### *Conjoint Tendon (Fig. 2.27)*

*Anatomy:* It is mainly formed by the lower part of the tendon of the transversus abdominis and the internal

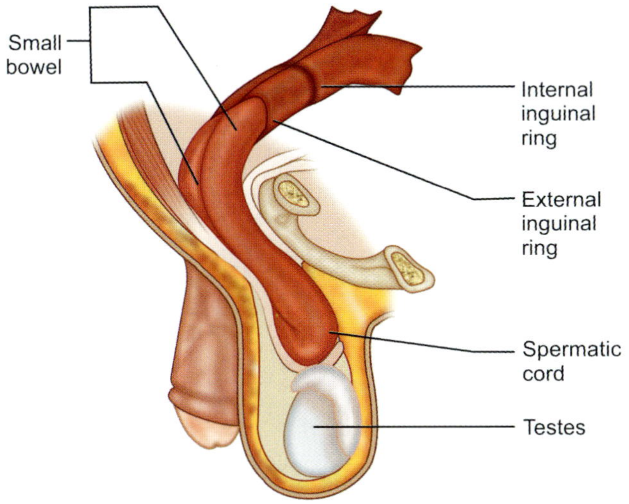


**Fig. 2.23:** Inguinal hernia

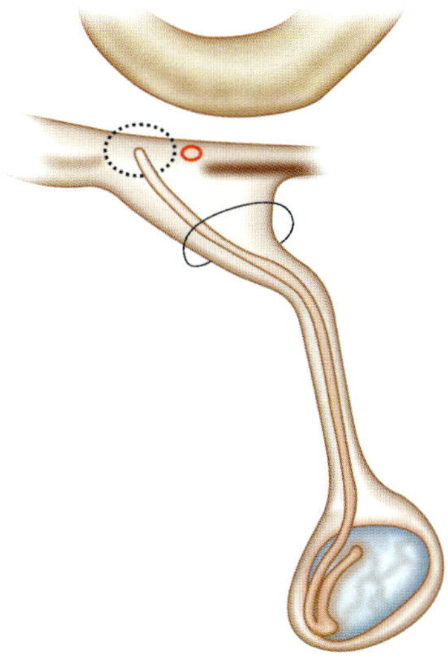

**Fig. 2.25:** Superficial inguinal ring

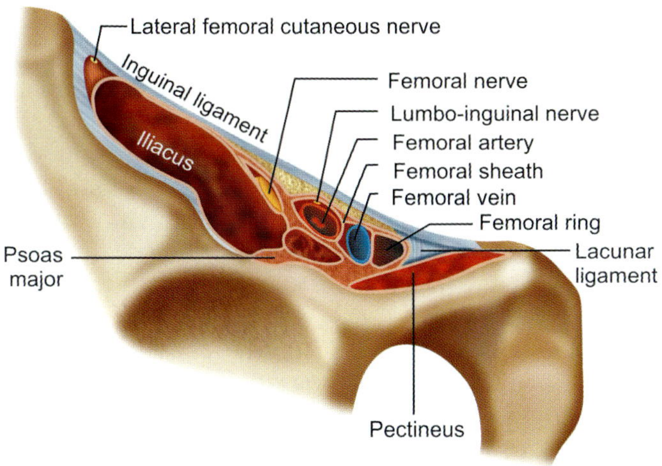


**Fig. 2.24:** Inguinal ligament

oblique muscle, and is inserted into the crest of the pubis and pectineal line immediately behind the subcutaneous inguinal ring, serving to protect what would otherwise be a weak point in the abdominal wall.

It forms the posterior wall of the inguinal canal, along with the transversalis fascia.

### *Clinical Significance*

A direct inguinal hernia will protrude through Hesselbach's triangle, whose borders are the linea semilunaris (medially), inferior epigastric artery and vein (superolaterally), and the inguinal ligament (inferiorly). The hernia will lie medial to the spermatic cord.

*Variations:* The conjoint tendon has a very variable structure and in 20% of subjects it does not exist as a discrete anatomic structure. It may be absent or only slightly developed, it may be replaced by a lateral extension of the tendon of origin of the rectus muscle., or it may extend laterally to the deep inguinal ring so that no interval is present between the lower border of transverses and the inguinal ligament. A shutter mechanism for the conjoint tendon can only be demonstrated when the lateral side of the tendon, that is transverses and internal oblique muscles, extend onto and are attached to the iliopectineal line.

### *Femoral Canal (See Fig. 2.13)*

The femoral canal lies below the inguinal ligament medially and lies medial to the femoral vessels. The femoral sheath is formed by the transversalis fascia and encloses the femoral vessels and the femoral canal. The lacunar ligament forms the medial border of the femoral canal. The femoral vein lies lateral to the femoral canal.

*The peritoneum:* In higher vertebrates and some invertebrates (annelids, for instance), the peritoneum is the serous membrane that forms the lining of the abdominal cavity or the coelom—it covers most of the intra-abdominal (or coelomic) organs. It is composed of a layer of mesothelium supported by a thin layer of

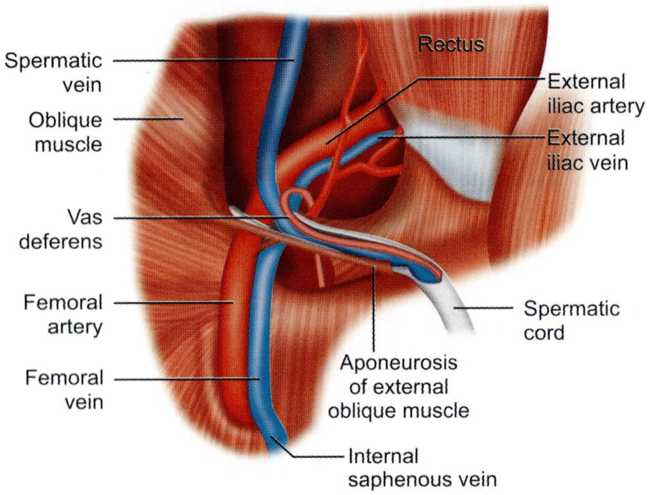


**Fig. 2.26:** Poupart's ligament

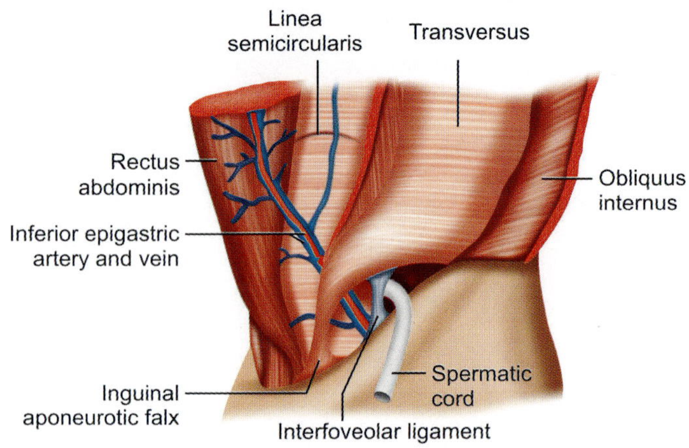


**Fig. 2.27:** The conjoint tendon

connective tissue. The peritoneum both supports the abdominal organs and serves as a conduit for their blood and lymph vessels and nerves (Figs 2.28A to D).

### Structure

*Layers:* The abdominal cavity (the space bounded by the vertebrae, abdominal muscles, diaphragm and pelvic floor) should not be confused with the intraperitoneal space (located within the abdominal cavity, but wrapped in peritoneum). For example, a kidney is inside the abdominal cavity, but is retroperitoneal.

Although they ultimately form one continuous sheet, two types or layers of peritoneum and a potential space between them are referenced:

- The outer layer, called the parietal peritoneum, is attached to the abdominal wall.
- The inner layer, the visceral peritoneum, is wrapped around the internal organs that are located inside the intraperitoneal cavity.
- The potential space between these two layers is the peritoneal cavity; it is filled with a small amount (about 50 ml) of slippery serous fluid that allows the two layers to slide freely over each other.
- The term mesentery is often used to refer to a double layer of visceral peritoneum. There are often blood vessels, nerves, and other structures between these layers. It should be noted that the space between these two layers is technically outside of the peritoneal sac, and thus not in the peritoneal cavity.

### Subdivisions

There are two main regions of the peritoneum, connected by the epiploic foramen:

- The greater sac (or general cavity of the abdomen), represented in red in the diagrams above.
- The lesser sac (or omental bursa), represented in blue. The lesser sac is divided into two "omenta":
  - The lesser omentum (or gastrohepatic) is attached to the lesser curvature of the stomach and the liver.
  - The greater omentum (or gastrocolic) hangs from the greater curve of the stomach and loops down in front of the intestines before curving back upwards to attach to the transverse colon. In effect it is draped in front of the intestines like an apron and may serve as an insulating or protective layer.

The mesentery is the part of the peritoneum through which most abdominal organs are attached to the abdominal wall and supplied with blood and lymph vessels and nerves.

### Development

The peritoneum develops ultimately from the mesoderm of the trilaminar embryo. As the mesoderm differentiates, one region known as the lateral plate mesoderm splits to form two layers separated by anintraembryonic coelom. These two layers develop later into the visceral and parietal layers found in all serous cavities, including the peritoneum.

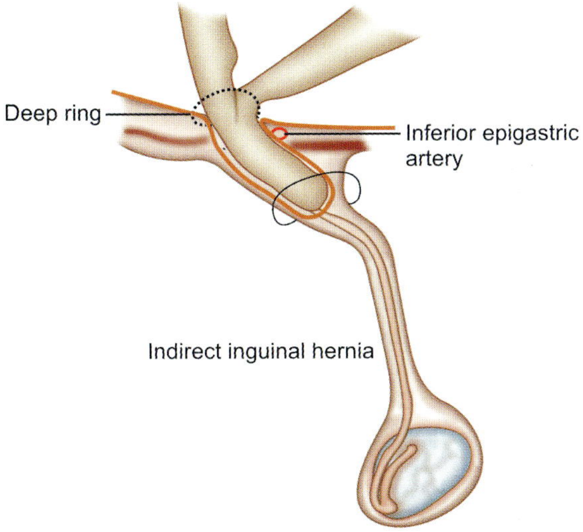


Fig. 2.28A

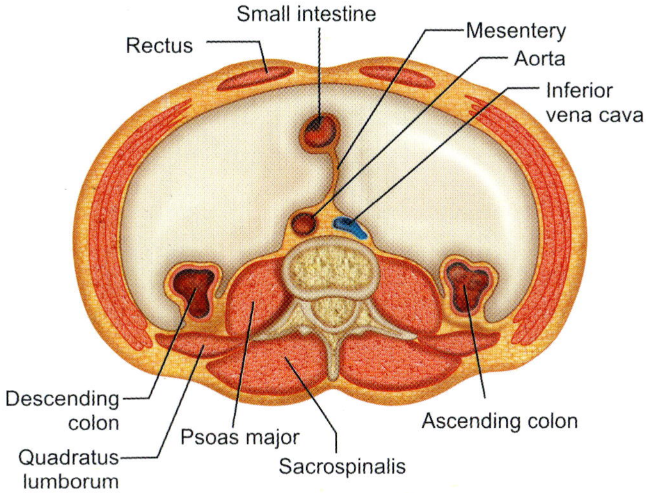


Fig. 2.28B

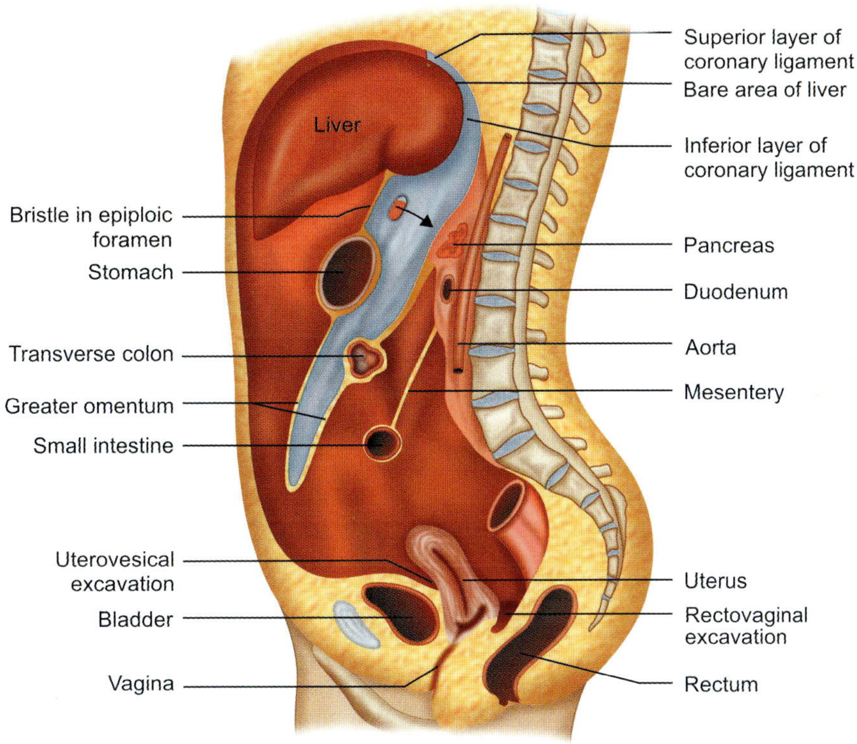


Fig. 2.28C

As an embryo develops, the various abdominal organs grow into the abdominal cavity from structures in the abdominal wall. In this process they become enveloped in a layer of peritoneum. The growing organs "take their blood vessels with them" from the abdominal wall, and these blood vessels become covered by peritoneum, forming a mesentery.

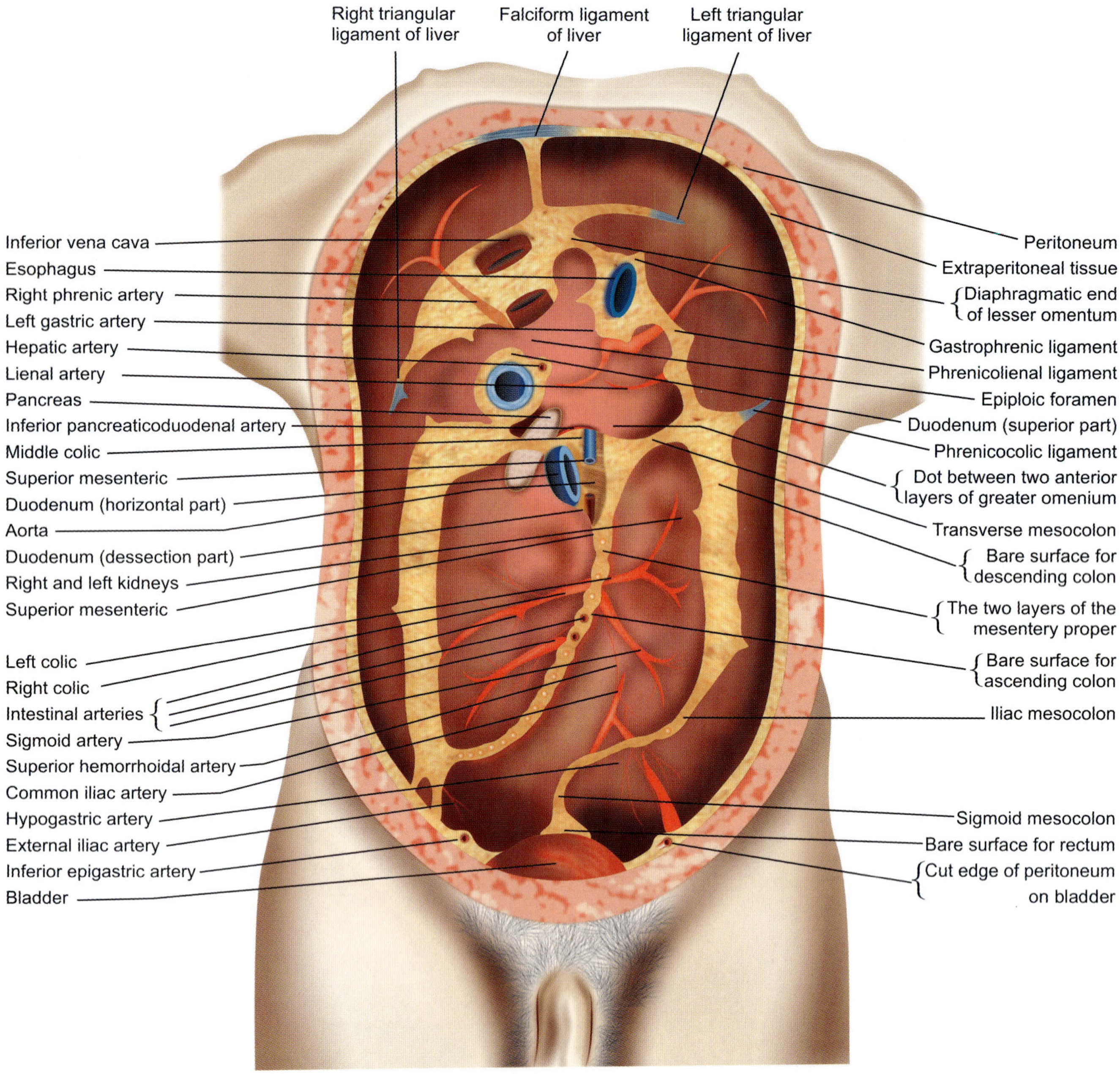


**Fig. 2.28D**

**Figs 2.28A to D:** The peritoneum

### *Importance*

Hernia sacs are composed of peritoneum and they may contain intra-abdominal viscera. From within they consist of the peritoneum, then a loose layer of extraperitoneal fat, then the deep membranous lamina of fascia transversalis, then the vessels such as epigastric vessels in the space of Bogros, then the stout anterior lamina of fascia transversalis, then the muscles and aponeurosis of the abdominal wall.

### *Radiological Anatomy*

The accurate knowledge of the radiological anatomy of abdomen is crucial in diagnosis of abdominal hernia as it may defeat clinical diagnosis.

For this many modalities like herniography, sonography, CT scans, MRI scan are available.

### *Herniography*

*Herniography:* Radiographic examination of suspected hernia in the pelvic region by injection of a positive contrast medium into the peritoneal cavity (peritoneography). The procedure is performed under sterile conditions with local anesthesia. The patient lies in the supine position, and the head-end of the examination table is slightly elevated. The urinary bladder must be empty. The anterior abdominal wall is punctured with a sheathed needle approximately 34 cm to the left of and 34 cm below the umbilicus, corresponding to the upper part of the left sacroiliac joint at fluoroscopy. The puncture of the peritoneum is facilitated by use of increased intra-abdominal pressure (Valsalva). A total of 60 to 70 ml of a water-soluble contrast medium is injected under fluoroscopic control; nonionic contrast media (200 mg iodine/ml) are recommended. The patient is turned prone, and the table further elevated (30) to promote filling of pelvic hernias. Frontal and oblique radiographs are taken with and without increased intra-abdominal pressure. Supplementary supine or erect views may be needed.

The contrast medium fills a right-sided direct inguinal hernia with a narrow neck, extending from the medial inguinal fossa.

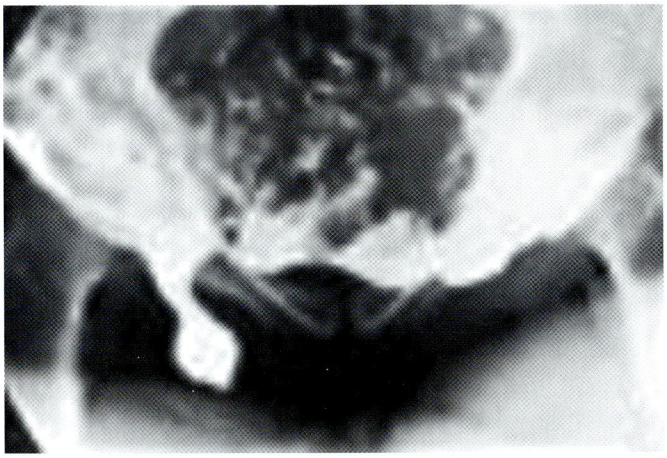

**Fig. 2.29:** The contrast medium fills a right-sided direct inguinal hernia with a narrow neck, extending from the medial inguinal fossa

## Diaphragm (Fig. 2.29)

### Anatomy

The diaphragm is a dome-shaped musculofibrous septum that separates the thoracic from the abdominal cavity, its convex upper surface forming the floor of the former, and its concave under surface the roof of the latter. Its peripheral part consists of muscular fibers that take origin from the circumference of the inferior thoracic aperture and converge to be inserted into a central tendon.

The muscular fibers may be grouped according to their origins into three parts (Table 2.4).

There are two lumbocostal arches, a medial and a lateral, on either side.

### Innervation

The diaphragm is innervated by the phrenic nerve. It is a branch of C3, C4, and C5.

You can remember that by the popular mnemonic "3, 4, 5 keeps the diaphragm alive".

### Crura and Central Tendon

At their origins the crura are tendinous in structure, and blend with the anterior longitudinal ligament of the vertebral column.

The central tendon of the diaphragm is a thin but strong aponeurosis situated near the center of the vault formed by the muscle, but somewhat closer to the front than to the back of the thorax, so that the posterior muscular fibers are the longer.

**Table 2.4**

**The muscular fibers may be grouped according to their origins into three parts**

| *Part* | *Origin* |
|---|---|
| Sternal | Two fleshy slips from the back of the xiphoid process |
| Costal | The inner surfaces of the cartilages and adjacent portions of the lower six ribs on either side, interdigitating with the transversus abdominis |
| Lumbar | Aponeurotic arches, named the lumbocostal arches, and from the lumbar vertebrae by two pillars or crura |

## Openings in the Diaphragm (Table 2.5 and Fig. 2.30)

Interior view of the human diaphragm, showing openings.

The diaphragm is pierced by a series of apertures to permit of the passage of structures between the thorax and abdomen. Three large openings—the aortic, the esophageal, and the vena cava—and a series of smaller ones are described.

## Esophageal Hiatus

In human anatomy, the esophageal hiatus is a hole in the diaphragm through which the esophagus passes. It is located in the right crus of the diaphragm.

It is located approximately at level of the tenth thoracic vertebra (T10).

The esophageal hiatus is situated in the muscular part of the diaphragm at the level of the tenth thoracic vertebra, and is elliptical in shape. It is placed superior, anterior,

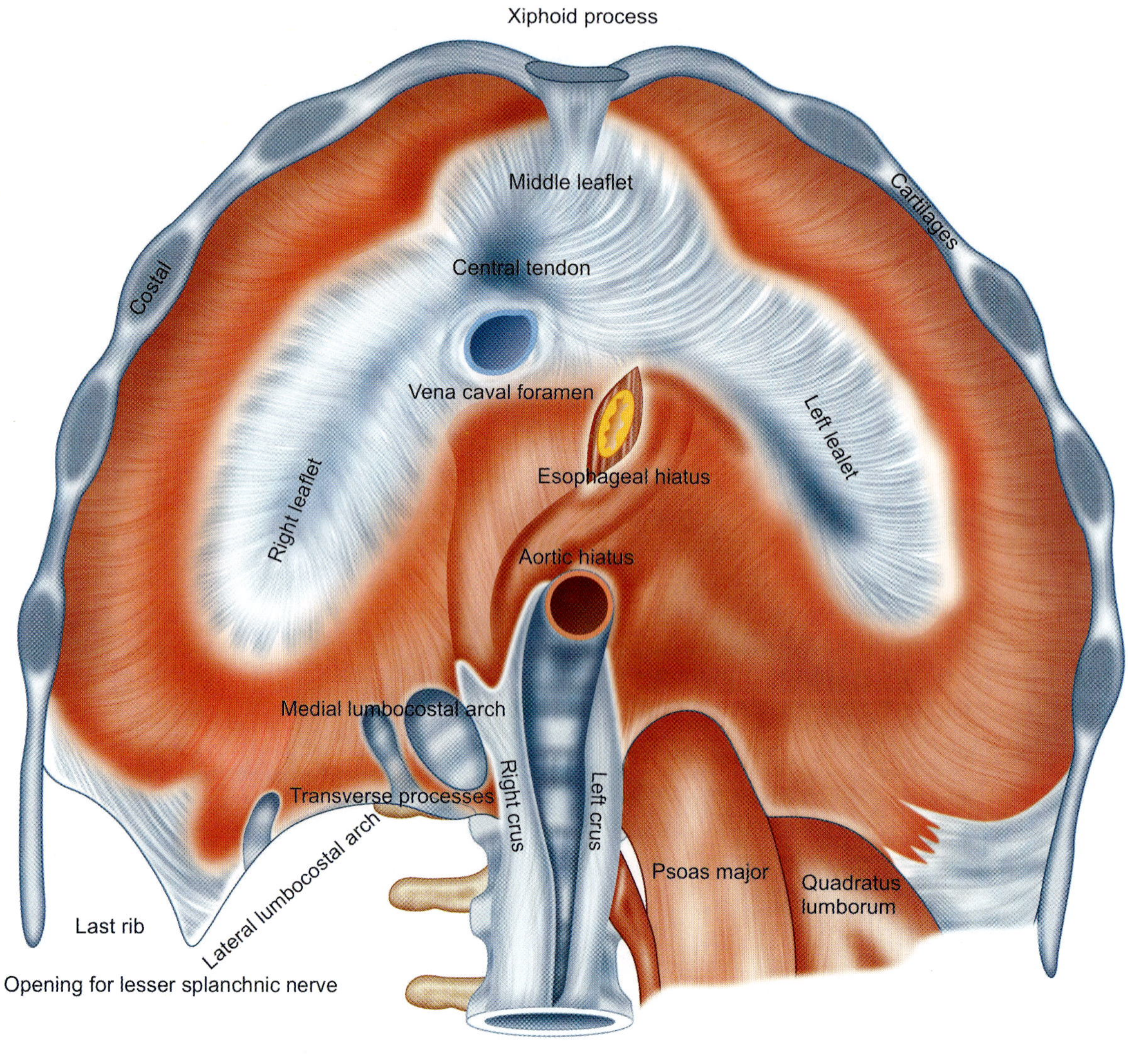


**Fig. 2.30:** Openings in the diaphragm

Table 2.5

| Openings in the diaphragm | | |
|---|---|---|
| *Opening* | *Level* | *Structures* |
| Caval opening | T8 | Inferior vena cava, and some branches of the right phrenic nerve |
| Esophageal hiatus | T10 | Esophagus, the anterior and posterior vagal trunks, and some small esophageal arteries |
| Aortic hiatus | T12 | The aorta, the azygos vein, and the thoracic duct |
| Two lesser aperture of right crus | | Greater and lesser right splanchnic nerves |
| Three lesser aperture of left crus | | Greater and lesser left splanchnic nerves and the hemiazygos vein |
| Behind the diaphragm, under the medial lumbocostal arches | | Sympathetic trunk |
| Areolar tissue between the sternal and costal parts (see also foramina of Morgagni) | | The superior epigastric branch of the internal mammary artery and somelymphatics from the abdominal wall and convex surface of the liver |
| Areolar tissue between the fibers springing from the medial and lateral lumbocostal arches | | This interval is less constant; when this interval exists, the upper and back part of the kidney is separated from the pleura by areolar tissue only. |

and slightly left of the aortic hiatus, and transmits the esophagus, the vagus nerves, and some small esophageal arteries. The right crus of the diaphragm loops around forming a sling around the diaphragm. Upon inspiration, this sling would constrict the diaphragm, forming an anatomical sphincter that prevents stomach contents from refluxing up the esophagus when intra-abdominal pressure rises during inspiration.

# Chapter 3

# Incidence, Prevalence of Hernia

## Incidence, Prevalence of Hernias (Abdominal)

### Inguinal Hernias in Adults

The true incidence of hernia is not known, but near accurate predictions are available. These are based on various surveys.

Inguinal hernias are more common in males than females (Fig. 3.1).

*Ratio:* There is always considerable under reporting of incidence of hernia.

In another survey this incidence comes out as Male: Female ratio (Fig. 3.2)

Inguinal hernias in males around age of 75 years (Fig. 3.3)

### Inguinal Hernias in Children

Inguinal hernias in children are 10 to 20 per 1000 births and male to female ratio is 4:1 (Figs 3.4 and 3.5).

Premature infants have more incidence of hernias in inguinal region.

The lifetime 'risk' of inguinal hernia repair is high: at currently prevailing rates we estimate it at 27% for men and 3% for women. There is significant elevation of mortality after emergency operations. Elective repair of inguinal hernia should be undertaken soon after the diagnosis is made to minimize the risk of adverse outcomes.

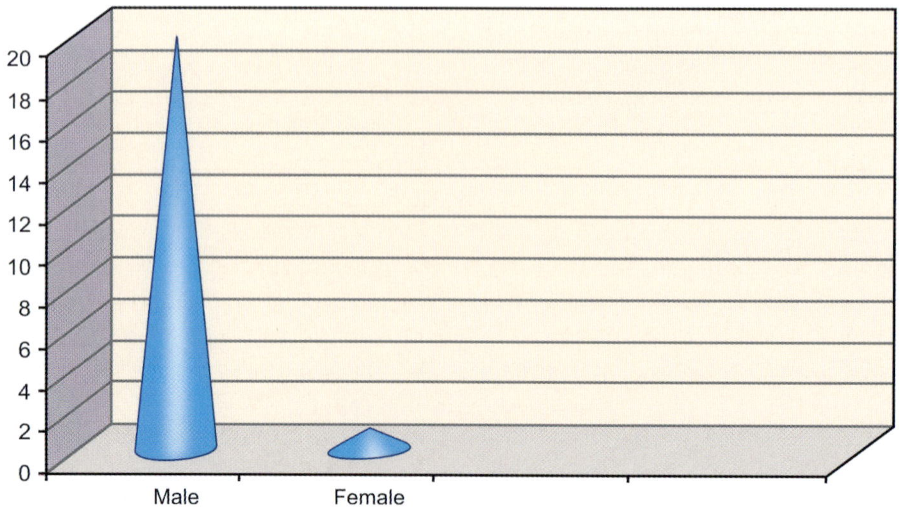


**Fig. 3.1:** Ratio of inguinal hernia

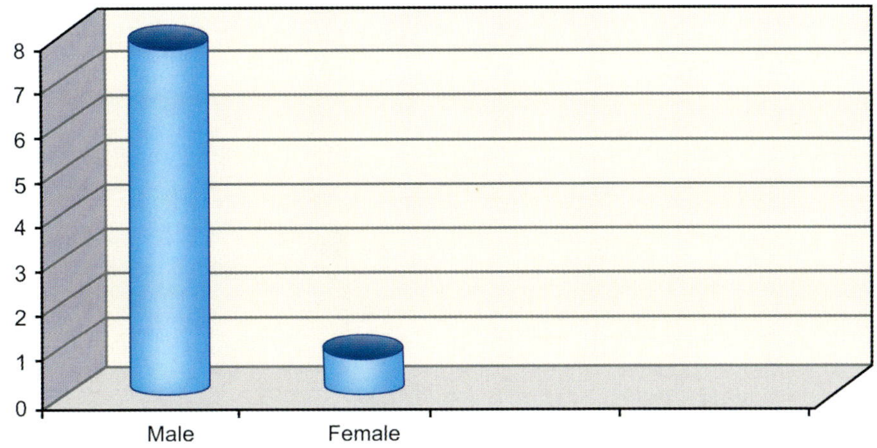


**Fig. 3.2:** Inguinal hernia ratio in another survey

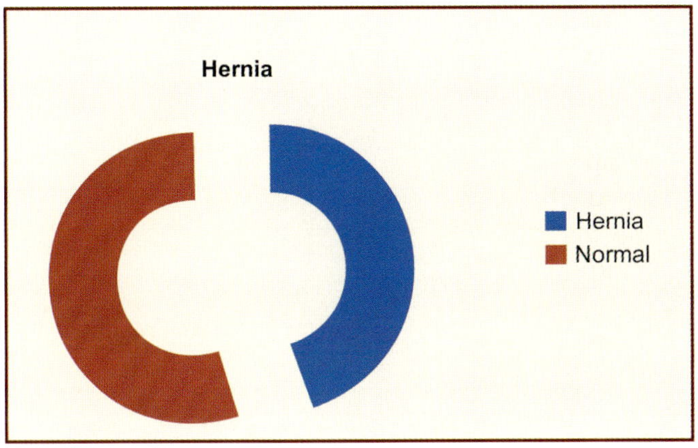


**Fig. 3.3:** Inguinal hernia in males around age of 75 years

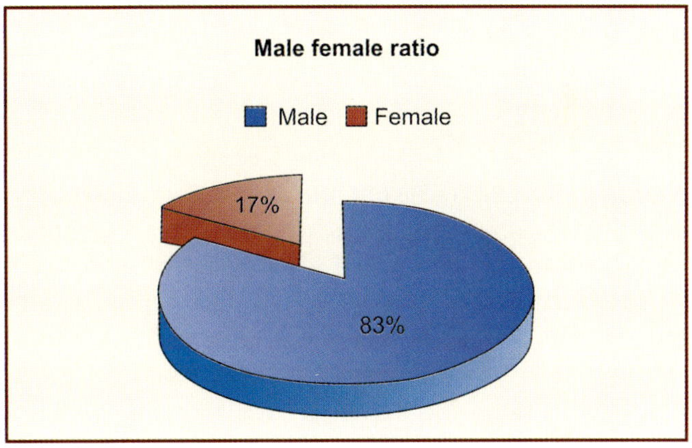


**Fig. 3.4:** Ratio of inguinal hernia in children of age 10 to 20 per 1000

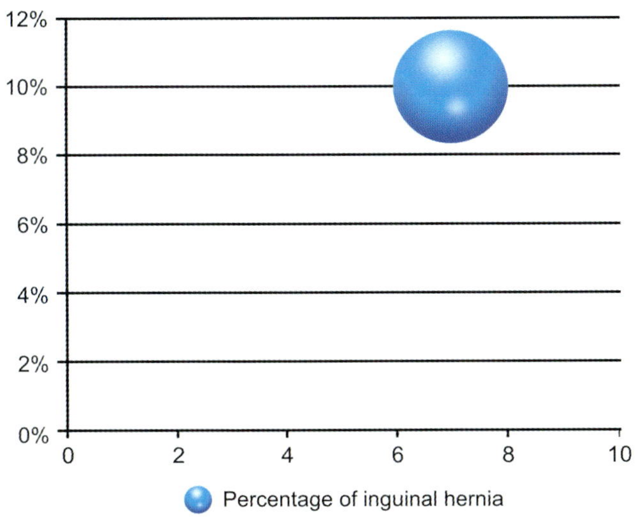


**Fig. 3.5:** Inguinal hernia in children of age 10 to 20 per 1000

## Femoral Hernias in Adults

Femoral hernias are a relatively uncommon type, accounting for only 3% of all hernias. While femoral hernias can occur in both males and females, almost all of them develop in females because of the wider bone structure of the female pelvis. Femoral hernias usually grow larger over time; any activity that involves straining, such as heavy lifting or a chronic cough, may cause the hernia to enlarge. Poor abdominal muscle tone, obesity, and pregnancy also increase a females risk of developing a femoral hernia. Most femoral hernias develop on only one side of the patient's abdomen, but about 15% of femoral hernias are bilateral. These bilateral hernias are more likely to become strangulated. An additional 20% of femoral hernias become incarcerated.

Femoral hernias are more common in adults than in children. Those that do occur in children are more likely

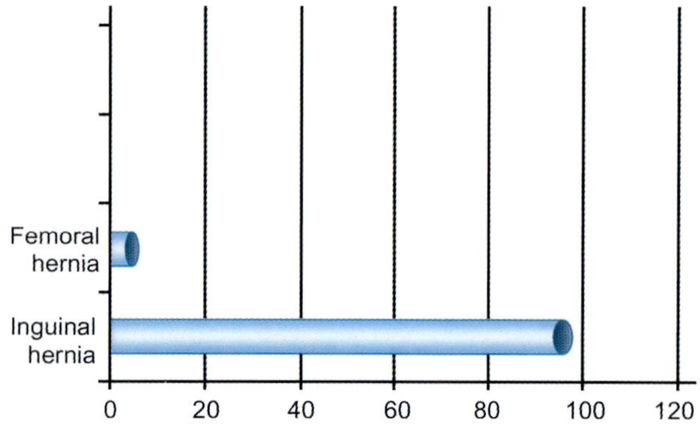


**Fig. 3.6:** Male: Female ratio

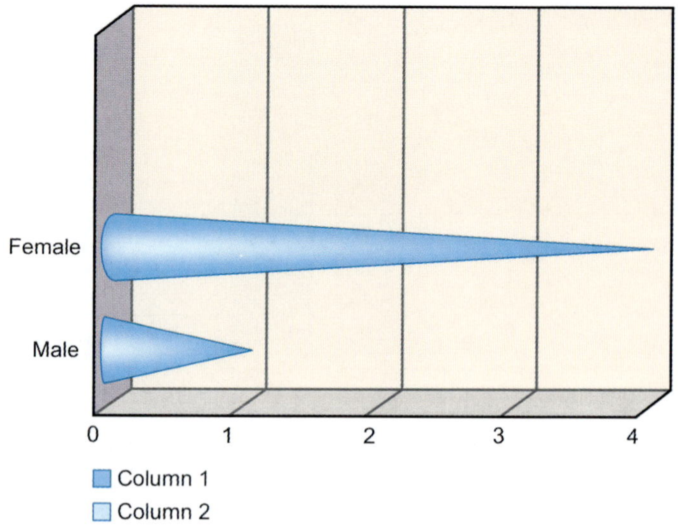


**Fig. 3.7:** Male: Female femoral hernia ratio

to be associated with a connective tissue disorder or with conditions that increase intra-abdominal pressure. Seventy percent of pediatric cases of femoral hernias occur in infants under the age of one.

## Epidemiology

Approximately 96% of groin hernias are inguinal and 4% are femoral (Fig. 3.6). Inguinal hernias are more common in males (ratio 9 to 1), while femoral hernias are more common in females (ratio 4 to 1), particularly elderly females (Fig. 3.7). The lifetime risk of developing a groin hernia is around 25% in males and less than 5 percent in females.

### Umbilical Hernia

The calculations of the incidence of umbilical hernia at birth vary greatly (Fig. 3.8).

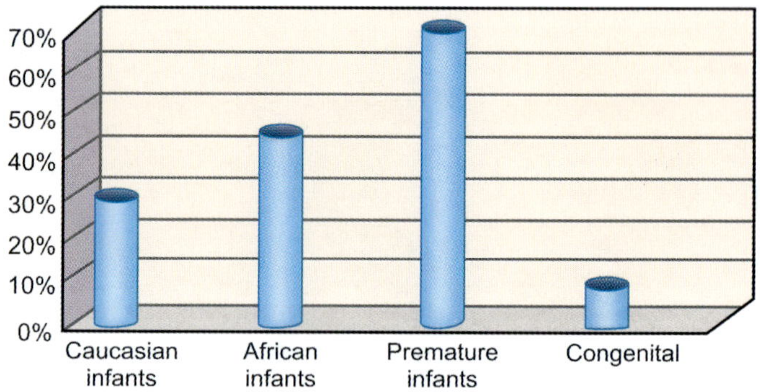


**Fig. 3.8:** Areawise occurrence of umbilical hernia

## Epigastric Hernia

The frequency of epigastric hernia in general population is 5%. It is occasionally found in infants and newborns (Fig. 3.9).

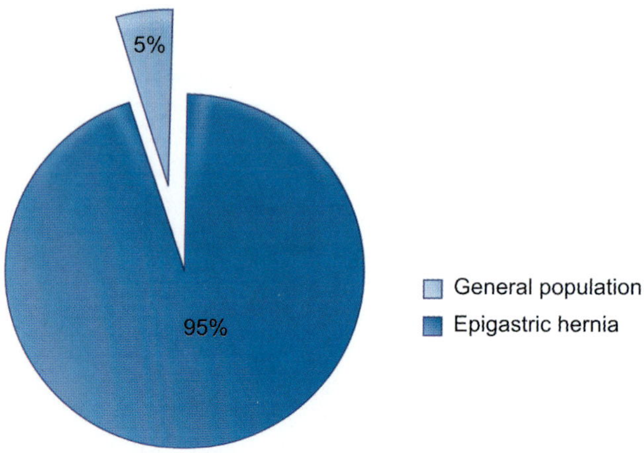


**Fig. 3.9:** Epigastric hernia

## Hiatal Hernia

### Frequency

#### *United States*

Hiatal hernias are more common in Western countries. The frequency of hiatus hernia increases with age, from

10% in patients younger than 40 years to 70% in patients older than 70 years.

## Frequency at a Glance

As much as 10% of the population develops some type of hernia during life. More than a half million hernia operations are performed in the United States each year. Fifty percent are for indirect inguinal hernias, with a male-to-female ratio of 7:1, while 25% are for direct inguinal hernias. Fourteen percent are umbilical (female-to-male ratio, 1.7:1), 5% are femoral (female-to-male ratio, 1.8:1), and 10% are incisional (female-to-male ratio, 2:1). The prevalence of all varieties of hernias increases with age.

Among inguinal hernias, a sliding component is found in 3%; they are overwhelmingly on the left side (left-to-right ratio, 4.5:1). Sliding hernias are much more common in males than in females, and the predominance increases with age. Female infants have a high incidence of sliding tube, ovary, or broad ligament hernias.

Umbilical hernias are much more common in persons of African ethnicity. The incidence of umbilical hernias is equal between male and female children, but, in adults, it is 3 times more common in females than in males. Epigastric hernias occur at a prevalence of 0.5% and are more common in males (male-to-female ratio, 3:1).

Spigelian hernias are rare and occur in persons aged approximately 50 years. No sex or side predilection exists for Spigelian hernias.

Interparietal, supravesical, lumbar, sciatic, and perineal hernias are rare.

Interparietal hernias are on the right side in 70% of cases, and a similar percentage has testicular maldescent (Denis-Browne pouch).

Reports of internal supravesical hernias are limited, but the literature suggests that they occur more often in males and in elderly people.

Primary perineal hernias occur most often in elderly multiparous females.

Obturator hernias occur most often in thin, elderly females and are more common on the right side.

Richter hernias present late in life, most often in females with femoral hernias.

Littre hernias have a much broader spectrum of hernia site and occur across all ages. The clinical presentation is umbilical, 30%; femoral, 25%; and inguinal, 50%.

In the case of congenital abdominal wall defects, the incidence of omphalocele has only slightly increased over the last few decades to about 1 to 2.5 in 5000 live births. In contrast, the incidence of gastroschisis has increased markedly over the past 25 years to a current level of 1 in 3600 live births. In addition, the prevalence of gastroschisis has increased by as much as 400% over the last two decades in some areas.

## Epidemiology of Inguinal Hernia Survey Results

Inguinal hernia is one of the most common surgical pathologies requiring operation (Fig. 3.10). A prevalence rate of 4.7% of inguinal hernia was found in males aged 25 years and older. Prevalence of inguinal hernia increased markedly with age. The lifetime prevalence rate reached 40 per 100 males between the ages of 65 to 74 years. The annual incidence of inguinal hernia was 13 per 10,000 population. The estimated lifetime risk of inguinal hernia repair was 27% for males. Optimal management

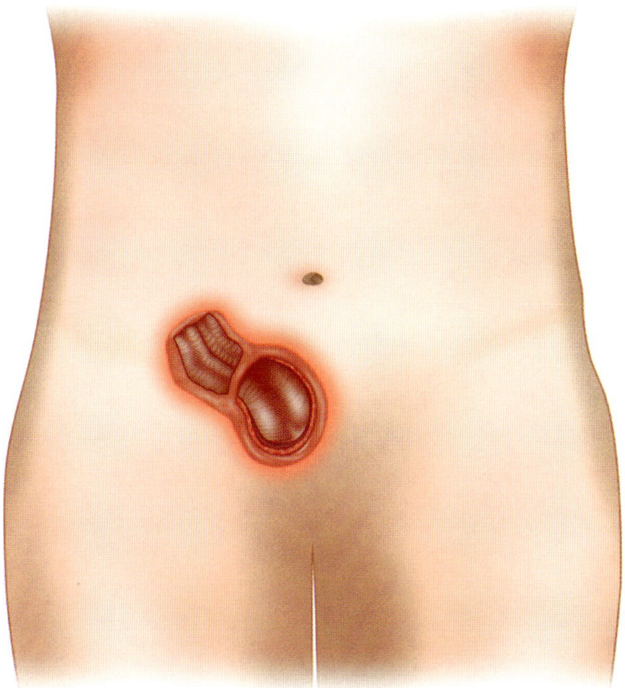

**Fig. 3.10:** Inguinal hernia is one of the most common surgical pathologies requiring operation

of inguinal hernia, the most frequent abdominal wall hernia, therefore carries significant socioeconomic impact on society.

The incidence of strangulation of groin hernias was reported in the literature to range from 1.3 to 5%. Mortality rate of strangulated inguinal hernia varied from 5 to 14%. Reported risk factors for strangulation of hernia included older age group, short duration of presentation, recurrent inguinal hernia, irreducibility of inguinal hernia and co-existing medical illness. As 40% of patients did not seek medical treatment before strangulation of their hernias and 10% of strangulation occurred in patients with no prior history of hernia, increased public awareness of this condition is, therefore, required to ensure that patients seek and receive prompt surgical treatment.

Chapter 4

# Etiology of Herniation

## Etiology

The embryology of the groin and of testicular descent largely explains indirect inguinal hernias. An indirect inguinal hernia is a congenital hernia regardless of the patient's age. It occurs because of protrusion of an abdominal viscus into an open processus vaginalis. If the processus contains viscera, it is called an indirect inguinal hernia. If peritoneal fluid fluxes between the space and the peritoneum, it is a communicating hydrocele. If fluid accumulates in the scrotum or spermatic cord without exchange of fluid with the peritoneum, it is a noncommunicating scrotal hydrocele or a hydrocele of the cord. In a girl, fluid accumulation in the processus vaginalis results in a hydrocele of the canal of Nuck.

The inguinal canal forms by mesenchyme condensation around the gubernaculum, which is Latin for rudder because it guides the testis into the scrotum. During the first trimester, the gubernaculum extends from the testis to the labioscrotal fold. The processus vaginalis and its fascial coverings also form during the first trimester. A bilateral oblique defect in the abdominal wall develops during the sixth or seventh week of gestation as the muscular wall develops around the gubernaculum. The processus vaginalis protrudes from the peritoneal cavity and lies anteriorly, laterally, and medially to the gubernaculum by the eighth week of gestation.

The testis produces many male hormones beginning at the eighth week of gestation. At the beginning of the seventh month, the gubernaculum begins a marked swelling influenced by a nonandrogenic hormone, probably a mullerian inhibiting substance. This results in expansion of the inguinal canal and the labioscrotal fold, forming the scrotum. The genitofemoral nerve also influences migration of the testis and gubernaculum into the scrotum under androgenic control. The female inguinal canal and processus is much less developed than the male equivalent. The inferior aspect of the gubernaculum is converted to the round ligament. The craniad part of the female gubernaculum becomes the ovarian ligament (Figs 4.1A to E).

Gonads develop on the medial aspect of the mesonephros during the fifth week of gestation. The kidney then moves cephalad, leaving the gonad to reside in the pelvis until the seventh month of gestation. During this time, it retains a ligamentous attachment to the proximal gubernaculum.

The gonads then migrate along the processus vaginalis, with the ovary descending into the pelvis and the testis being enwrapped within the distal processus, known as the tunica vaginalis. The processus fails to close adequately at birth in 40 to 50% of boys. Therefore, other factors play a role in the development of a clinical indirect hernia. A familial tendency exists, with 11.5% of patients having a family history. The relative risk of inguinal hernia is 5.8 for brothers of male cases, 4.3 for brothers of female cases, 3.7 for sisters of male cases, and 17.8 for sisters of female cases.

### Theories for Hernia Formation

1. Russell's theory—preformed sac.
2. Reid's metastatic emphysema theory—do not smoking.
3. Cloquet's lipoma theory—pile driver action of fat.
4. Fruchaud's theory—big opening in the lower abdomen-between the pubic bone and conjoint tendon. Divided into two by inguinal ligament.

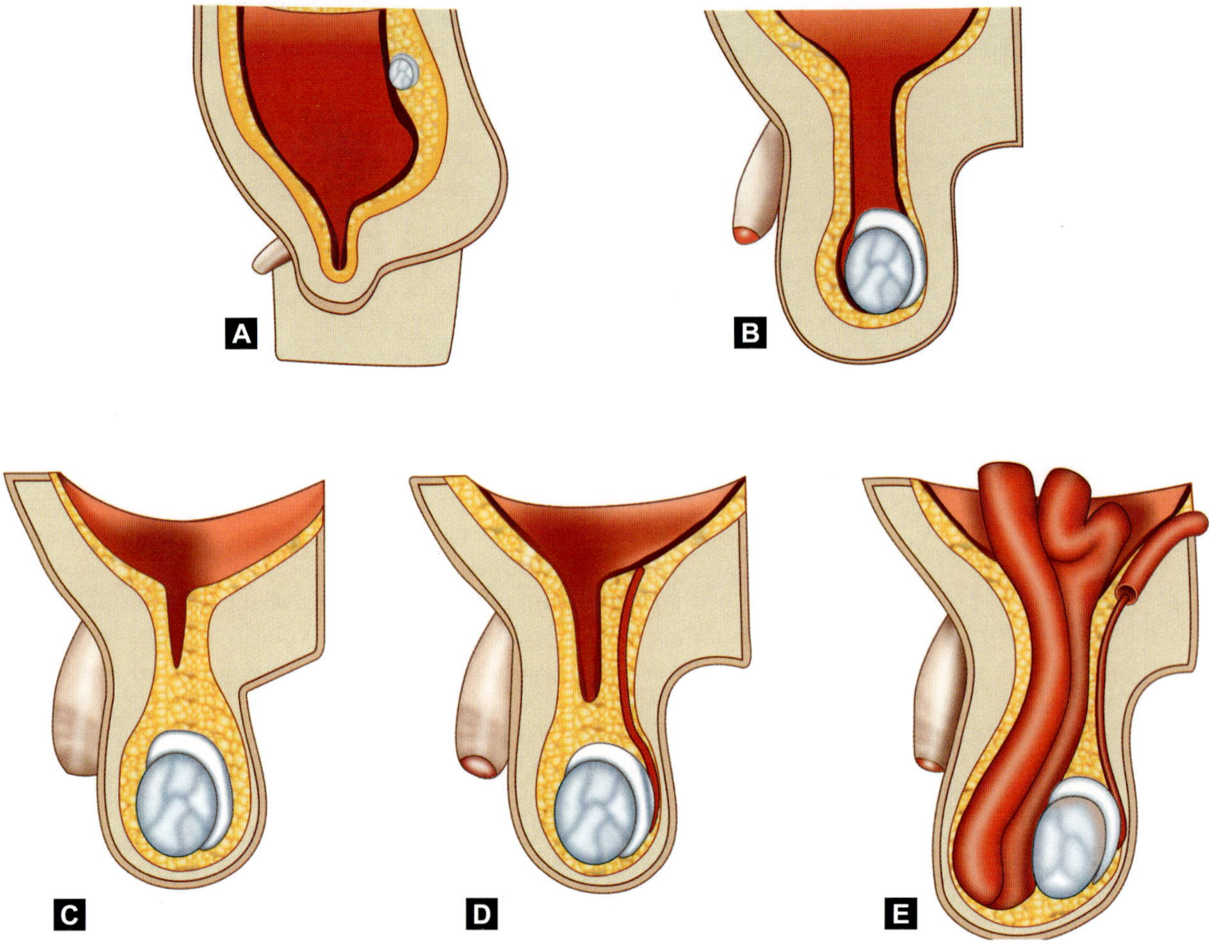


**Figs 4.1A to E:** Descent of testis in embryonic life

Through the upper part passes the inguinal hernia, while through the lower part passes the femoral hernia.

5. Denervation theory—ilioinguinal nerve especially after appendectomy.
6. Oblique pelvis—high arch of the internal oblique-inefficient shutter mechanism-prone to inguinal hernia.
7. Wide female pelvis—lower arch of internal oblique-more efficient shutter mechanism-indirect inguinal hernias are uncommon in females. Results in wider femoral ring-femoral hernias most common in females.
8. Uglavasky theory—chronic increased IAP.
9. Peacock's theory—defective collagen synthesis.
10. Walk's theory—weakness of abdominal wall at exit of neurovascular bundle.
11. Keith's theory—stress related degeneration of connective tissue, especially in the fascia transversalis.
12. Deficient insertion of the conjoint tendon seen in males-especially white males—predisposes to direct inguinal hernia-less support to posterior inguinal canal wall. Attachment quite wide in females-direct hernia almost never occurs in females.
13. Dr Desarda's theory adynamic and weak posterior wall due to absent or deficient aponeurotic extensions is the main cause of hernia formation. Loss of shielding action of the muscles and binding action of the interparietal connective tissue are also important factors (Fig. 4.2).

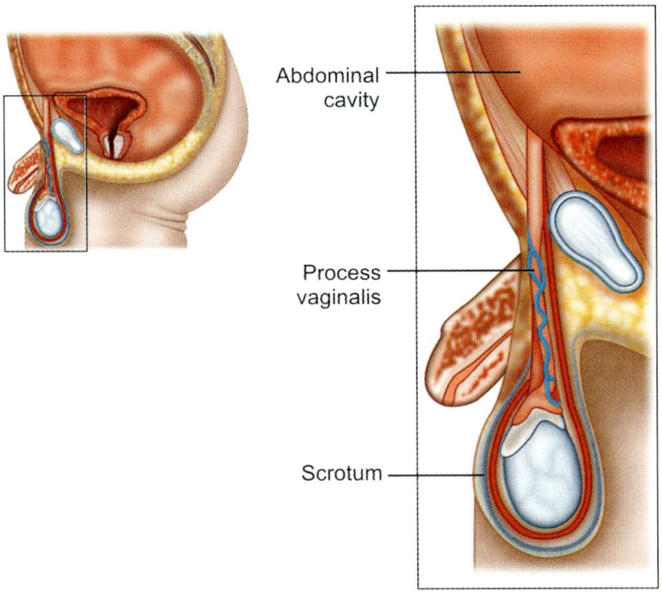


**Fig. 4.2:** Completely descended testis

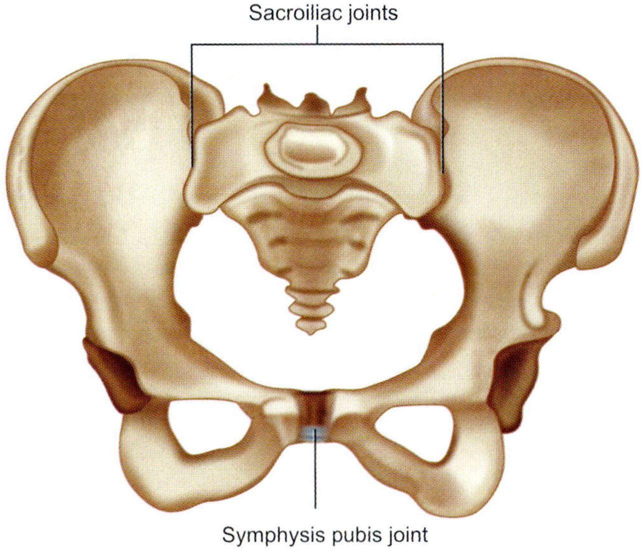


**Fig. 4.3:** Negro pelvis

## Pathophysiology

### Inguinal Hernias

The pinchcock action of the musculature of the internal ring during abdominal muscular straining prohibits protrusion of the intestine into a patent processus. Paralysis or injury to the muscle can disable the shutter effect. In addition, the transversus abdominis aponeurosis flattens during tensing, thus reinforcing the inguinal floor. A congenitally high position of the aponeurotic arch might preclude the buttressing effect. Neuropraxic or neurolytic sequelae of appendectomy or femoral vascular procedures may contribute to a greater incidence of hernia in these patients.

Repetitive stress as a factor in hernia development is suggested by clinical presentations. Increased intra-abdominal pressure is seen in a variety of disease states and seems to contribute to hernia formation in these populations. Elevated intra-abdominal pressure is associated with chronic cough, ascites, increased peritoneal fluid from biliary atresia, peritoneal dialysis or ventriculoperitoneal shunts, intraperitoneal masses or organomegaly, and obstipation. Other conditions with increased incidence of inguinal hernias are extrophy of bladder, neonatal intraventricular hemorrhage, myelomeningocele, and undescended testes. A high incidence (16–25%) of inguinal hernias occurs in premature infants; this incidence is inversely related to weight.

The rectus sheath adjacent to groin hernias is thinner than normal. The rate of fibroblast proliferation is less than normal, while the rate of collagenolysis appears increased. Sailors who developed scurvy had an increased incidence of hernia. Aberrant collagen states, such as Ehlers-Danlos syndrome, fetal hydantoin syndrome, Freeman-Sheldon syndrome, Hunter-Hurler syndrome, Kniest syndrome, Marfan syndrome, and Morquio syndrome, have increased rates of hernia formation, as do osteogenesis imperfecta, pseudo-Hurler polydystrophy, and Scheie syndrome. Acquired elastase deficiency also can lead to increased hernia formation. In 1981, Cannon and Read found that increased serum elastase and decreased $\alpha$1-antitrypsin levels in people who smoke contribute to an increase in the rate of hernia in those who smoke heavily. The contribution of biochemical or metabolic factors in the creation of inguinal hernia remains speculative.

### Mechanism of Hernia of the Groin

Utilitarian aspects of hernia pathogenicity are envisaged to assist comprehension of surgical gestures, the choice of effective techniques and the abandon of those which

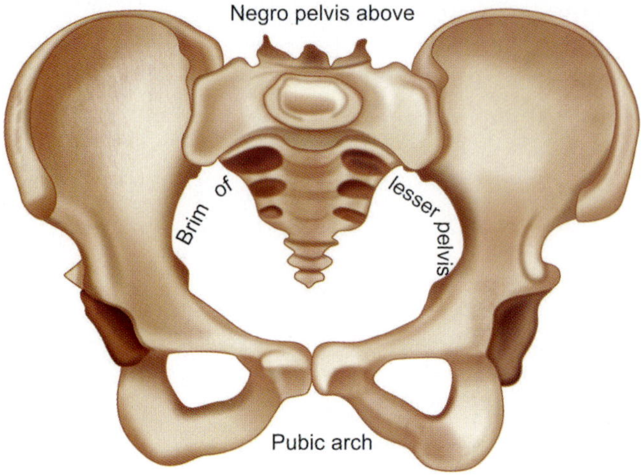


**Fig. 4.4:** European pelvis

are not and may be of medicolegal interest: all inguinal hernias are due to parietal weakness. Anatomical factors are studied based on data from dissection, from in front backwards and then from behind forwards, from which certain major notions are drawn: that of role of transverse fascia in imperviousness to intra-abdominal pressure; that of uniqueness of inguinal hernias, all of which cross the transverse fascia in the region of the regional osteomuscular framework; that of the necessary degradation of musculofascial plane for a hernia to develop, with as a corollary the need for inguinal imperviousness at the transverse fascia level to be restored. Factors may be present that increase the "natural weakness" of the groin: anatomical variations affecting inguinal triangle; biological disorders affecting inguinal structures (aponeurotic and fascial senescence, collagen diseases, musculo-tendino-aponeurotic dystrophy). A breakdown in mechanisms of protection against increased intra-abdominal pressure promoted a summary of features defining intra-abdominal pressure under physiologic conditions and classical herniogenic circumstances. A summary of pathogenic mechanisms of inguinal hernia is presented while emphasizing the two principal theories: the saccular theory and that of musculofascial weakness, with their consequences for choice of therapies to be opposed to the polymorphism of hernial lesions.

The European pelvis is relatively wide with a less deep arch than the Negro pelvis. This ensures that the internal oblique muscle origin from the lateral inguinal ligament is broad, so that the internal oblique muscle protects the deep ring.

The Negro pelvis is narrower than the European, which means that the lowness of the arch of the pelvis is greater in the Negro and the origin of the internal oblique relatively narrower. Hence, the internal oblique will not cover the deep ring during straining and the shutter mechanism of the inguinal canal is deficient. Negros have a ten times greater incidence of indirect inguinal hernia than Europeans (Figs 4.3 and 4.4).

### *List of Causes of Inguinal Hernia*

Following is a list of causes or underlying conditions that could possibly cause inguinal hernia includes:

- Obesity
- Pregnancy
- Heavy lifting
- Straining to pass stool, urine
- Enlarged prostate

### *Inguinal Hernia as a Complication of other Conditions*

Other conditions that might have inguinal hernia as a complication may, potentially, be an underlying cause of inguinal hernia. List includes the following as having Inguinal hernia as a complication of that condition:

- Cutis laxa
- Marfan syndrome
- Whooping cough

### *Inguinal Hernia as a Symptom*

Conditions listing inguinal hernia as a symptom may also be potential underlying causes of inguinal hernia. list includes the following as having inguinal hernia as a symptom of that condition:

- Aarskog syndrome
- Achondrogenesis
- Achondroplasia regional-dysplasia abdominal muscle
- Acrocallosal syndrome (Schinzel Type)
- Acrofacial dysostosis Catania form
- Alport syndrome
- Amyloidosis, familial cutaneous
- Aniridia-absent patella
- Anophthalmia—megalocornea-cardiopathy skeletal anomalies
- Arterial tortuosity syndrome

- Arthrogryposis-ophthalmoplegia-retinopathy
- Arthrogryposis multiplex with deafness, inguinal hernias, and early death
- Blepharophimosis telecanthus microstomia
- Bosma-Henkin-Christiansen syndrome
- Bruck syndrome 2
- Chitty Hall Baraitser syndrome
- Chromosome 1, deletion *q21 q25*
- Chromosome 1, partial trisomy
- Chromosome *11q* duplication syndrome
- Chromosome *12p* deletion
- Chromosome *12p* deletion syndrome
- Chromosome 13 trisomy syndrome
- Chromosome *15q* duplication syndrome
- Chromosome *15q*, trisomy
- Chromosome 17, deletion *17q23 q24*
- Chromosome *17p*, partial duplication
- Chromosome 2 trisomy syndrome
- Chromosome *20p*, partial duplication
- Chromosome *21q* deletion syndrome
- Chromosome *22q* duplication syndrome
- Chromosome 3, monosomy *3p25*
- Chromosome 4, trisomy *4q*
- Chromosome *4q* duplication syndrome
- Chromosome *5q* deletion syndrome
- Chromosome 6, monosomy *6q*
- Chromosome *6p* deletion syndrome
- Chromosome *6q* deletion syndrome
- Chromosome 8, monosomy *8p*
- Chromosome 8, monosomy *8p2*
- Chromosome 8, monosomy *8p21*-pter
- Chromosome 8, monosomy *8q*
- Chromosome *8p* deletion syndrome
- Chromosome *8p* duplication syndrome
- Chromosome *8p* inverted duplication syndrome
- Chromosome 9, monosomy *9p*
- Collins-Pope syndrome
- Davis-Lafer syndrome
- Deafness–epiphyseal dysplasia–short stature
- Dermatocardioskeletal syndrome, Boronne type
- Ectodermal dysplasia, sensorineural hearing loss, and distinctive facial features
- Edward syndrome
- Ehlers-Danlos syndrome Type IX
- Ehlers-Danlos syndrome Type VI
- Ehlers-Danlos syndrome, *6B*
- Ehlers-Danlos syndrome, Beasley Cohen Type
- Ehlers-Danlos syndrome, cardiac valvular form
- Ehlers-Danlos syndrome, kyphoscoliosis Type
- Ehlers-Danlos syndrome, VIIB
- Elliott-Ludman-Teebi syndrome
- Emanuel syndrome
- Exstrophy of the bladder
- Facioskeletalgenital syndrome, Rippberger Type
- Faciothoracogenital syndrome
- Femoral facial syndrome
- Fetal Hydantoin syndrome
- Focal dermal hypoplasia
- Freeman-Sheldon syndrome
- Furlong-Kurczynski-Hennessy syndrome
- Gangliosidosis generalized *GM1*, Type 1
- GM1 gangliosidosis
- Grix-Blankenship-Peterson syndrome
- Hajdu-Cheney syndrome
- Hermaphroditism
- Herrmann opitz arthrogryposis syndrome
- Hydrocephaly low insertion umbilicus
- Kniest dysplasia
- Krieble Bixler syndrome
- Lambert syndrome
- Lenz Majewski hyperostotic dwarfism
- Lindstrom syndrome
- Lowry-Maclean syndrome
- Mental retardation, Wolff Type
- Mental retardation, X-linked, Armfield Type
- Microspherophakia with hernia
- Montefiore syndrome
- Mucopolysaccharidosis Type 2 Hunter syndrome-mild form
- Mucopolysaccharidosis Type 6
- Mucopolysaccharidosis Type 7 Sly syndrome
- Mucopolysaccharidosis Type I Hurler syndrome
- Mucopolysaccharidosis Type I Hurler/Scheie syndrome
- Mucopolysaccharidosis Type I Scheie syndrome
- Mullerian derivatives, persistent
- Osteogenesis imperfecta Type I
- Osteogenesis imperfecta, Type 1A
- Osteogenesis imperfecta, Type 1B
- Osteogenesis imperfecta, Type 2
- Osteogenesis imperfecta, Type 2A
- Osteogenesis imperfecta, Type 4
- Osteogenesis imperfecta, Type IIB
- Oto-facio-osseous-gonadal syndrome
- Palmer-Pagon syndrome
- Persistent Mullerian duct syndrome (PMDS)
- Polydactyly-myopia syndrome
- Rubella congenital syndrome

- Rudiger syndrome
- Rüdiger syndrome 2
- Sakati syndrome
- SCARF syndrome
- Schwartz-Jampel syndrome
- SHORT syndrome
- Simpson-Golabi-Behmel syndrome
- Subaortic stenosis-short stature syndrome
- Supraumbilical midabdominal raphe and facial cavernous hemangiomas
- Trigonocephaly-bifid nose-acral anomalies
- Trisomy 13 mosaicism
- Weaver syndrome

### Causes for Inguinal Hernia

*Causes:* Inguinal hernia—obesity, pregnancy, heavy lifting, and straining to pass stool can cause the intestine to push against the inguinal canal.

### Inguinal Hernia—Risk Factors Prematurity

- *Urologic conditions:* Cryptorchidism, hypospadia, epispadia, bladder exstrophy
- *Abdominal wall defects:* Gastroschisis, omphalocele
- Conditions that increase intra-abdominal pressure: Ascites, peritoneal dialysis, ventriculoperitoneal shunt
- Meconium peritonitis
- Cystic fibrosis
- Congenital dislocation of the hip
- *Connective tissue disease:* Marfan syndrome, Ehlers-Danlos syndrome
- Mucopolysaccharidoses
- Family history

### Inguinal Hernia—Pathophysiology

- In boys, during the seventh month of gestation, the testes begin their descent from the peritoneal cavity, where they developed, through the inguinal canal and down into the scrotum.
- Between the 7th and 9th months of gestation, the testes reach the scrotum, at which point the processus vaginalis—an outpouching of the peritoneum attached to the testes—begins to obliterate spontaneously, leaving a small potential space adjacent to the testes, called tunica vaginalis.
- In girls, although the ovaries do not leave the abdomen, the round ligament (part of the gubernaculum) travels through the inguinal ring into labium majus. When the processus vaginalis remains open, it is called the canal of Nuck.
- Incomplete obliteration of the processus vaginalis leaves a sac of peritoneum extending all the way from the internal inguinal ring to the scrotum or labium majus, from which an inguinal hernia may develop.
  - An inguinal hernia may be indirect or direct. An indirect inguinal hernia, the more common form, results from weakness in the fascial margin of the internal inguinal ring. In an indirect hernia, abdominal viscera leave the abdomen through the inguinal ring and follow the spermatic cord (in males) or round ligament (in females); they emerge at the external ring and extend down the inguinal canal, commonly into the scrotum or labia. An indirect inguinal hernia may develop at any age, is more common in males, and is especially prevalent in infants younger than age 1. According to the American Academy of Pediatrics, about 5 out of 100 children have inguinal hernias.
  - A direct inguinal hernia results from a weakness in the fascial floor of the inguinal canal. Instead of entering the canal through the internal ring, the hernia passes through the posterior inguinal wall, protrudes directly through the transverse fascia of the canal (in an area known as *Hesselbach's triangle*), and comes out at the external ring.
  - In males, during the seventh month of gestation, the testicle normally descends into the scrotum, preceded by the peritoneal sac. If the sac closes improperly, it leaves an opening through which the intestine can slip. In either sex, a hernia can result from weak abdominal muscles (caused by congenital malformation, trauma, or aging) or increased intra-abdominal pressure (due to heavy lifting, pregnancy, obesity, or straining).
  - About 10% of people develop some type of hernia during their lifetime, and more than 500,000 hernia operations are performed in the United States each year. Hernias are seven times more common in males than in females.
  - *Inguinal hernia and appendisectomy:* Hoguet in 1911 described the occurrence of inguinal hernia in few patients who had undergone appendisectomy. The cause specified is injury to iliohypogastric nerve and denervation of transversus abdominis which leads to disruption of the abdominal shutter mechanism.

- Hernias are related with trauma and pelvic fractures. The complete disruption of inguinal canal and rupture of conjoint tendon are possible causes.
- Hernias are the outcomes of erect posture of humans.
- Smoking causes the inguinal hernia. The nicotine is absorbed in blood and weakens the abdominal musculature which reduces the function of shutter mechanism, thereby causing inguinal hernia.

## Umbilical Hernias

Umbilical hernias in children are secondary to failure of closure of the umbilical ring, but only 1 in 10 adults with umbilical hernias reports a history of this defect as a child. The adult umbilical hernia occurs through a canal bordered anteriorly by the linea alba, posteriorly by the umbilical fascia, and laterally by the rectus sheath. Proof that umbilical hernias persist from childhood to present as problems in adults is only hinted at by an increased incidence among black Americans. Multiparity, increased abdominal pressure, and a single midline decussation are associated with umbilical hernias.

Congenital hypothyroidism; fetal hydantoin syndrome; Freeman-Sheldon syndrome; Beckwith-Wiedemann syndrome; and disorders of collagen and polysaccharide metabolism, such as Hunter-Hurler syndrome, osteogenesis imperfecta, or Ehlers-Danlos syndrome, should be considered as possibilities in children with large umbilical hernias.

### *Causes of Umbilical Hernia that are Very Rare*

Congenital hypothyroidism—umbilical hernia

### *Causes of Umbilical Hernia without any Prevalence Information*

The following causes of umbilical hernia are ones for which we do not have any prevalence information:

- Achondrogenesis–umbilical hernia
- Achondroplasia regional–dysplasia abdominal muscle-umbilical hernia
- Acrocallosal syndrome–umbilical hernia
- Amastia, bilateral, with ureteral triplication and dysmorphism–umbilical hernia
- Ampola syndrome–umbilical hernia
- Anophthalmia–megalocornea–cardiopathy–skeletal anomalies–umbilical hernia
- Athyrotic hypothyroidism sequence–umbilical hernia
- Aural atresia–multiple congenital anomalies–mental retardation–umbilical hernia
- Brachycephalofrontonasal dysplasia–umbilical hernia
- Carpenter syndrome–umbilical hernia
- Chitty Hall Baraitser syndrome–umbilical hernia
- Chromosome 1, monosomy *1p32*–umbilical hernia
- Chromosome *10p* deletion syndrome–umbilical hernia
- Chromosome *10p* duplication/*10q* deletion syndrome–umbilical hernia
- Chromosome 13 trisomy syndrome–umbilical hernia
- Chromosome *1p* duplication syndrome–umbilical hernia
- Chromosome *20p*, partial duplication–umbilical hernia
- Chromosome 21, tetrasomy *21q*–umbilical hernia
- Chromosome 22 Ring-umbilical hernia
- Chromosome 3, monosomy *3p*–umbilical hernia
- Chromosome 3, monosomy *3p25*–umbilical hernia
- Chromosome 4, trisomy *4q*–Umbilical hernia
- Chromosome *4q* duplication syndrome-umbilical hernia
- Chromosome 6, monosomy *6q*–Umbilical hernia
- Chromosome *6p* deletion syndrome–umbilical hernia
- Chromosome *6q* deletion syndrome–umbilical hernia
- Chromosome *8p* inverted duplication syndrome-umbilical hernia
- Chromosome 9, monosomy *9p*–umbilical hernia
- Chromosome *9p* tetrasomy syndrome–umbilical hernia
- Chromosomes 1 and 2, monosomy *2q* duplication 1p-umbilical hernia
- Congenital hypothyroidism–umbilical hernia
- Craniofacial dyssynostosis–umbilical hernia
- Deafness–epiphyseal dysplasia–short stature–umbilical hernia
- Deafness–mental retardation, Martin-Probst type–umbilical hernia
- Deletion *3p*–umbilical hernia
- Deletion *6q*–umbilical hernia
- Duplication 13–umbilical hernia
- Duplication 18–umbilical hernia
- Dysostosis acral with facial and genital abnormalities-umbilical hernia

- Edward syndrome–umbilical hernia
- Ehlers-Danlos syndrome, VIIB–umbilical hernia
- Elliott-Ludman-Teebi syndrome–umbilical hernia
- Facioskeletalgenital syndrome, Rippberger type–umbilical hernia
- Fetal Hydantoin syndrome–umbilical hernia
- Fetal minoxidil syndrome–umbilical hernia
- Focal dermal hypoplasia–umbilical hernia
- Gangliosidosis generalized GM1, Type 1–umbilical hernia
- GAPO syndrome–umbilical hernia
- GM1 gangliosidosis–umbilical hernia
- Gonadal dysgenesis XY Type associated anomalies–umbilical hernia
- Hajdu-Cheney syndrome–umbilical hernia
- Hypertrichotic osteochondrodysplasia–umbilical hernia
- Hypothyroidism–dermoid cyst-cleft palate–umbilical hernia
- Idaho syndrome–umbilical hernia
- Intracranial aneurysms-multiple congenital anomaly–umbilical hernia
- Kniest dysplasia–umbilical hernia
- Kosztolanyi syndrome–umbilical hernia
- Lateral meningocele syndrome–umbilical hernia
- Marshall-Smith syndrome–umbilical hernia
- Medrano-Roldan syndrome–umbilical hernia
- Mental retardation, Buenos Aires Type–umbilical hernia
- Mucopolysaccharidosis Type 6–umbilical hernia
- Mucopolysaccharidosis Type 7 Sly syndrome–umbilical hernia
- Mucopolysaccharidosis Type I Hurler syndrome–umbilical hernia
- Mucopolysaccharidosis Type I Scheie syndrome–umbilical hernia
- Osteogenesis imperfecta Type I–umbilical hernia
- Osteogenesis imperfecta Type 1A–umbilical hernia
- Osteogenesis imperfecta Type 1B–umbilical hernia
- Osteogenesis imperfecta Type 4–umbilical hernia
- Petty-Laxova-Wiedemann syndrome-umbilical hernia
- SCARF syndrome–umbilical hernia
- Schwartz-Jampel syndrome–umbilical hernia
- Simpson-Golabi-Behmel syndrome–umbilical hernia
- Stiff baby syndrome–umbilical hernia
- Tetra-amelia with pulmonary hypoplasia–umbilical hernia
- Triploid syndrome–umbilical hernia
- Trisomy 13 mosaicism–umbilical hernia
- Unusual facies, short webbed neck, mental retardation, short stature–umbilical hernia
- Urban Roger Meyer syndrome–umbilical hernia
- Weaver syndrome–umbilical hernia
- Whelan syndrome–umbilical hernia

#### *All Causes of Umbilical Hernia*

The full list of all possible causes for umbilical hernia described in various sources is as follows:

- Achondrogenesis–umbilical hernia
- Achondroplasia regional–dysplasia abdominal muscle–umbilical hernia
- Acrocallosal syndrome–umbilical hernia
- Amastia, bilateral with ureteral triplication and dysmorphism–umbilical hernia
- Ampola syndrome–umbilical hernia

## Congenital Abdominal Wall Defects

The underlying embryogenic factor in both omphalocele and gastroschisis is deficient closure of the developing anterior wall at the umbilical stalk. Variations in lateral fold migration can result in both omphalocele and gastroschisis. In addition, most children with omphalocele and all children with gastroschisis have intestinal malrotation as their extracoelomic location precludes normal attachment of the intestines to the posterior peritoneum.

Improper development of other portions of the abdominal wall leads to specific anomalies. In 1967, Duhamel proposed that maldevelopment of the superior (cephalad) of the 4 folds producing the abdominal wall leads to the thoracic, sternal and diaphragmatic, and abdominal wall defects that make-up the upper midline syndrome or pentology of Cantrell. In this syndrome, there is a bifid sternal cleft, anterior diaphragmatic defect, anterior pericardial defect, epigastric omphalocele, and congenital cardiac defects. Maldevelopment of the inferior (caudal) fold produces pelvic, hindgut, sacral, genital, and bladder defects. Lower midline syndrome includes a hypogastric omphalocele, extrophy of the bladder or cloaca, vesicointestinal fissure, colonic atresia, imperforate anus, sacral vertebral defects, and often meningoceles.

Lateral fold maldevelopment results in omphalocele and gastroschisis. It has been postulated that an omphalocele results from persistence of the umbilical stalk in the somatopleure. Approximately 20% of infants with omphaloceles have associated chromosomal abnormalities, such as trisomy 13, trisomy 18, trisomy 21, and Klinefelter syndrome. Over 50% of infants with omphaloceles have associated neurologic, urinary tract, cardiac, and skeletal anomalies. The liver is present in the omphalocele sac in 35% of patients. In small omphaloceles, there is a high coincidence of Meckel diverticulum. Maternal smoking is associated with an increased prevalence of omphalocele and gastroschisis.

Gastroschisis is thought to be the result of a failure of the umbilical coelom to develop to an appropriate size. The intestine then ruptures out of the body wall to the right of the umbilicus, where a slight weakness exists secondary to resorption of the right umbilical vein early in gestation. Gastroschisis is associated with intestinal atresias in 10 to 15% of cases, likely due to an interruption of the vascular supply to the intestine. Experimentally, administration of the insecticide methylparathion has produced gastroschisis. Transplacental transmission of such teratogens helps explain gastroschisis in siblings with different fathers.

## Other Hernias

Aberrant formation of the decussations of the linea alba, leading to a midline pattern of single anterior and posterior lines, predisposes to the formation of epigastric hernias (epiploceles). Abnormal orientation of the semilunar and semicircular lines, in combination with obesity, increased intra-abdominal pressure, aging, and rapid weight loss, leads to the production of spigelian hernias.

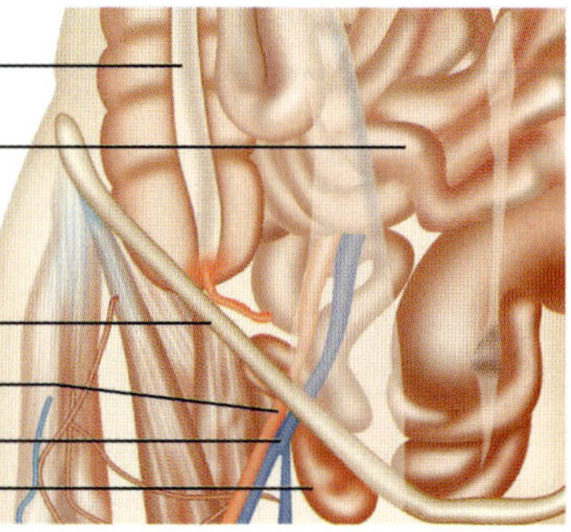


**Fig. 4.5:** Femoral hernia

Internal supravesical hernias probably arise from congenital deficiency in the fasciae. The perihernial fasciae or musculature may be malformed in lumbar, femoral, and other abdominal hernias. Interparietal hernias are often a product of ectopic testicular descent. Multiparity and age produce laxity of the pelvic floor to cause obturator hernias and perineal hernias.

## Femoral Hernia (Fig. 4.5)

### *Causes of Femoral Hernia*

A femoral hernia can simply occur of its own accord, but anything which increases pressure on this part of body can also cause a hernia. This can include:

- Coughing
- Straining to pass feces or to pass urine
- Pregnancy
- Straining to lift heavy objects
- Stresses and straining of muscles due to physical exercise.

# Chapter 5

# Prosthesis Used in Hernioplasty

In the last 30 years with the introduction of the "tension-free" techniques in hernia repair based on the use of alloplastic, nonabsorbable prosthetic materials, we have witnessed to a significant reduction in postoperative pain degree and incidence of hernia recurrences when confronted with the older nonprosthetic hernioplasties.

The use of nonabsorbable prosthetic materials such as polypropylene, polyester, and ePTFE, have hence expanded and are now widely used in reparative surgery for abdominal wall hernias. When implanted, these nonabsorbable materials—although extremely biocompatible-stimulate a foreign-bodies reaction within the host.

It is important to remember that prosthetic repair has been proven to have a significant less risk of recurrence than repair with direct sutures.

Recently, new "biologic" prosthetic materials have been developed and proposed for the clinical use in infected fields. These materials can be called "remodeling" for the way by which they are replaced after their placement within the patient. The "remodeling" process is made possible through a process of incorporation, where a reproduction of a site-specific tissue similar to the original host tissue is created.

After the initial inflammatory phase, the reaction is followed by an intense deposition of nonspecific fibrotic tissue and concluded by a permanent encapsulation of the alloplastic material in the host's tissues.

If these are the physiopathological bases that explain the success of alloplastic nonabsorbable prosthetic materials in hernia surgery, they are also the reasons for not uncommon complications such as infections.

Surgical meshes today represent a group of implants used mainly for hernia repair. Modern hernia surgery is no longer imaginable without the application of these special biomaterials, leading to about 1 million implantations each year, worldwide. The net-like alloplastic mesh is used to close the hernial gap and, with extended overlap, to reinforce the abdominal wall. Since the introduction of surgical meshes for hernia repair in 1959 by Usher, the main interest of hernia surgeons in the past decades was focused on surgical techniques to optimize hernia repair and the application of the mesh. The surgical mesh itself, however, seemed to have little impact on the clinical outcome after hernia repair. The meshes themselves were regarded as biologically inert, can be observed in about half of the patients. Serious complications such as recurrence, chronic and persisting pain as well as infection, including fistula formation are rare, but sometimes force a surgeon to remove the surgical mesh. Nevertheless, these complications have been the rationale to examine the role of the mesh in hernia repair in detail and to begin to investigate the biocompatibility of different mesh modifications and to challenge old mesh concepts.

## Use of Prosthetics in Hernia Repair

The need for a satisfactory prosthesis for hernia repair has been recognized for more than a century. Various materials, including autografts (the patient's own tissue), have been tried. The most successful of the autografts is fascia lata, which has been used as suture material, a pedicle graft, and as a free transplanted graft. However,

**Table 5.1**

| Characteristics of an ideal prosthesis |
|---|
| *The ideal prosthetic mesh should* |
| Not be physically modified by tissue fluids |
| Be chemically inert |
| Not excite inflammatory or foreign body reaction |
| Be noncarcinogenic |
| Not produce allergy or hypersensitivity |
| Be capable of resisting mechanical strain |
| Be capable of being fabricated in the form required, and constructed in a way such that sutures or cutting will not cause the mesh to unravel or fray |
| Be sterilizable |
| Be permeable and allow tissue ingrowth within it |
| Stimulate fibroblastic activity to allow incorporation into tissue rather than sequestration or encapsulation |
| Be sufficiently pliable so as not to cause stiffness or to be felt by the patient |
| Strong enough to resist bursting by the maximum forces that can be created by intra-abdominal pressure or from an outer force |

**Table 5.2**

| Metal prosthetic graft material | |
|---|---|
| Silver filigree mesh (1900) | Became brittle and fractured and eventually extruded causing multiple sinuses and fistulas |
| | Fractured and caused sinus formation |
| Toilinox (stainless steel) | Setup electrolyte reactions between ingredients if composition varied |

in addition to requiring a second operation to harvest it, fascia lata weakens and fails over time and dissolves in the presence of infection.

Artificial prostheses. Many authors have attempted to define characteristics of the ideal prosthetic material for hernia repairs (Table 5.1), although attempts to achieve this "ideal" have met with varying degrees of success (Tables 5.2 and 5.3). No currently available prosthesis is perfect or free of problems, and the choice of material thus requires compromise. Surgeons do, however, have a large array of products from which to choose.

Any area in which surgery with a possible risk of bacterial contamination is performed (bowel resections, cholecystectomy, operations on bile duct, parastomal hernias, etc.), is potentially at risk for prosthetic repair. On one side there is a common consensus on what should be done in frankly contaminated areas such as in peritonitis. In fact the opinion is not to position any kind of nonabsorbable prosthetic material due to a very high risk of infection (do not use nonabsorbable materials). On the other side it is not demonstrated that there is an increased risk of contamination of the mesh in case that simultaneous operations on the digestive tract are performed (potentially contaminated surgical fields).

Some authors report prosthetic repair of the abdominal wall after colonic resection (potentially contaminated surgical field) with good results. Many other perform prosthetic inguinal hernia repair in emergencies in which intestinal resection has to be made (strangulated hernias, another potentially contaminated surgical field).

All these problems can be avoided with the use of absorbable prosthetic materials such as those composed of lactic acid polymers or lactic and glycolic acid copolymers.

**Table 5.3**

| Nonmetal synthetic prosthesis | |
|---|---|
| Nylon (1944) | Replaced rubber, metals and animal products. Initially used for sutures, later knitted or woven into patches for hernia repair; disintegrates in tissue and loses most of its tensile strength within 6 months |
| Polyethylene mesh (1958)<br>Polypropylene mesh (1962) | High-density polyethylene mesh (*Marlex*, 1958) resistant to chemicals and sterilizable, but unraveled after being cut. Modified to polypropylene mesh (1962). Available under various trade names (*Hertra-2, Marlex, Prolene, Surgipro, Tramex, Trelex*). Available as a flat mesh as well as three-dimensional devices (*Altex, Hermesh3, PerFix Plug, Prolene Hernia System*) |
| Polyester mesh (*MERSILENE*) (1984) | Composed of polyester fiber with the characteristics of filigree; can be inserted into narrow spaces without distortion |
| Expanded polytetrafluoroethylene | Teflon product; produces minimal adhesions when placed intraperitoneally. Does not allow significant fibroblastic or angiogenic ingrowth; must be removed if infection occurs |
| Polyglycolic acid mesh (*Dexon*)<br>Polyglactin 910 mesh (*Vicryl*) | Absorbable mesh; loses strength after 8–12 weeks; should not be used as a sole prosthesis for the repair of abdominal or groin hernias |

However, the use of these absorbable prosthesis exposes the patient to a rapid and inevitable hernia recurrence as these materials, once implanted, are attacked by an inflammatory reaction that, through a hydrolytic reaction, removes and digests the implanted prosthetic material completely. In this case, the high risk of hernia recurrence is explained by the complete dissolution of the prosthetic support.

It is already possible however, to identify clear indications to the use of this biomaterial when considering its peculiarities in the emergency hernia repair of infected or potentially infected fields or in patients with high risk of infection of the nonabsorbable prosthesis (i.e. immune-depressed subject).

## Indications for Use of Prosthesis in Hernia Repair

1. The reason for the increased use of mesh is because primary (suture, without mesh) repair of abdominal wall hernias has a significant recurrence rate that can be as high as 52%
2. Mesh repair has been shown to reduce recurrence rates in a well-controlled trial
3. Mesh is used to decrease the tension placed on tissues and sutures, which, in turn, is thought to decrease the incidence of recurrence.
   - Replacement of lost musculofascial tissue caused by trauma
   - Infection
   - Reinforcement of native tissue weakness
   - Aging (Laxity of tissues)
   - Neurological deficit (Denervation).

### *Causes of Loss of Musculofascial Tissue*

1. Weakness developed after laparotomy
2. Abdominal incisions
3. Gunshot wounds
4. Weight gain
5. Increased abdominal pressure
6. Reduced nutrition
7. Protein loss
8. Nicotine (smoking)
9. Emphysema
10. Chronic bronchitis
11. Fasciitis
12. Gangrene
13. Postoperative wound infection

### *Aging Effects*

1. Loss of fascial strength
2. Diastasis recti.

*Diastasis recti* (also known as abdominal separation) is a disorder defined as a separation of the rectus abdominis muscle into right and left halves. Normally, the two sides of the muscle are joined at the linea alba at the body midline. Diastasis of this muscle occurs principally in two populations: newborns and pregnant women. In the newborn, the rectus abdominis is not fully developed and may not be sealed together at midline. Diastasis recti is more common in premature and African American newborns. In pregnant or postpartum women, the defect is caused by the stretching of the rectus abdominis by the growing uterus. It is more common in multiparous women due to repeated episodes of stretching. When the defect occurs during pregnancy, the uterus can sometimes be seen bulging through the abdominal wall beneath the skin.

### *Denervation Effect*

- In nephrectomy incision
- In lumbar sympathectomy incision

### *What makes the Ideal Prosthetic?*

Good handling characteristics

- Compatible with infection
- Strong enough to prevent failure
- Invokes favorable host response (biocompatible)
- Does not limit postimplant function
- Does not restrict future access
- Does not shrink or degrade over time
- Easy to manufacture
- Inexpensive
- Does not transmit infectious disease.

## Prosthetics for Inguinal Hernia Repair

### *Prosthetic Biomaterial—Absorbable Type*

1. Knitted vicryl mesh
2. Woven vicryl mesh
3. Dexon mesh.

### *Collagen Containing Mesh*

1. Surgisis (Enhanced strength)
2. Surgisis Gold
3. FortaPerm

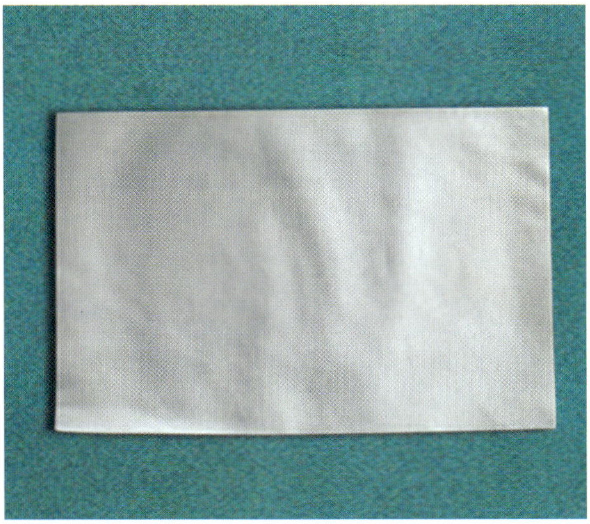

**Fig. 5.1:** Permacol is a sheet of acellular porcine collagen

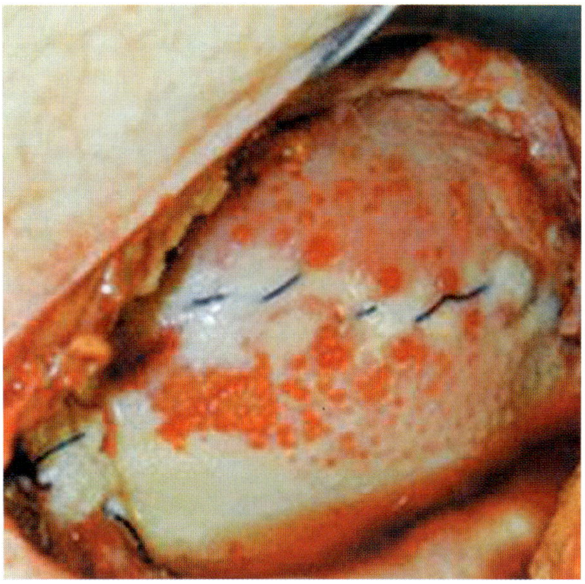

**Fig. 5.2:** AlloDerm® tissue matrix

4. FortaGen
5. Permacol
6. AlloDerm.

## Permacol (Fig. 5.1)

Permacol is a sheet of acellular porcine collagen and is very effective in managing contaminated and complex abdominal wounds. The highly developed architecture makes the sheet resistant to collagenase and its longer durability makes it a safe and acceptable alternative to prosthetic mesh.

Permacol can be used to manage open and complex laparotomy wounds and abdominal wall defects as it becomes incorporated by tissue ingrowth and neovascularization. Permacol has been a successful prosthetic material in closing complex abdominal wounds.

## AlloDerm Mesh (Fig. 5.2)

AlloDerm® Tissue Matrix is derived from cadaveric dermis and undergoes nondamaging proprietary processing that removes cells. AlloDerm® Tissue Matrix provides a strong and safe hernia repair and may minimize the risk of short- and long-term complications. AlloDerm® Tissue Matrix may keep patients from undergoing additional surgical interventions.

- Supports rapid revascularization which can minimize the risk of infection
- Rapid revascularization through existing vascular channels and new blood vessel formation
- Rapid revascularization allows white blood cells to migrate to the site.

### AlloDerm

Resists adhesion formations to bowel:

- Minimizes complications such as bowel obstructions and fistula formations
- Allows for simpler future surgeries in the abdominal area.

AlloDerm mesh is an acellular matrix derived from the donated cadaveric human skin. It provides a complex, three-dimensional array of proteins that interact with each other and with the host cells. These proteins include networks of collagen, elastin, hyaluronan, and proteoglycans. Rapid revascularization, repopulation, and remodeling of the matrix occur on contact with the patient's own tissue. As a result, the mesh gets completely incorporated into the host fascial tissue. Acellular human dermis is capable of significant revascularization of its compact collagen composition in the early postoperative period (Figs 5.3 and 5.4).

### Surgisis Mesh (Figs 5.5 and 5.6)

Surgisis mesh is derived from a natural biomaterial harvested from porcine small intestine submucosa (SIS).

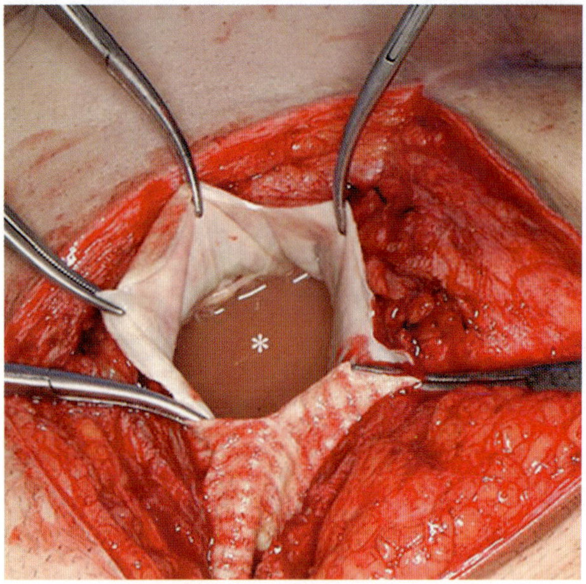

Fig. 5.3: Alloderm mesh is an acellular matrix derived from the donated cadaveric human skin

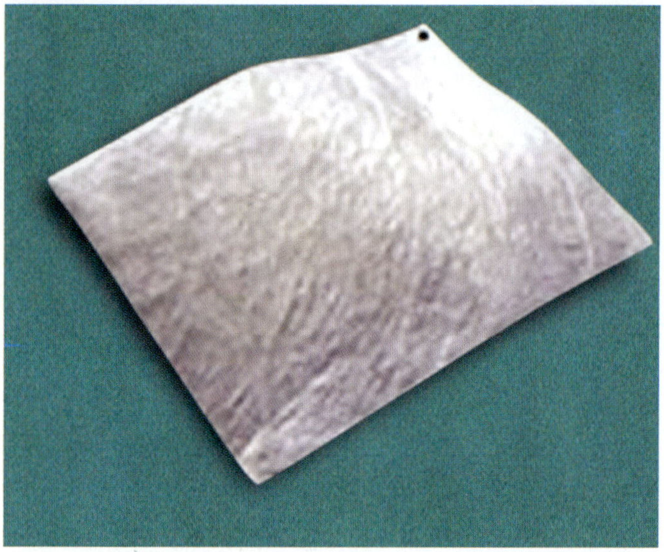

Fig. 5.5: Surgisis ES (Enhanced strength)

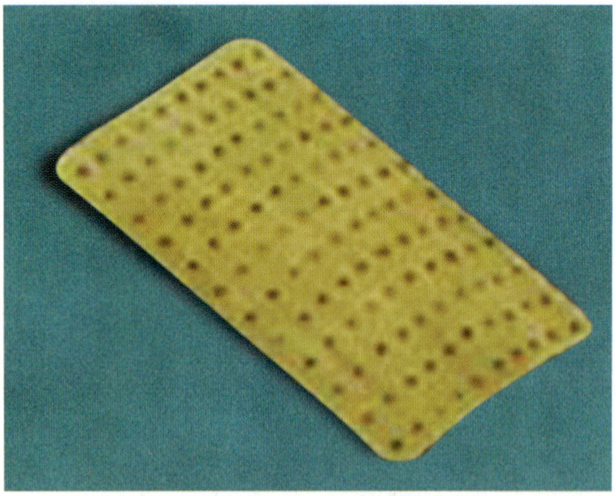

Fig. 5.4: Gold type

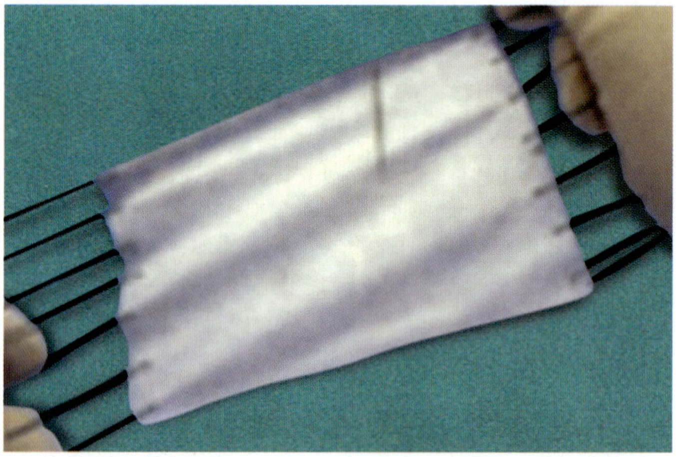

Fig. 5.6: FortaPerm mesh

The three-dimensional, extra-cellular matrix (ECM) comprises of collagen and noncollagenous proteins and biomolecules, including glycosaminoglycans, proteoglycans, and glycoproteins. Material is then vacuum-dried and sterilized. When implanted, host tissue cells and blood vessels readily infiltrate the graft. Connective and epithelial tissue growth and differentiation, as well as deposition and maturation of the host ECM components, occur. Finally, tissue remodeling takes place and the graft and the host tissue become indistinguishable.

## Flat Nonabsorbable/Partially Absorbable Mesh

In modern hernia surgery, there are two competing mesh concepts which often lead to controversial discussions, on the one hand the heavyweight small porous model and on the other, the lightweight large porous hypothesis (Figs 5.7 and 5.8). Furthermore, the new mesh concept reveals an optimized foreign body reaction based on reduced amounts of mesh material and, in particular,

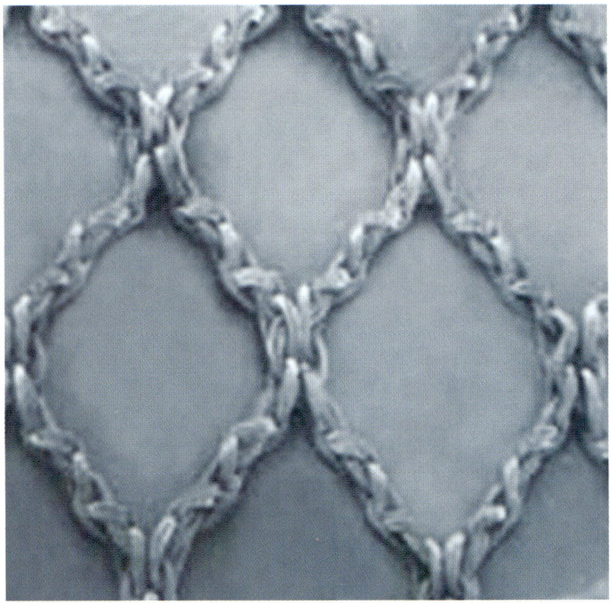

Fig. 5.7: Large pores

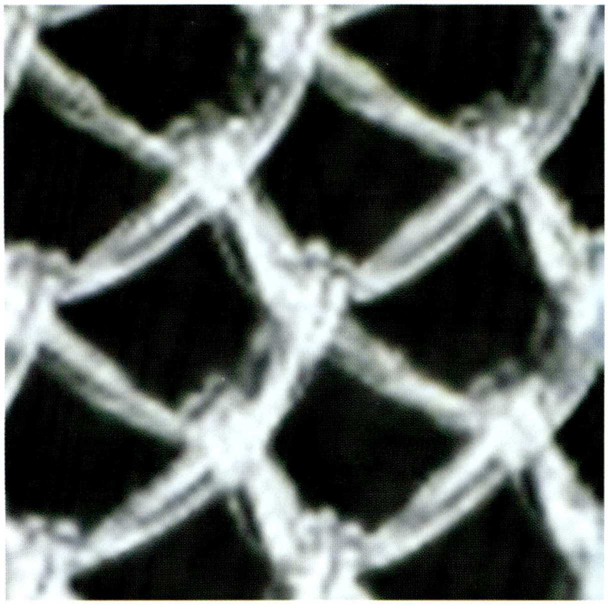

Fig. 5.9: Prolene mesh

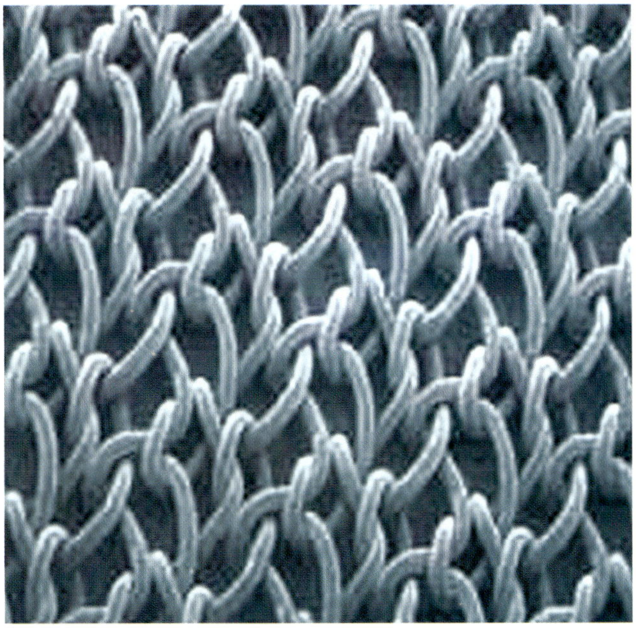

Fig. 5.8: Small pores

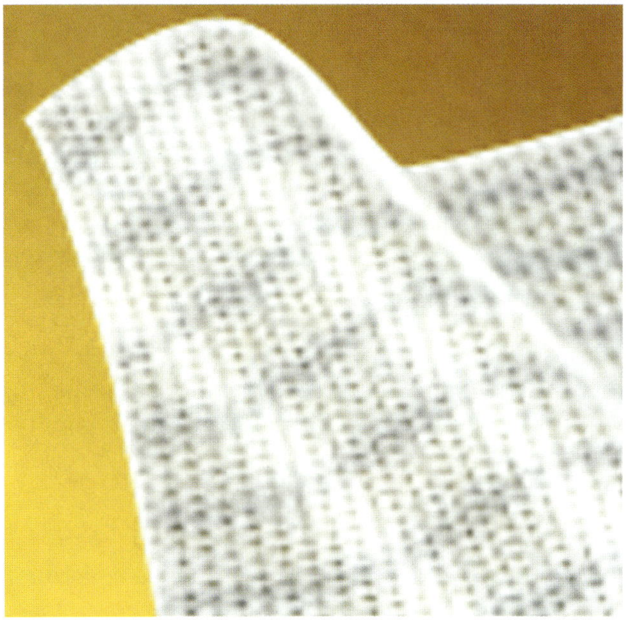

Fig. 5.10A

a significantly decreased surface area in contact with the recipient host tissues by the large porous model. Finally, recent data demonstrate that alterations in the extracellular matrix of hernia patients play a crucial role in the development of hernia recurrence. In particular, long-term recurrences months or years after surgery and implantation of mesh can be explained by the extracellular matrix hypothesis.

However, if the altered extracellular matrix proves to be the weak area, the decisive question is whether the

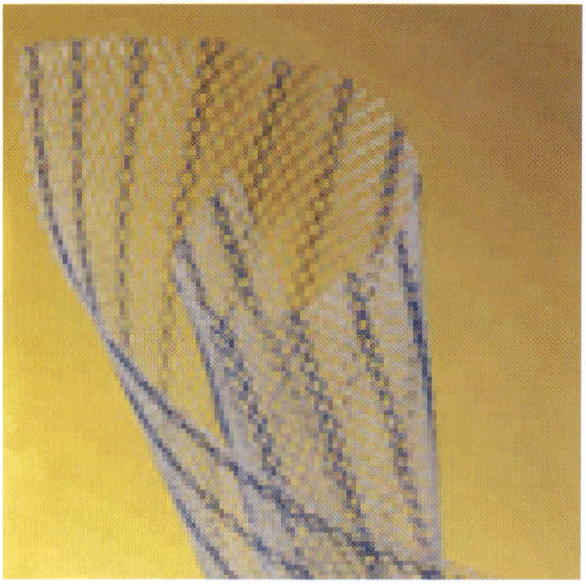

Fig. 5.10B

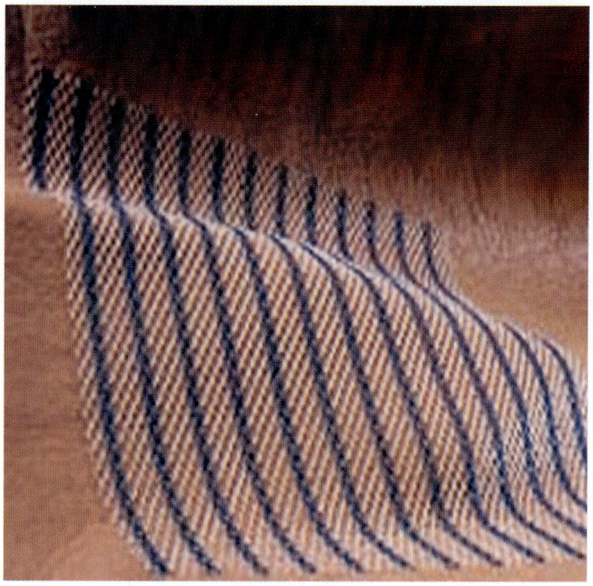

Fig. 5.10C

**Figs 5.10A to C:** Ultrapro mesh

amount of material as well as mechanical and tensile strength of the surgical mesh are really of significant importance for the development of recurrent hernia. All experimental evidence and first clinical data indicate the superiority of the lightweight and large porous mesh concept with regard to a reduced number of long-term complications and particularly, increased comfort and quality of life after hernia repair.

Implant materials very quickly absorb a layer of host proteins after implantation—in a process lasting a few seconds, which occurs well before an initial cellular response to the biomaterial can be observed.

## Polypropylene Prosthetic Mesh (Flat Type)

*Prolene mesh*: Prolene polypropylene mesh is constructed of knitted filaments of extruded polypropylene identical in composition to that used in prolene* Polypropylene Suture, Nonabsorbable Surgical Sutures, USP (Ethicon, Inc.) (Fig. 5.9).

The mesh is approximately 0.020 inches thick. This material, when used as a suture, has been reported to be nonreactive and to retain its strength indefinitely in clinical use. Prolene mesh is knitted by a process which interlinks each fiber junction and which provides for elasticity in both directions.

This construction permits the mesh to be cut into any desired shape or size without unraveling. The fiber junctions are not subject to the same work fatigue exhibited by more rigid metallic meshes. This bi-directional elastic property allows adaption to various stresses encountered in the body.

## Actions

Prolene mesh is a nonabsorbable mesh used to span and reinforce traumatic or surgical wounds to provide extended support during and following wound healing. Animal studies show that implantation of Prolene mesh elicits a minimum to slight inflammatory reaction, which is transient and is followed by the deposition of a thin fibrous layer of tissue which can grow through the interstices of the mesh, thus incorporating the mesh into adjacent tissue. The mesh remains soft and pliable, and normal wound healing is not noticeably impaired. The material is not absorbed nor is it subject to degradation or weakening by the action of tissue enzymes.

## Indications

This mesh may be used for the repair of hernia and other fascial deficiencies that require the addition of a reinforcing or bridging material to obtain the desired surgical result.

### Contraindications

When this mesh is used in infants or children with future growth potential, the surgeon should be aware that this mesh will not stretch significantly as the patient grows.

Prolene mesh in contaminated wounds should be used with the understanding that subsequent infection may require removal of the material.

Ethicon ultrapro mesh is the only partially absorbable mesh. It is constructed of polypropylene (nonabsorbable) and poliglecaprone 25 (absorbable) monofilament materials.

- Strong, secure repair
- Flexible scar lets abdominal wall move naturally
- Trusted, proven materials.

## Ultrapro (Poliglecaprone-25/ Polypropylene)Synthetic Partially Absorbable Mesh

Ultrapro mesh (Figs 5.10A to C) incorporates the three most important characteristics of lightweight design: thin filament size, large pore construction, and absorbable materials.

- Leaves behind 65% less foreign materials than traditional weight polypropylene mesh
- Withstands four times the maximum abdominal pressure (Fig. 5.11)
- Excellent tissue in-growth.

*Proceed mesh*: Ethicon's Proceed® Surgical Mesh-Multilayer tissue-separating mesh for open and laparoscopic incisional hernia repair. New Proceed® Surgical Mesh features a thin, bioresorbable fabric layer that effectively separates its strong, supportive mesh from underlying viscera. A composite of proven products from Ethicon Products, Proceed® Mesh can be placed both below the muscle layer and outside of the peritoneum, or in the intra-abdominal cavity and offers the following benefits:

- Effectively seperates mesh from underlying viscera
- Does not harbor bacteria that can lead to infection
- Lightweight monofilament construction for patient comfort.

Proceed® is now the preferred mesh in the repair of incisional hernias.

### Open-Skirted Flap for Increased Rigidity and Accessible Fixation

Parietex™ Composite OS Series skirted mesh provides a new level of control during open ventral repair. based on clinically proven Parietex™ Composite mesh, the OS Series design has increased rigidity for easier handling

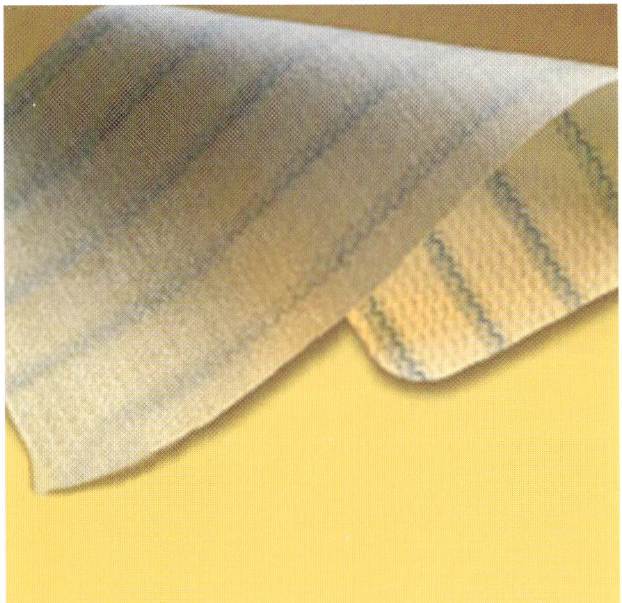

**Fig. 5.11:** Ultrapro mesh

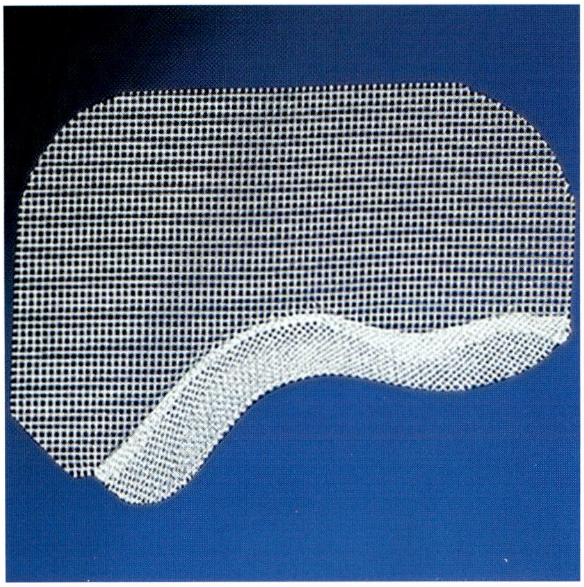

**Fig. 5.12:** Parietex mesh (Right/Left sided for inguinal hernias)

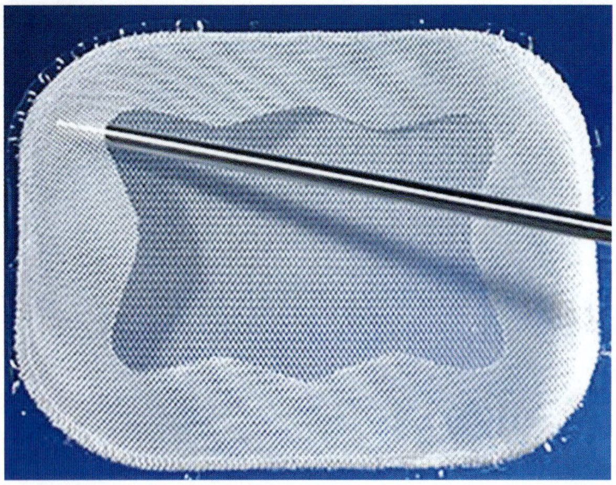

**Fig. 5.13:** Parietex mesh (for ventral hernia)

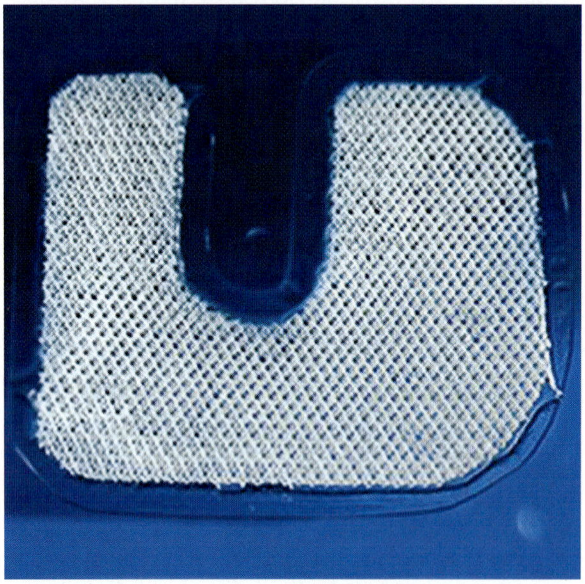

**Fig. 5.14:** Parietex mesh (for hiatus hernia)

during implantation. The skirted flap on the parietal side of the mesh provides more easily accessible fixation points in the open approach (Fig. 5.12).

- Parietex™ Composite dual-sided mesh provides optimal tissue in-growth and fewer visceral attachments
- The skirt on parietal side provides accessible, secure fixation points
- Increased rigidity during implantation allows superior handling
- The polyester material softens and conforms to the anatomy once implanted
- Protects viscera from fixation points (Fig. 5.13).

### Reliable Treatment for Paraesophageal and Hiatal Hernia (Fig. 5.14)

The Parietex™ Composite 2H Series makes surgical treatment of gastroesophageal reflux disease (GERD) and hiatal hernia viable. While ordinary meshes carry the risk of in-growth into the esophagus, Parietex™ Composite is coated on one side with a protective collagen-based barrier to help prevent tissue attachment. The 2H Series is created in the shape of the hiatus to buttress the primary repair by reinforcing the approximation of the crus on either side of the esophagus.

- Non-resorbable polyester mesh allows fast and complete tissue in-growth on one side for efficient reinforcement
- Resorbable hydrophilic film provides a temporary barrier, minimizing tissue attachment to mesh
- Polyester mesh is easy to place and manipulate around the esophagus.

## Devices for Inguinal Hernioplasty

### Prolene* Polypropylene Hernia System (Fig. 5.15)

The Prolene* polypropylene hernia system (PHS) is a sterile, preshaped, three dimensional device constructed of an onlay patch connected by a mesh cylinder to an oblong or circular underlay patch. The material is undyed PROLENE* Polypropylene Mesh constructed of knitted nonabsorbable polypropylene filaments.

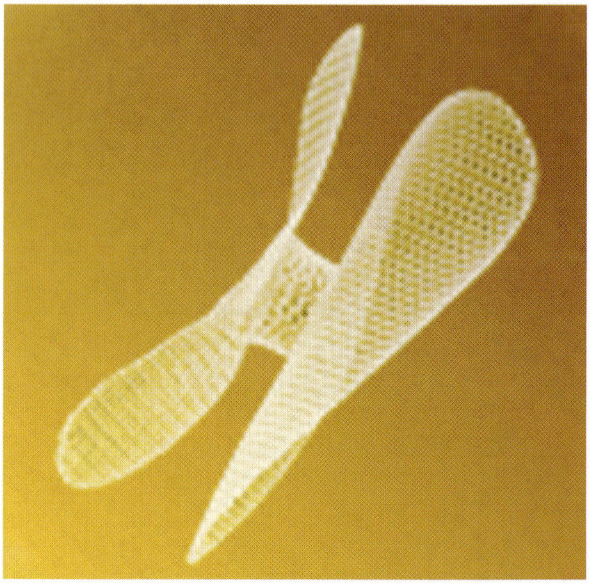

**Fig. 5.15:** Polypropylene hernia system

The Prolene Hernia System is a nonabsorbable mesh used to reinforce or bridge inguinal hernia deficiencies to provide extended support during and following wound healing. Animal studies show that implantation of Prolene Mesh elicits a minimum to slight inflammatory reaction, which is transient and is followed by the deposition of a thin fibrous layer of tissue which can grow through the interstices of the mesh, thus incorporating the mesh into adjacent tissue. The mesh remains soft and pliable, and normal wound healing is not noticeably impaired. The material is neither absorbed nor is it subject to degradation or weakening by the action of tissue enzymes.

### *Using the Sytem*

For indirect hernia repair, a high dissection of the neck of the hernia sac to utilize the potential of the preperitoneal space can be performed to insert the Prolene Hernia System. The oblong/circular or bottom underlay portion of the Prolene Hernia System is folded and is inserted through the internal ring allowing the mesh to expand to the underlay position.

Surgical manipulation may be used to facilitate the expansion of the device to the underlay position. No sutures are necessary in the bottom underlay patch. The top onlay patch, which is designed to cover the posterior wall (floor of the canal), is then modified as needed to accommodate the cord structures. If one end of the oval onlay patch is longer than the other, the Prolene Hernia System is positioned so that the longer end covers the posterior wall (floor of the canal) and overlaps the pubic tubercle. Sutures or clips may be used to secure the top onlay patch in place. The cord structures then lie on top of the medial portion of the onlay patch. For direct hernia, the defect is circumscribed at its base, the contents fully reduced, and the preperitoneal space is actualized prior to the insertion of the Prolene Hernia System. The circular, or bottom underlay portion of the Prolene Hernia System is folded and is inserted through the defect or the internal ring allowing the mesh to expand to the underlay position. The underlay portion should expand under the defect in the floor of the inguinal canal. Surgical manipulation may be used to facilitate the expansion of the device to the underlay position. Sutures or clips may be used to secure the top onlay patch in place.

For repair of ventral/incisional or umbilical hernias the sac is dissected free down to the abdominal fascia. Dissection then proceeds under the anterior abdominal fascia to create a submuscular space that is anterior to the posterior fascia and peritoneum. An additional space is created anterior to the rectus muscle and posterior to the anterior rectus sheath. A Prolene Hernia System of appropriate size for the defect is then selected. The hernia sac is reduced and the underlay mesh is placed posterior to the rectus muscle and anterior to the posterior rectus sheath. Adequate overlap with the rectus muscle is assured. The overlap mesh is then positioned anterior to the rectus muscle and posterior to the anterior rectus sheath. Sutures or clips may be used to secure the top onlay and/or the bottom underlay patch in place.

## Ultrapro* Hernia System (Fig. 5.16)

The Ultrapro* Hernia System (UHS) is a sterile, pre-shaped, three dimensional device constructed of an undyed onlay patch: (1) connected by a mesh cylinder (connector), (2) to an underlay patch, (3) which is reinforced by a flat undyed absorbable film of Poliglecaprone-25 (Monocryl). The underlay patch is marked with dyed polypropylene fibers to be clearly distinguishable from the onlay patch. The onlay patch, connector and underlay patch are manufactured from approximately equal parts of absorbable Poliglecaprone-25 monofilament fiber and non-absorbable polypropylene monofilament fiber. The polymer of the undyed and dyed polypropylene fibers (phthalocyanine blue, color index no.: 74160) is identical to the material used for dyed/undyed Prolene* suture material. Poliglecaprone-25 fiber consists of a copolymer containing glycolide and e-caprolactone. This copolymer

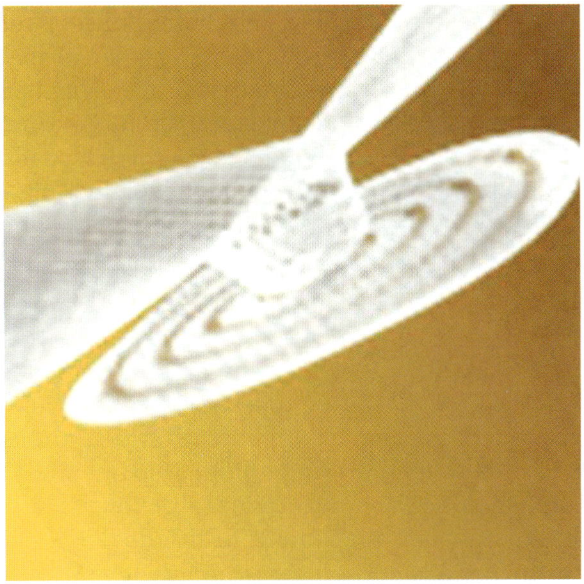

**Fig. 5.16:** Ultrapro hernia system

is also used for Monocryl* suture material. After absorption of the Poliglecaprone-25 components only the polypropylene mesh remains. The structure and size of this remaining mesh are designed for the physiological stresses to which the abdominal wall is subject.

For indirect hernia, a high dissection of the neck of the hernia sac can be performed to utilize the preperitoneal space for insertion of the UHS. The underlay patch of the device (marked with blue threads) is folded and inserted through the internal ring, allowing the underlay patch to deploy in the preperitoneal space (beneath the epigastric vessels) and cover the entire myopectineal orifice. Correct expansion of the underlay patch may be supported by surgical manipulation, if necessary, to ensure that it is free of folds.

For direct hernia, the defect is circumscribed at its base, the contents fully reduced, and the preperitoneal space is entered. After adequate dissection, the underlay patch of the device (marked with blue threads) is folded and inserted through the defect allowing the underlay patch to expand and to cover the myopectineal orifice. Correct expansion of the underlay patch may be supported by surgical manipulation, if necessary, to ensure that it is free of folds. For indirect as well as for direct hernia the onlay patch of the device is designed to cover the floor of the canal. It is necessary to modify the onlay patch as needed to accommodate the cord structures.

This can be done by creating a slit in the mesh. The longer side of the onlay patch should be positioned parallel to the inguinal ligament. The onlay patch should be positioned without folds, and should be adequately fixed (e.g. sutures, staples) in order to avoid edge rollup and/or folding and to minimize the risk of hernia recurrence. It is recommended that points of fixation be placed at a distance approximately 1 cm (0.4") from the edge of the mesh. The tails created to accommodate the cord structures need to be fixated.

### Ventral/Incisional or Umbilical Hernias

The hernia sac is dissected free down to the abdominal fascia. Dissection then proceeds to create a preperitoneal space. An additional space is created anterior to the rectus sheath. A UHS of appropriate size for the defect is then selected. The hernia sac is reduced and the underlay patch is deployed in the preperitoneal space. The onlay patch is then positioned anterior to the rectus sheath. After tension-free placement of the device without folds, the onlay patch should be adequately fixed (e.g. sutures, staples) in order to avoid edge rollup and/or folding and to minimize the risk of hernia recurrence. It is recommended that points of fixation be placed at a distance approximately 1 cm (0.4") from the edge of the mesh. The patches can be cut to size as required using scissors or a scalpel; do not use thermal devices.

## Ultrapro* Plug (Figs 5.17A to D)

### Prolene 3D Patch

It is a polypropylene three-dimensional system consisting of a flat onlay patch, securely linked to a diamond-shaped plug, which can be deployed through the use of

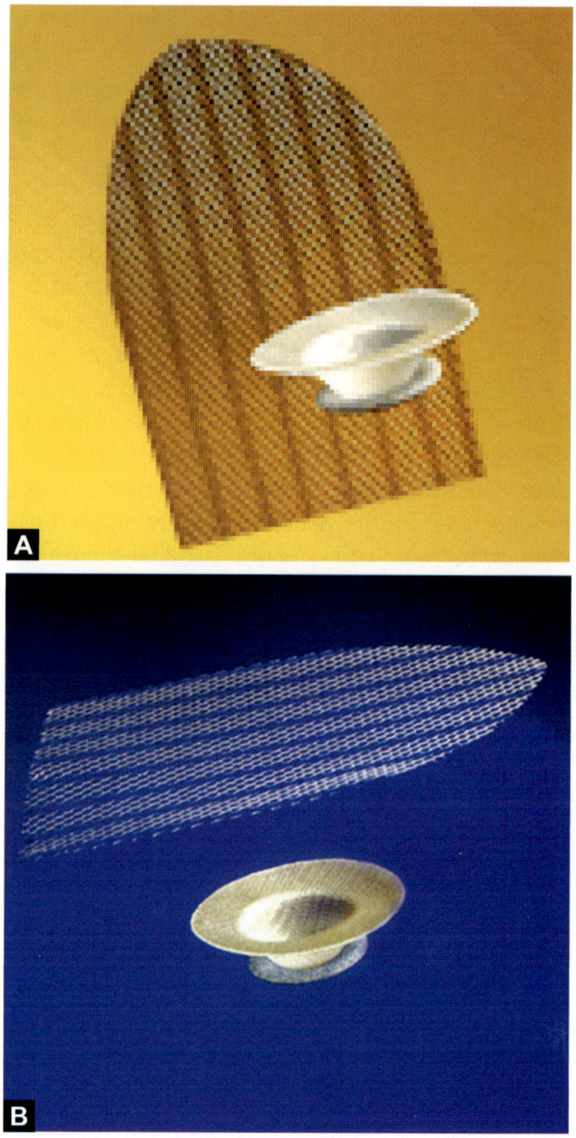

Figs 5.17A and B

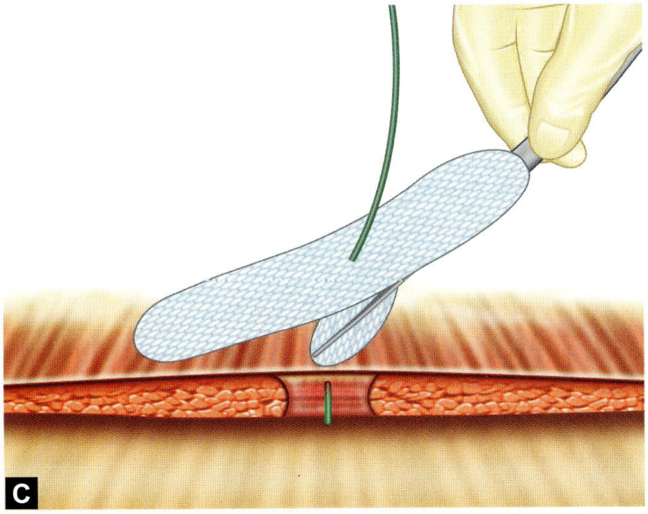

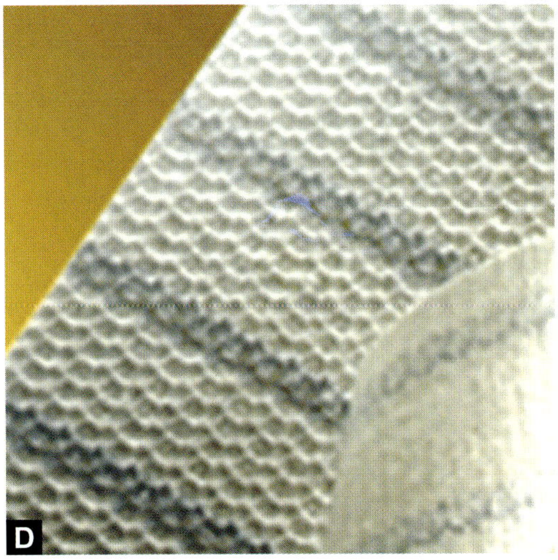

**Figs 5.17C and D**

**Figs 5.17A to D:** Ultrapro plug, prolene 3D patch

an integrated looped non-absorbable suture. The new mesh, measuring 12.5 × 5.5 cm, is available in two types: the Extended Overlay type which is lozenge-shaped and mainly used for, but not limited to, direct hernia and women's hernia, and the Preshaped

Overlay type, with its opening and hole specific for men's spermatic cord. The plug is hollow and available in two sizes: medium size measuring 4.8 × 2.3 cm, and small size measuring 3.5 × 1.9 cm. The plug must be placed in the preperitoneal space through the deep inguinal ring or through the direct defect, while the flat onlay patch, either the Extended or Preshaped Overlay type, shall lie on the inguinal floor; pulling the suture will cause the deployment of the plug, which will expand flattened in the opposite side. In the new 3D patch system, the onlay portion is not a rigid mesh but flexible, with good memory and, at the same time, well resistant; which is already an advantage as it fits quite well the groin area, thus reducing, in our view, all troubles linked to patient's movement and his postural changes. The plug is diamond-shaped and this ergonomic form makes the insertion easier into the deep inguinal ring or the direct defect, without the need to dissect the preperitoneal space; besides it's hollow and this implies an overall reduction of the prosthetic material used.

The plug, once inserted, is flattened by pulling the looped suture, therefore the deep repair becomes "bidimensional"and more subject to tissue ingrowth by fibroblasts, if compared to the various non-flat type plugs; furthermore, since the two parts of the new device are joint together, the plug migration is duly prevented.

## Proceed* Surgical Mesh

Proceed* Surgical Mesh is a sterile, thin, flexible laminate mesh designed for the repair of hernias and other fascial deficiencies. The mesh product is comprised of an oxidized regenerated cellulose (ORC) fabric, and Prolene* Soft Mesh, a nonabsorbable polypropylene mesh, which is encapsulated by a polydioxanone polymer. The polypropylene mesh side of the product allows for tissue ingrowth while the ORC side provides a bioresorbable layer that physically separates the polypropylene mesh from underlying tissue and organ surfaces during the wound-healing period to minimize tissue attachment to the mesh. The polydioxanone provides a bond to the ORC layer.

The Prolene Soft Mesh component is constructed of knitted filaments of extruded polypropylene identical in composition to that used in Prolene* Polypropylene Suture, nonabsorbable surgical sutures, USP (Ethicon, Inc.). This material, when used as a suture, has been reported to be nonreactive and to retain its strength indefinitely in clinical use. The Prolene Soft Mesh affords excellent strength, durability and surgical adaptability, with a porous structure to enable mesh incorporation into surrounding tissues.

The ORC component is an absorbable off-white knitted fabric prepared by the controlled oxidation of regenerated cellulose. The ORC layer is absorbed from the site of implantation within four (4) weeks. Absorption rate depends upon several factors including the amount used and implantation site. The polydioxanone components made from the polyester, poly (p-dioxanone) polymer that is identical to the polymer used in PDS* II (polydioxanone) Suture, Synthetic Absorbable Suture, USP (ETHICON, Inc.). The polydioxanone polymer has been found to be nonantigenic, nonpyrogenic and to elicit only a mild tissue reaction during absorption. The polydioxanone component is absorbed within six (6) months.

### Actions/Performance

Proceed Mesh is a laminate mesh, whose Prolene Soft Mesh component is knitted with nonabsorbable fibers, used to reinforce or bridge traumatic or surgical wounds to provide extended support during and following wound healing. The ORC is intended to physically separate the mesh from underlying tissue and organ surfaces during the critical wound healing period, thereby reducing the severity and extent of tissue attachment to the mesh.

Animal studies show that implantation of PROCEED Mesh elicits a transient inflammatory reaction that does not interfere with integration of the mesh into adjacent tissue. The mesh remains soft and pliable, and normal wound healing is not noticeably impaired.

The ORC and polydioxanone components are essentially absorbed within six (6) months, whereas the polypropylene material is not absorbed, nor is it subject to degradation or weakening by the action of tissue enzymes.

Minimal visceral tissue attachment has been demonstrated in animal studies that show reduction in the extent and severity of adhesions to the mesh.

### Indications

Proceed Mesh is used for the repair of hernias and other fascial deficiencies that require the addition of a reinforcing or bridging material to obtain the desired surgical result.

### Instructions

Correct surface orientation is critical for Proceed Mesh to function as intended. The polypropylene mesh side (side with the blue stripes) of the product should be placed adjacent to those tissues where tissue ingrowth is desired. The other surface, the ORC side, should be placed adjacent to those tissues where minimal tissue attachment is desired (i.e. visceral surfaces). The orientation is essential.

Uncontrolled and/or active bleeding should be controlled prior to placement of the Proceed Mesh.

The mesh should be shaped in such a way that sufficient overlap of the fascial defect on all sides is achieved, thereby allowing adequate stabilization of each of the fascial borders.

To avoid dislodging, crinkling or curling of the edges, a sufficient number of fixation points should be placed along the borders of the Proceed Mesh.

Fixation may be accomplished with devices such as tackers, anchors, staples or nonabsorbable sutures. It is recommended that points of fixation be placed 6.5 mm to 12.5 mm (1/4" to 1/2") apart at a distance approximately 6.5 mm (1/4") from the edge of the mesh. Fixation of this product with tissue adhesives has not been evaluated.

## Proceed* Ventral Patch

Partially Absorbable Mesh Device.

### Description

Proceed* ventral patch (PVP) is a sterile, self-expanding, partially absorbable, flexible laminate mesh device designed for the repair of hernias and other fascial deficiencies such as those caused by trocar use. The mesh patch is comprised of multiple layers of absorbable and nonabsorbable materials, laminated together with an absorbable polydioxanone polymer. The bottom layer of the patch, facing underlying tissue and organ surfaces is comprised of an oxidized regenerated cellulose (ORC) fabric bonded to Prolene* Soft Mesh, a nonabsorbable, macroporous polypropylene mesh. The polypropylene mesh side of the product allows for tissue ingrowth. The ORC side of the patch provides a bioresorbable layer that physically separates the polypropylene mesh from underlying tissue and organ surfaces while minimizing tissue attachment to the polypropylene mesh during the critical wound healing period. The polypropylene mesh layer is encapsulated with layers of PDS* film.

The parietal side of the patch contains a polydioxanone polymer reinforcement film and positioning ring, which provide memory to the patch. These patch reinforcements offer stability to help the clinician achieve proper placement. Vicryl* Mesh is placed on top of the polydioxanone polymer reinforcement film to facilitate placement of the mesh. The Vicryl Mesh layer is encapsulated with layers of PDS film. Anchoring straps of the patch are designed to facilitate placement and fixation of the mesh device. An Ethibond* polyester suture is attached to each anchoring strap enabling tension to be placed on the patch prior to fixation. After the patch has been fixated, the sutures should be removed and discarded.

The ORC component is an absorbable off-white knitted fabric prepared by the controlled oxidation of regenerated cellulose. The ORC layer is absorbed from the site of implantation within four (4) weeks. Absorption rate depends upon several factors including the amount used and implantation site. The Prolene Soft Mesh components are constructed of knitted filaments of extruded polypropylene, identical in composition to that used in Prolene* Polypropylene Suture, nonabsorbable surgical suture, USP (Ethicon, Inc.).

This material, when used as a suture, has been reported to be nonreactive and to retain its strength indefinitely in clinical use. The Prolene Soft Mesh affords excellent strength, durability and surgical adaptability, with a porous structure to enable mesh incorporation into surrounding tissues.

The polydioxanone components are made from poly (p-dioxanone) polymer that is identical to the polymer used in PDS* II Polydioxanone Suture, Synthetic Absorbable Suture, USP (ETHICON, Inc.). The polydioxanone polymer has been found to be nonantigenic, nonpyrogenic, and to elicit only a mild tissue reaction during absorption. The polydioxanone component is essentially absorbed within six (6) months.

The Vicryl Mesh component is prepared from polyglactin 910, a synthetic absorbable copolymer of glycolide and lactide, derived respectively from glycolic acid and lactic acids. Polyglactin 910 polymer is identical to the polymer used in Vicryl* Polyglactin 910 Synthetic Absorbable Suture, USP (Ethicon, Inc.). The polyglactin 910 polymer has been found to be nonantigenic, nonpyrogenic, and to elicit only a mild tissue reaction during absorption. The polyglactin 910 component is essentially absorbed within 56 to 70 days.

## Actions/Performance

Proceed ventral patch (PVP) is a laminate mesh device, whose Prolene Soft Mesh component is knitted with nonabsorbable fibers, used to reinforce or bridge traumatic or surgical wounds to provide extended support during and following wound healing. The ORC is intended to physically separate the mesh from underlying tissue and organ surfaces during the critical wound healing period, thereby reducing the severity and extent of tissue attachment to the mesh.

An animal model shows that implantation of PVP elicits a mild inflammatory reaction that does not interfere with integration of the mesh into adjacent tissue. The mesh remains soft and pliable, and normal wound healing is not noticeably impaired.

The ORC, VICRYL Mesh, and polydioxanone components are essentially absorbed within six (6) months, whereas the polypropylene material is not absorbed, nor is it subject to degradation or weakening by the action of tissue enzymes.

Minimal visceral tissue attachment has been demonstrated in an animal model that shows reduction in the extent and severity of adhesions to the mesh.

## Indications

Proceed ventral patch (PVP) is intended for the repair of hernias or other abdominal fascial defects that require the addition of a reinforcing or bridging material to obtain the desired surgical result. PVP is also indicated for the repair of tissue deficiencies caused by trocar use.

## Instructions for Use

Correct surface orientation is critical for PROCEED Ventral Patch to function as intended. The VICRYL Mesh side (side with straps) should be placed adjacent to those tissues where tissue ingrowth is desired. The ORC side (uniformly off-white) should be placed adjacent to those tissues where minimal tissue attachment is desired (e.g. visceral surfaces).

Uncontrolled and/or active bleeding should be controlled prior to placement of PROCEED Ventral Patch.

## Hernia Repair Technique

Just prior to insertion, dip mesh patch in saline for ease of use and to avoid attachment of tissue during insertion. Fold the mesh patch into a semi-circle with the ORC side facing outward (straps folded in) for insertion into the defect.

During insertion, secure suture loops with a clamp or fingers. When using a mesh clamp, be certain to avoid kinking the mesh. Be sure to refold as previously described if re-insertion is needed. Once the mesh patch has been inserted into the defect, manipulate the suture loops to facilitate proper positioning of the patch. Pulling up on the suture loops allows the mesh patch to flatten itself against the abdominal wall. Pull the device with sufficient tension to assure tight seating against the abdominal wall as demonstrated in Figure 5.19.

It is important to manually ensure that no tissue is trapped between the device and the abdominal wall. Secure the patch to the margins of the defect through the mesh straps to anterior fascia (Fig. 5.20). Excess length of the straps should be cut off and discarded. The incision should then be closed.

It is recommended that non-absorbable sutures be used to fixate the patch. Alternative means of fixation (i.e. tissue adhesives, staples, tackers) have not been evaluated.

### Polytetrafluoroethylene

Prosthetics of this material are typically solid but can be woven. Tissue response to polytetrafluoroethylene (PTFE) is characteristic of mesothelialization along with a lesser chronic inflamatory response than heavyweight polypropylene. On rare occasions, a membrane can form around the polymer and secrete serous fluid, leading to persistent seroma on both sides of the prosthesis. When reoperating through PTFE, one should take care to avoid pulling the prosthetic off the abdominal wall to minimize the risk of subsequent infection. If mesh infection is present, the entire prosthetic generally needs to be removed.

### Prosthetics without a Barrier

The product with the most data for intraperitoneal use is DualMesh (WL Gore, Inc). This pure, expanded PTFE mesh has been used in thousands of repairs with excellent clinical results and an acceptable cost profile.18 Another solid, pure PTFE product is Dulex Mesh (Davol, Inc). Both prosthetics are smooth on the viscera side and more porous on the abdominal wall side. However,their handling, pore size, and configuration differ significantly.

### Prosthetics with Absorbable Barriers

Absorbable barriers are designed to protect the viscera from adhering to the polymeric prosthetic long enough for the body to cover the mesh with a mesothelial layer. Most absorbable barriers are polymeric and degrade within two weeks, but the optimal absorption rate is unknown. Barriers can be on one or both sides. The former run the risk of exposing the bare prosthetic to the viscera along the edges. The latter have a theoretic risk of slowing abdominal wall tissue in-growth.

Available products include Parietex (Sofradim Corporation), Proceed (Ethicon, Inc), Sepramesh-IP (Genzyme Corporation, Cambridge, MA), and C-Qur (Atrium Medical, Hudson, NH). The latter is a promising new product coated on both sides with a nonpolymeric, omega-3 fatty acid coating derived from fish oil.

## Preshaped Mesh Device for Inguinal Hernia

### Bard® 3DMax® Mesh (Figs 5.18 to 5.20)

The Bard 3DMax mesh is a three-dimensional, anatomically formed prosthesis for use in laparoscopic inguinal hernia repair. The Bard 3DMax mesh has been designed based on careful and precise anatomical research of the inguinal canal. The result is a truly unique prosthesis for laparoscopic hernia surgery. The Bard 3DMax mesh was developed by Dr Philippe Pajotin, a prominent laparoscopic surgeon. After years of performing transabdominal preperitoneal (TAPP)

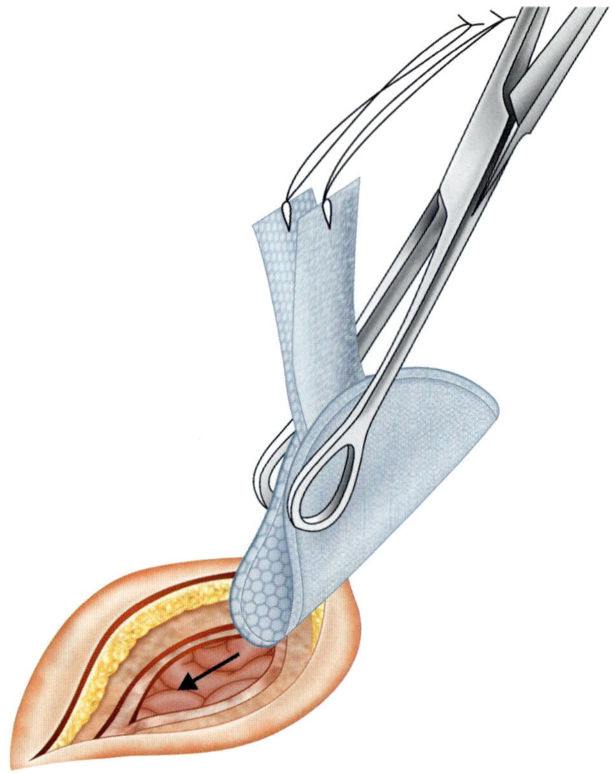

Fig. 5.18A

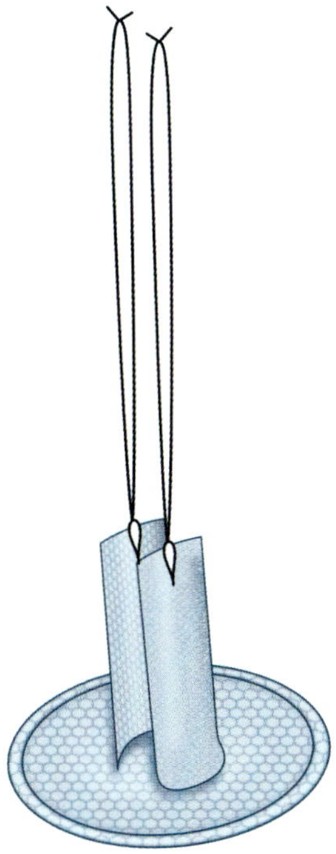

Fig. 5.18B

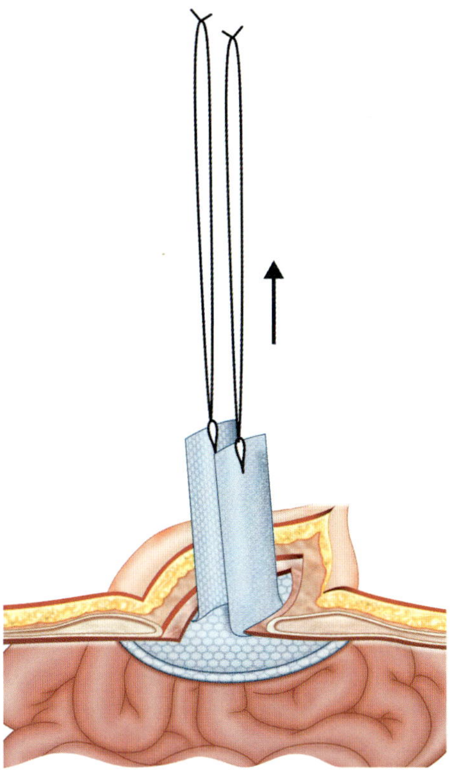

Fig. 5.18C

**Figs 5.18A to C:** Bard 3D max mesh

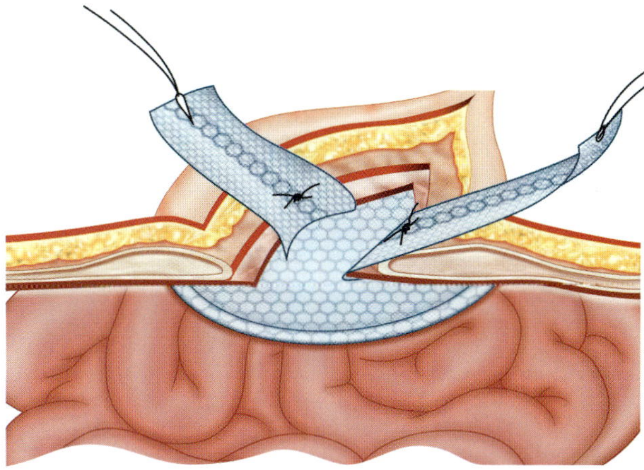

**Fig. 5.19:** Device on abdominal wall

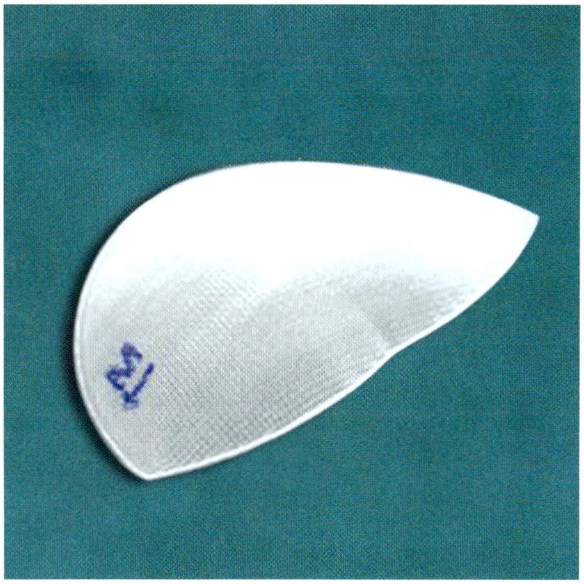

**Fig. 5.20:** Mesh strap

repair, Dr Pajotin came to the realization that a flat sheet of mesh may not be the ideal configuration for a laparoscopic repair. After all, the inguinal anatomy was anything but the two-dimensional image seen on the monitor. After careful cadaver research and molding, Dr Pajotin developed what he believed to be the ideal prosthetic—one that was anatomically formed and shaped to the inguinal anatomy. The Bard 3DMax mesh offers significant advantages over current laparoscopic mesh alternatives:

- *Anatomically formed:* The Bard 3DMax mesh is perfectly suited to the inguinal anatomy. It is a three-

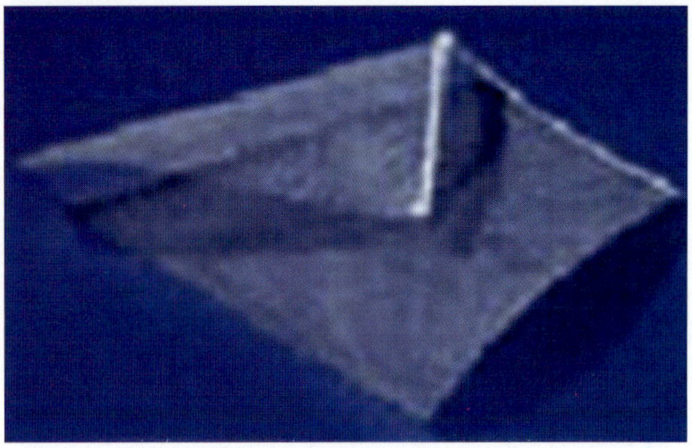

**Fig. 5.21:** Bard visilex mesh

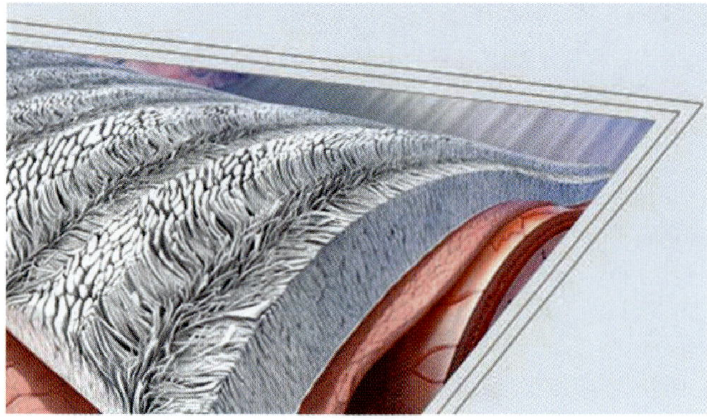

**Fig. 5.22:** Gore Dualmesh® biomaterial

dimensional, anatomically shaped mesh for use in laparoscopic inguinal hernia repair.

- *Comes in left and right orientations:* Due to its precise anatomical form, the Bard 3DMax mesh is offered in a left and right orientation. This allows for precise and specific mesh positioning for any inguinal hernia.
- *Reinforced edge:* A reinforced edge helps to maintain the curved, three-dimensional shape of the Bard 3DMax mesh. Additionally, this edge allows for easier mesh positioning and overall fixation.

### Bard Visilex Mesh (Fig. 5.21)

Bard Visilex mesh is the first polypropylene mesh specifically designed for laparoscopic hernia repair. Visilex mesh directly addresses the critical issues associated with laparoscopic procedures. More specifically, it delivers maximum visibility, enhanced maneuverability and retains a flat profile after insertion through the trocar. Visilex mesh is the culmination of input and insight from laparoscopic surgeons. With a myriad of clinical benefits, it will change the way you look at laparoscopic hernia repair. The Visilex reinforced edge can be easily grasped and manipulated with standard laparoscopic instruments, eliminating the need for additional instruments to assist in mesh positioning. The Visilex reinforced edge also helps the mesh easily return to its original flat shape after simple insertion through the trocar. During placement, the mesh maintains flexibility necessary to conform to the anatomy—without ever losing the integrity of its shape. Visilex mesh is the first laparoscopic mesh to offer the clinical advantage of a patented reinforced edge. Visilex Mesh Comes with one other significant advantage: monofilament polypropylene.

Visilex mesh is constructed with monofilament polypropylene. This proven material is inert in the presence of infection, will not harbor bacteria, and promotes tissue ingrowth. Furthermore, the unique knit construction of Visilex mesh will not unravel.

## Gore Dualmesh® Biomaterial (Fig. 5.22)

### Indications

Reconstruction of hernias and soft tissue deficiencies and for the temporary bridging of fascial defects.

### Surface Orientation

Correct surface orientation is extremely important for Gore Dualmesh® Biomaterial to function as intended. One surface of the product has been textured for identification. This textured surface should be placed adjacent to those tissues where tissue ingrowth is desired. The other, smoother surface should be placed adjacent to those tissues where minimal tissue attachment is desired (i.e. serosal surfaces).

### Suturing

Use only nonabsorbable sutures, such as Gore-Tex® Suture, with a noncutting needle (such as taper or piercing point) of appropriate size to anchor the mesh. The use of absorbable sutures may lead to inadequate anchoring of Gore Dualmesh® Biomaterial to the host tissue and necessitate reoperation. For best results, use monofilament sutures. Suture size should be determined by surgeon preference and the nature of the reconstruction. When suturing Gore Dualmesh® Biomaterial to the host tissue, a bite and spacing ratio of 1:1 in both Gore Dualmesh® Biomaterial and the host tissue is recommended. The same ratio applies when suturing two pieces of Gore Dualmesh® Biomaterial together. Follow the curve of the needle when piercing the material and pierce through the full thickness of the material to ensure adequate mechanical strength of the material. Interrupted sutures can provide additional security against recurrence due to suture failure. Mattress suturing can provide additional strength to the suture line.

### Other Fixation Devices

Staples or helical tacks (also known as helical coils) can be used as an alternative to sutures. Staple size and staple or tack spacing should be determined by surgeon preference to provide for adequate tissue fixation and to prevent reherniation.

## Complications Related to the Use of Prosthetics

Materials composed of polypropylene and polyester insight a prompt and strong fibroblastic tissue response with minimal inflammation. This response consists of macrophages and giant cells, most of which eventually disappear. Fibroblastic activity allows rapid integration of the prosthesis into tissues; however, contraction of the enveloping scar tissue creates undesirable deformation of unsecured pieces of the monofilament; its free margins tend to curl, and small pieces roll up. There also have been some reports in the literature of freeform and preformed prosthetic mesh products migrating.

Serum or blood that accumulate in dead spaces surrounding any prosthesis becomes an excellent media for infection. Suction drainage is therefore advisable to eliminate dead space as well as to remove serum collections. Intestinal obstruction and fistula formation are serious complications and often require removal of the mesh/prosthesis. When a prosthesis is placed inside the peritoneal cavity, various degrees of visceral adhesions form depending upon the type of material used. When this is unavoidable, omentum or an absorbable prosthesis should be interposed between the mesh and the bowel.

Treatment of infection involves the application of basic surgical principles. Although most infections occur acutely, delayed infections involving nonabsorbable prostheses can occur months or years later. In the case of an acute infection of a groin hernia repair, it is advisable to quickly and widely open the wound (including the subcutaneous layer down to the external oblique) to avoid chronic sinus formation. A specimen should be taken for culture and sensitivity, irrigation and antibiotics started and healing observed by secondary intention. Frequent wound check to remove accumulated fluid is advisable.

If a prosthetic mesh had been used in the repair, it can usually be left in place if the above measures are employed promptly. If the wound closes, but a sinus continues to drain, it is likely that the mesh and all old suture material will need to be removed. Unlike early infection, when the mesh can be salvaged, late infection involving mesh requires the complete removal of the unincorporated material, although the incorporated mesh may be left undisturbed.

If the surgeon encounters an inflammatory granuloma in the course of repairing a recurrent inguinal hernia, it is prudent to avoid using a new prosthesis. Gram staining of the inflammatory granuloma at the time of surgery is not sufficiently reliable to exclude subsequent infection. In most cases of persistent infection related to a prior prosthetic repair, the culprit is the nature of the suture material rather than the graft itself. Multifilament and braided sutures, such as silk and cotton should be avoided.

Although there are vast armamentarium of surgical mesh available in market as of today, we have compiled a few mesh from the market. There are still more mesh available globally. This is the information up-to-date till going to press. The surgeon should analyze the need of the mesh for the particular patient and proceed for the choice of mesh.

Chapter 6

# Classification of Hernia

## Classification of Abdominal Hernia

All groin hernia classifications are somewhat arbitrary and artificial. Currently, there is no consensus among either general surgeons or hernia specialists as to a preferred system. A survey by Zollinger in 1998 of hernia specialists in North American and Europe showed, that although the Nyhus, Gilbert, and Schumpelick-Arit systems were commonly used, the majority of these specialists still used the traditional classification for groin hernias. It is apparent that only the traditional classification of groin hernias has stood the test of time. As stated by Fitzgibbons, "the primary purpose of a classification system for any disease is to stratify for severity so that reasonable comparisons can be made between various treatment strategies." Given the multiplicity of operative techniques and approaches for the repair of groin hernias, it appears that no one classification system can satisfy all. With time, it is likely that we will settle upon a given operation for a specific type of inguinal hernia. For that given operation to be accepted as proven best, however, it is essential the competing operations be applied to similar (classified) groups of groin hernia patients.

Numerous classifications for groin and ventral hernias have been proposed over the past five to six decades. The old, simple classification of groin hernia in to direct, inguinal and femoral components is no longer adequate to understand the complex pathophysiology and management of these hernias.

### Classification of Groin Hernias

#### *The Most Popular Classifications*

Casten divided hernias into three stages:

- *Stage 1:* An indirect hernia with a normal internal ring.
- *Stage 2:* An indirect hernia with an enlarged or distorted internal ring.
- *Stage 3:* All direct or femoral hernias.

Halverson and McVay classification divided hernias into four classes:

- *Class 1:* Small indirect hernia.
- *Class 2:* Medium indirect hernia.
- *Class 3:* Large indirect hernia or direct hernia.
- *Class 4:* Femoral hernia.

Ponka's system defined two types of indirect hernia:

1. Uncomplicated indirect inguinal hernia
2. Sliding indirect inguinal hernia.

Three types of direct hernias:

1. Small defect in the medial aspect of Hesselbach's triangle near the pubic tubercle
2. Diverticular hernia in the posterior wall with an otherwise intact inguinal floor
3. A large diffuse direct inguinal hernia of the entire floor of Hesselbach's triangle.

Gilbert designed a classification for primary and recurrent inguinal hernias done through an anterior approach (Fig. 6.1). It is based on evaluating three factors:

1. Presence or absence of a peritoneal sac
2. Size of the internal ring
3. Integrity of the posterior wall of the canal.

Types 1, 2 and 3 are indirect hernias; types 4 and 5 are direct hernia:

- Type 1 hernias have a peritoneal sac passing through an intact internal ring that will not admit 1 fingerbreadth (i.e. < 1 cm); the posterior wall is intact.
- Type 2 hernias (the most common indirect hernia) have a peritoneal sac coming through

| Classification for inguinal hernias | | | | | |
|---|---|---|---|---|---|
| Type | 1 | 2 | 3 | 4 | 5 |
| Internal ring | <IFB | IFB | >IFB | Norm | Norm |
| Peritoneal sac | Y | Y | Y | N | N |
| Canal floor | I | I | DES | DES | DES (IFB) |

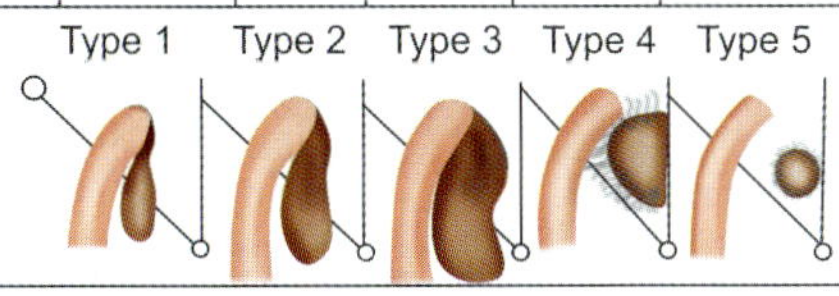


**Fig. 6.1:** Gilbert classification. Five types of primary and recurrent inguinal hernias

a 1-fingerbreadth internal ring (i.e. ≤2 cm); the posterior wall is intact.

- Type 3 hernias have a peritoneal sac coming through a 2-fingerbreadth or wider internal ring (i.e. >2 cm).
- Type 3 hernias frequently are complete and often have a sliding component. They begin to break down a portion of the posterior wall just medial to the internal ring.
- Type 4 hernias have a full floor posterior wall breakdown or multiple defects in the posterior wall. The internal ring is intact, and there is no peritoneal sac.
- Type 5 hernias are pubic tubercle recurrence or primary diverticular hernias. There is no peritoneal sac and the internal ring remains intact. In cases where double hernias exist, both types are designated (e.g. Types 2/4).
- In 1993, Rutkow and Robbins added a Type 6 to the Gilbert classification to designate double inguinal hernias and a Type 7 to designate a femoral hernia.

Nyhus developed a classification designed for the posterior approach based on the size of the internal ring and the integrity of the posterior wall. According to this scheme:

- Type 1 is an indirect hernia with a normal internal ring
- Type 2 is an indirect hernia with an enlarged internal ring
- Type 3a is a direct inguinal hernia
- Type 3b is an indirect hernia causing posterior wall weakness
- Type 3c is a femoral hernia
- Type 4 represents all recurrent hernias.

Of these and other classifications that have been proposed, a recent survey indicated that the most commonly used classifications by members of the American Hernia Society are the classical indirect/direct designation, that of Nyhus, and that of Gilbert/Rutkow and Robbins. Most recently, Zollinger proposed a unified classification of groin hernias that combines one of the most commonly used individual classifications and is applicable to the anterior and posterior approaches. The principal feature of Zollinger's combined classification is the recognition that a large indirect hernia defect also imposes on the posterior wall, and in effect becomes a combined defect.

## Endoscopic/Laparoscopic Classification of Hernia

### Classification of Inguinal Hernia for Total Extraperitoneal Repair

This functional classification grades groin hernias according to the preoperative predictive level of difficulty of endoscopic surgery. For multiple or pantaloon (direct and indirect components) hernias, grading is according to the dominant hernia. Bowel obstruction and strangulation are unsuitable for the total extraperitoneal (TEP) approach. Intraoperatively, the factors considered as predictors of the grade of difficulty include: Reducibility, degree of descent of the hernial sac, previous hernia repair.

*Grade I:* Small, direct, reducible hernia.
*Grade II:* Small, indirect, incomplete, reducible hernia.
*Grade III:* Moderate-size indirect, reducible inguinal hernia.
*Grade IV:* Large reducible indirect inguinoscrotal hernia.
*Grade V:* Large, complete, indirect inguinal hernia.

### Classification of Ventral Hernia

*Grade I:* Primary, small, completely reducible ventral hernia.
*Grade II:* Completely reducible incisional hernia.
*Grade III:* Primary hernia-partially reducible or irreducible.
*Grade IV:* Primary hernia containing bowel, which is partially reducible or irreducible.

*Grade V:* Incisional hernia containing bowel-partially reducible or irreducible.

*Grade VI:* Multiple scarred abdomen, multiple previous incisions, previous hernia repair (recurrent incisional hernia).

## Types of Abdominal Hernia

- Inguinal hernia
- Femoral hernia
- Umbilical hernia

*Incisional hernia:* An incisional hernia occurs when the defect is the result of an incompletely healed surgical wound. When these occur in median laparotomy incisions in the linea alba, they are termed ventral hernias. These can be the most frustrating and difficult to treat, as the repair utilizes already attenuated tissue.

*Diaphragmatic hernia:* Higher in the abdomen, an internal "diaphragmatic hernia" results when part of the stomach or intestine protrudes into the chest cavity through a defect in the diaphragm.

A hiatus hernia is a particular variant of this type, in which the normal passageway through which the esophagus meets the stomach (esophageal hiatus) serves as a functional "defect", allowing part of the stomach to (periodically) "herniate" into the chest. Hiatus hernias may be either "sliding," in which the gastroesophageal junction itself slides through the defect into the chest, or nonsliding (also known as paraesophageal), in which case the junction remains fixed while another portion of the stomach moves up through the defect. Nonsliding or paraesophageal hernias can be dangerous as they may allow the stomach to rotate and obstruct.

A congenital diaphragmatic hernia is a distinct problem, occurring in up to 1 in 2000 births, and requiring pediatric surgery. Intestinal organs may herniate through several parts of the diaphragm, posterolateral (in Bochdalek's triangle, resulting in Bochdalek's hernia), or anteromedial-retrosternal (in the cleft of Larrey/ Morgagni's foramen, resulting in Morgagni-Larrey hernia, or Morgagni's hernia).

## Other Abdominal/Inguinal Hernias

Since many organs or parts of organs can herniate through many orifices, it is very difficult to give an exhaustive list of hernias, with all synonyms and eponyms.

- *Cooper's hernia:* A femoral hernia with two sacs, the first being in the femoral canal, and the second passing through a defect in the superficial fascia and appearing immediately beneath the skin.
- *Epigastric hernia:* A hernia through the linea alba above the umbilicus.
- *Hiatal hernia:* A hernia due to "short esophagus"-insufficient elongation-stomach is displaced into the thorax.
- *Littre's hernia:* A hernia involving a Meckel's diverticulum. It is named after the French anatomist Alexis Littre (1658-1726).
- *Lumbar hernia:* A hernia in the lumbar region (not to be confused with a lumbar disk hernia), contains the following entities:
  - *Petit's hernia:* A hernia through Petit's triangle (inferior lumbar triangle). It is named after French surgeon Jean Louis Petit (1674-1750).
  - *Grynfeltt's hernia:* A hernia through Grynfeltt-Lesshaft triangle (superior lumbar triangle). It is named after physician Joseph Grynfeltt (1840-1913).
- *Obturator hernia:* Hernia through obturator canal.
- *Pantaloon hernia:* A combined direct and indirect hernia, when the hernial sac protrudes on either side of the inferior epigastric vessels.
- *Paraumbilical hernia:* A type of umbilical hernia occurring in adults.
- *Perineal hernia:* A perineal hernia protrudes through the muscles and fascia of the perineal floor. It may be primary but usually, is acquired following perineal prostatectomy, abdominoperineal resection of the rectum, or pelvic exenteration.
- *Properitoneal hernia:* Rare hernia located directly above the peritoneum, for example, when part of an inguinal hernia projects from the deep inguinal ring to the preperitoneal space.
- *Richter's hernia:* A hernia involving only one sidewall of the bowel, which can result in bowel strangulation leading to perforation through ischemia without causing bowel obstruction or any of its warning signs. It is named after German surgeon August Gottlieb Richter (1742-1812).
- *Sliding hernia:* Occurs when an organ drags along part of the peritoneum, or, in other words, the organ is part of the hernia sac. The colon and the urinary bladder are often involved. The term also frequently refers to sliding hernias of the stomach.

- *Sciatic hernia:* This hernia in the greater sciatic foramen most commonly presents as an uncomfortable mass in the gluteal area. Bowel obstruction may also occur. This type of hernia is only a rare cause of sciatic neuralgia.
- *Spigelian hernia:* It also known as spontaneous lateral ventral hernia.
- *Sports hernia:* A hernia characterized by chronic groin pain in athletes and a dilated superficial ring of the inguinal canal.
- *Velpeau hernia:* A hernia in the groin in front of the femoral blood vessels.

# Chapter 7

# Diagnosis of Hernia

## Presentation of Hernia

History and physical examination remain the best means of diagnosing hernias.

### Inguinal Hernia

#### *Examination of an Adult*

- Surgeon in seated position with the patient standing
- Surgeon visualizes the inguinal canal areas for the bulge
- A provocative cough is necessary to expose the hernia.

Do the following (Fig. 7.1):

1. Ask patient to repeat cough.
2. Invaginate scrotum.
3. Try to feel impulse in inguinal region.
4. Assess the diameter of internal ring.
5. Palpate the cord structure by finger rolling perpendicular to long axis of cord just medial to internal ring (Look for the thickening of cord structures).
6. Put your index finger on internal ring, middle finger on external ring and ring finger on the femoral ring. Ask the patient to cough. Read the impression of the test. If you feel impulse at index finger then this is indirect inguinal hernia; impulse at middle finger suggests direct inguinal hernia; while obvious impulse at ring finger denotes femoral hernia.

   When attempting to identify a hernia, look for a swelling or mass in the area of the fascial defect.
7. Place a fingertip into the scrotal sac and advance up into the inguinal canal. If the hernia is elsewhere on the abdomen, attempt to define the borders of the fascial defect.
8. If the hernia comes from superolateral to inferomedial and strikes the distal tip of the finger, it most likely is an indirect hernia.
9. If the hernia strikes the pad of the finger from deep to superficial, it is more consistent with a direct hernia.

### In Children

Palpation of the cord—may reveal thickened cord, particularly during straining.

There is sensation of rubbing two layers of silk together (the Silk sign).

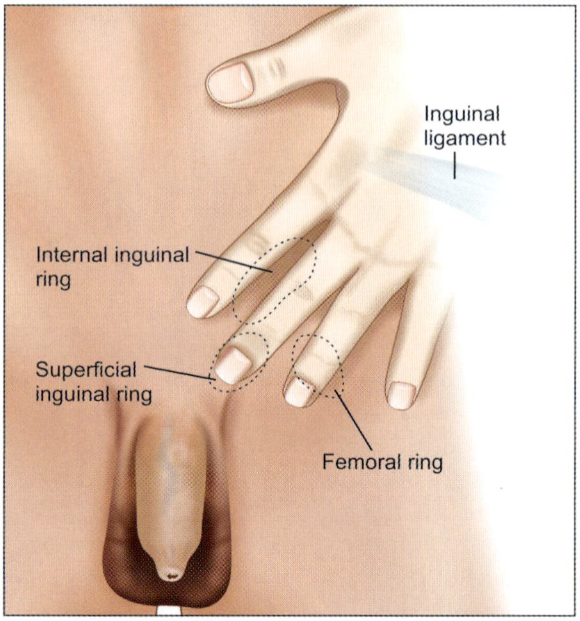


**Fig. 7.1:** Examination of adult groin hernia

Examine the child in the upright position by applying intermittent manual pressure to the abdomen.

Indirect hernias are most common.

### Incarcerated Hernia

If the visceral contents of a hernial sac do not easily reduce into the peritoneal cavity, the hernia is incarcerated.

Strangulated hernias are differentiated from incarcerated hernias by the following:

- Pain out of proportion to examination findings
- Fever or toxic appearance
- Pain that persists after reduction of hernia.

### Strangulated Hernia

- Symptoms of an incarcerated hernia present combined with a toxic appearance.
- Systemic toxicity secondary to ischemic bowel is possible.
- Strangulation is probable if pain and tenderness of an incarcerated hernia persist after reduction.
- Suspect an alternative diagnosis in patients who have a substantial amount of pain without evidence of incarceration or strangulation.

### Reducible Hernia

If the contents can be reduced, the hernia is reducible.

### Irreducible Hernia

If the contents cannot be reduced at all, the hernia is irreducible.

## Other Hernias

### Spigelian Hernia

A Spigelian hernia (or lateral ventral hernia) is a hernia through the spigelian fascia, which is the aponeurotic layer between the rectus abdominis muscle medially, and the semilunar line laterally. These hernias almost always develop at or below the linea arcuata, probably because of the lack of posterior rectus sheath. These are generally interparietal hernias, meaning that they do not lie below the subcutaneous fat but penetrate between the muscles of the abdominal wall; therefore, there is often no notable swelling.

Spigelian hernias are usually small and therefore risk of strangulation is high. Most occur on the right side. Most develop around age 50 (4th–7th decade of life). Compared to other types of hernias they are rare.

Patients typically present with either an intermittent mass, localized pain, or signs of bowel obstruction. Ultrasonography or a CT scan can establish the diagnosis, although CT scan provides the greatest sensitivity and specificity.

### Femoral Hernia

They typically present as a groin lump. They may or may not be associated with pain. Often, they present with a varying degree of complication ranging from irreducibility through intestinal obstruction to frank gangrene of contained bowel. The incidence of strangulation in femoral hernias is high. A femoral hernia has often been found to be the cause of unexplained small bowel obstruction.

The obvious finding may be a lump in the groin. Cough impulse is often absent and should not be relied on solely when making a diagnosis of femoral hernia. The lump is more globular than the pear shaped lump of the inguinal hernia. The bulk of a femoral hernia lies below an imaginary line drawn between the anterosuperior iliac spine and the pubic tubercle (which essentially represents the inguinal ligament) whereas an inguinal hernia starts above this line. Nonetheless, it is often impossible to distinguish the two preoperatively.

## Diagnosis

The diagnosis is largely a clinical one, generally done by physical examination of the groin. However, in obese patients, imaging in the form of ultrasonography, CT or MRI may aid in the diagnosis. An abdominal X-ray showing small bowel obstruction in a female patient with a painful groin lump needs no further investigation.

Several other conditions have a similar presentation and must be considered when forming the diagnosis: inguinal hernia, an enlarged inguinal lymph node, aneurysm of the femoral artery, saphena varix, and an abcess of the psoas.

Prevascular femoral hernia is rare and manifests as a bulge. It may be mistaken for a femoral aneurysm. External femoral hernias pass beneath the inguinal ligament to lie lateral to the femoral vessels and deep to the iliopubic tract. The hernia of Laugier traverses a defect in the lacunar ligament. A hernia of Cloquet results from an abnormal insertion of the pectineus muscle, which allows perforation of the aponeurosis as the hernia sac courses over the femoral canal. The retrovascular hernia sac descends in the posterior sheath of the femoral vein.

### Epigastric Hernia

An epigastric hernia is a type of hernia which may develop in the epigastrium. Epigastric hernias are most common in infants but may occur in humans of any age. They typically result from a minor defect of the linea alba between the rectus abdominis muscles. This allows tissue from inside the abdomen to herniate anteriorly. On infants, this may manifest as an apparent 'bubble' under the skin of the belly between the umbilicus and xiphisternum

### Umbilical Hernia

Umbilical hernia is a congenital malformation, especially common in infants of African descent, and more frequent in girls. An acquired umbilical hernia directly results from increased intra-abdominal pressure and are most commonly seen in obese individuals.

## Presentation

A hernia is present at the site of the umbilicus in the newborn; although sometimes quite large, these hernias tend to resolve without any treatment by around the age of 5 years. Obstruction and strangulation of the hernia is rare because the underlying defect in the abdominal wall is larger than in an inguinal hernia of the newborn. The size of the base of the herniated tissue is inversely correlated with risk of strangulation (i.e. narrow base is more likely to strangulate). An umbilical hernia presents as a central, midabdominal bulge.

Babies are prone to this malformation because of the process during fetal development by which the abdominal organs form outside the abdominal cavity, later returning into it through an opening which will become the umbilicus.

## Differential Diagnosis

Importantly this type of hernia must be distinguished from a paraumbilical hernia which occurs in adults and involves a defect in the midline near to the umbilicus, and from omphalocele.

### Paraumbilical Hernia

The name paraumbilical hernia applies when this defect is adjacent to the umbilicus.

### Hiatus Hernia

A hiatus hernia or hiatal hernia is the protrusion (or herniation) of the upper part of the stomach into the thorax through a tear or weakness in the diaphragm.

## Symptoms

The symptoms include acid reflux and pain, similar to heartburn, in the chest, and upper stomach.

In most patients, hiatus hernias cause no symptoms. Sometimes patients experience heartburn and regurgitation, when stomach acid refluxes back into the esophagus.

## Diagnosis

The diagnosis of a hiatus hernia is typically made through an upper gastrointestinal (GI) series or endoscopy (Fig. 7.2).

### Incisional Hernia

An incisional hernia occurs in an area of weakness caused by an incompletely-healed surgical wound. Since median

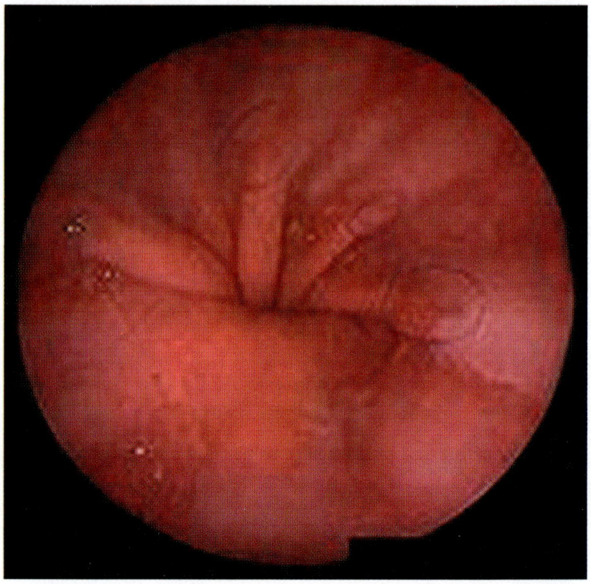

**Fig. 7.2:** Upper gastrointestinal (GI) endoscopy depicting hiatus hernia

incisions in the abdomen are frequent for abdominal exploratory surgery, ventral incisional hernias are termed ventral hernias.

Clinically, incisional hernias present as a bulge or protrusion at or near the area of a surgical incision. Virtually any prior abdominal operation can develop an incisional hernia at the scar area (provided adequate healing does not occur), from large abdominal procedures (intestinal surgery, vascular surgery), to small incisions (appendix removal, or abdominal exploratory surgery). While these hernias can occur at any incision, they tend to occur more commonly along a straight line from the xiphoid process of the sternum straight down to the pubic bone, and are more complex in these regions.

## Obturator Hernia

An obturator hernia is a rare type of abdominal wall hernia in which abdominal content protrudes through the obturator foramen. Because of differences in anatomy, it is much more common in females than in males, especially multiparous and older women who have recently lost a lot of weight. The diagnosis is often made intraoperatively after presenting with bowel obstruction. A gynecologist may come across this type of hernias as a secondary finding during gynecological open surgery or laparoscopy. The Howship-Romberg sign is suggestive of an obturator hernia, exacerbated by thigh extension, medial rotation and adduction. It is characterized by lancilating pain in the medial thigh/obturator distribution, extending to the knee; caused by hernia compression of the obturator nerve.

Obturator hernias have intermittent, acute, and severe hyperesthesia or pain in the medial thigh or in the region of the greater trochanter. The symptoms are usually relieved by flexion of the thigh and are worsened by medial rotation, adduction, or extension at the hip. Rarely, there is a palpable mass in the medial upper thigh.

## Perineal Hernia

Perineal hernia is a hernia involving the perineum. The hernia may contain fat, any part of the intestine, the rectum, or the bladder. It appears as a sudden swelling to one side (sometimes both sides) of the anus.

## Petit's Hernia

Petit's hernia is the one that protrudes through lumbar triangle. This triangle lies in the posterolateral abdominal wall bounded in front by free margin of external oblique muscle, behind by latissimus dorsi and below by iliac crest. The neck is large, so chances of strangulating are small. Occurs more often in males on the left side. Protrudes when the child cries.

## Grynfeltt-Lesshaft Hernia

Grynfeltt-Lesshaft hernia is a herniation of abdominal contents through the back, specifically through the superior lumbar triangle, which is defined by the quadratus lumborum muscle, twelfth rib, and internal oblique muscle.

## Sciatic Hernia

A tender mass in the gluteal area that is increasing in size is suggestive of a sciatic hernia. Sciatic neuropathy and symptoms of intestinal or ureteral obstruction can also occur. Perineal hernias generally present as a perineal mass with discomfort on sitting and occasionally have obstructive symptoms with incarceration.

## Diastasis Recti

Diastasis recti or a widened linea alba has no clinical significance and does not require operative repair. However, there may be small openings in the linea alba through which preperitoneal fat can protrude.

## Interparietal Hernia

The term "interparietal hernia" is used collectively to designate a group of rather unusual hernias which are located in the inguinal region between the various layers of the abdominal parietes. Anatomically, these hernias may be classified as follows:

1. Properitoneal hernia, that type in which the hernial sac lies between the peritoneum and the transversalis fascia.
2. Interstitial hernia, in which the sac lies between the transversalis fascia and the transversalis, internal oblique, or external oblique muscles.
3. Superficial hernia, in which the sac is situated between the aponeurosis of the external oblique muscle and the integument.

# Monolocular Properitoneal Hernia

Properitoneal hernia (Figs 7.3 to 7.8), in both the monolocular and the bilocular forms, may be classified as follows:

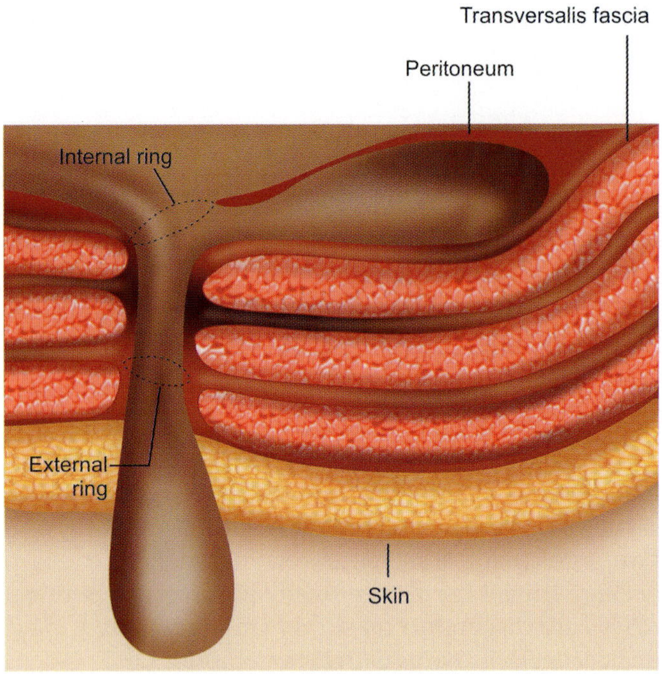


**Fig. 7.3:** Bilocular properitoneal hernia

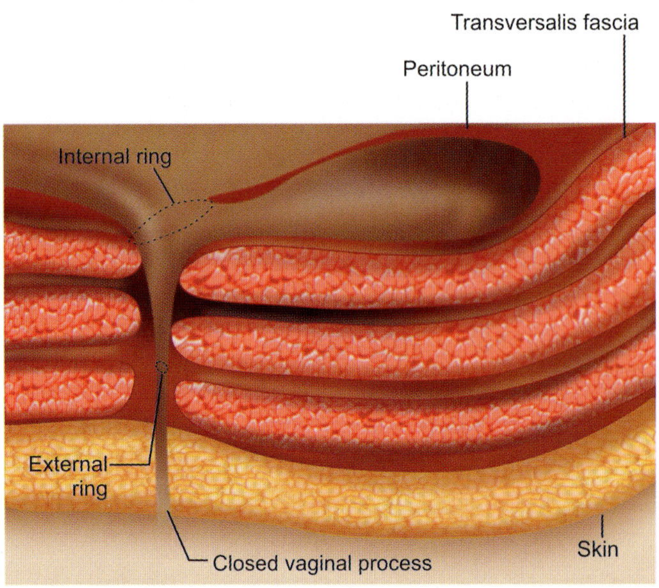


**Fig. 7.4:** Monolocular properitoneal hernia

1. Inguinoproperitoneal hernia, which occurs as a diverticulum from a pre-existing inguinal hernia.
2. Cruroproperitoneal hernia, which occurs as an outpouching of a femoral hernia.
3. Simple properitoneal hernia which is independent of the inguinal or femoral canals.

## Symptoms

There is no pathognomonic sign or symptom that will lead to the diagnosis of properitoneal hernia. Fully 90% of the patients will present themselves with the clinical syndrome of acute intestinal obstruction. They may have had a reducible inguinal or femoral hernia of long standing. Following an apparent reduction, the patient becomes nauseated and vomits, the abdomen becomes distended, and the bowels constipated. On examination, an irreducible inguinal or femoral hernia may be found, with some tenderness over the region of the internal inguinal ring, but as a rule no swelling occurs above Poupart's ligament.

## Interstitial Hernia

### *Superficial Hernia*

In superficial hernia the sac lies between the skin and the aponeurosis of the external oblique muscle.

## Diaphragmatic Hernia

A diaphragmatic hernia is a birth defect, which is an abnormality that occurs before birth as a fetus is forming

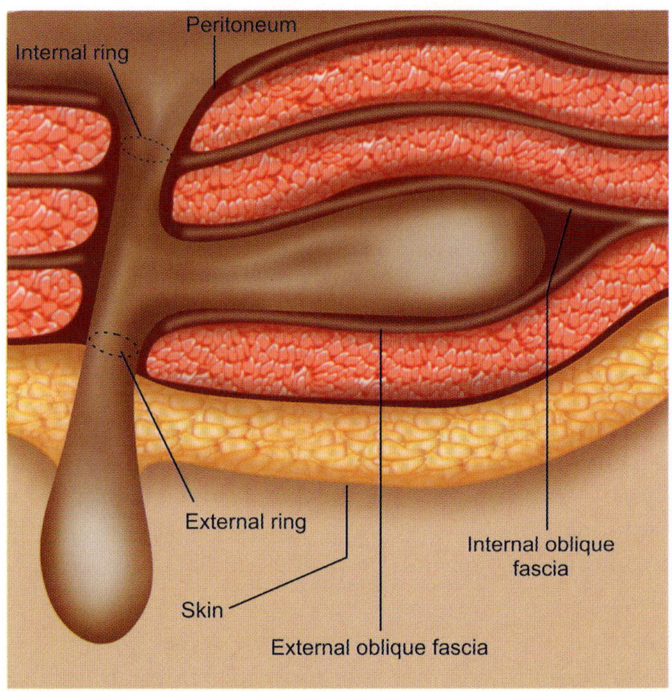


**Fig. 7.5:** Bilocular interstitial hernia

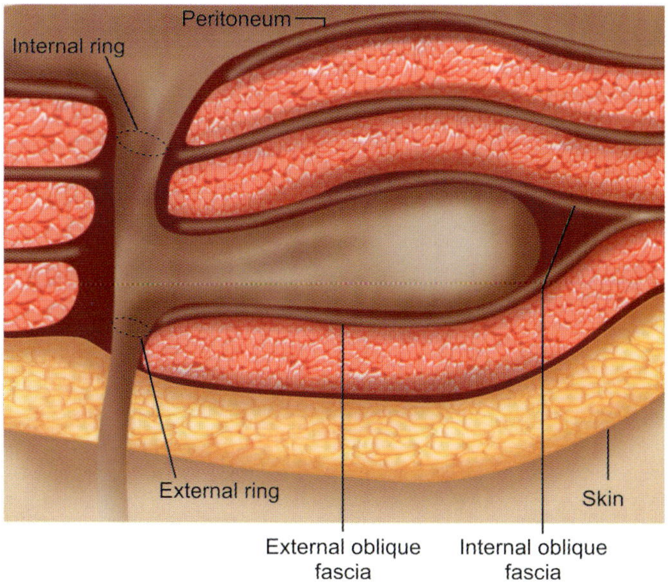


**Fig. 7.6:** Monolocular interstitial hernia

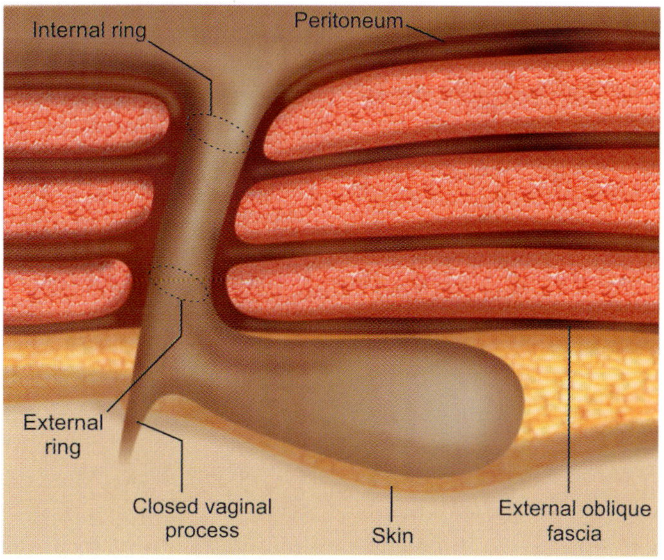


**Fig. 7.8:** Monolocular

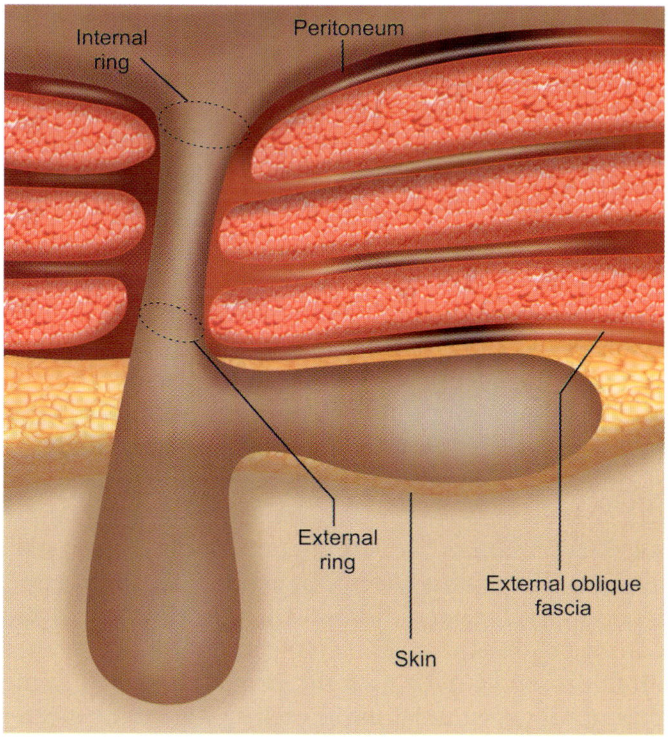


**Fig. 7.7:** Bilocular

in the mother's uterus. An opening is present in the diaphragm. With this type of birth defect, some of the organs that are normally found in the abdomen move up into the chest cavity through this abnormal opening.

There are two types of diaphragmatic hernia:

1. *Bochdalek hernia:* A Bochdalek hernia involves an opening on the left side of the diaphragm. The stomach and intestines usually move up into the chest cavity.
2. *Morgagni hernia:* A Morgagni hernia involves an opening on the right side of the diaphragm. The liver and intestines usually move up into the chest cavity.

## Congenital Abdominal Wall Defects

Maternal serum alpha-fetoprotein screening can help identify ventral wall defects in the fetus during the second trimester. Prenatal ultrasonography can define the location of the abdominal wall defect, the status of the viscera, its involvement with associated structures, and the presence of additional malformations. Recognition of a small omphalocele or hernia of the umbilical cord stalk may not occur until after delivery. This may result in compromise of the small bowel or damage to an omphalomesenteric duct as the cord is clamped. Therefore, the cord should be clamped well away from the abdomen in an infant with an unusual cord base or widened umbilical cord base to prevent iatrogenic injury to the intestine (Fig. 7.9).

## Radiology in Hernia Diagnosis

Sometimes hernia may not be obvious as it may be on many occasions. For the complete diagnosis of hernia the

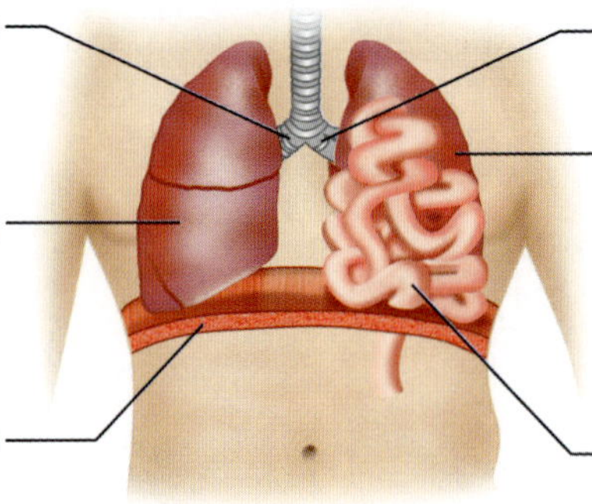


**Fig. 7.9:** Congenital diaphragmatic hernia

surgeon has to undertake some investigations to prove the diagnosis of hernia. Some hernias are well hidden in the abdomen or pelvis like obturator hernia. It becomes difficult to diagnose these hernias clinically. For instance epigastric hernia may also be misleading to diagnosis of lipoma. As the swelling is soft in epigastric hernia; it confuses the surgeon. Here some special investigations are helpful to the surgeon like CT scan, ultrasonography, barium swallow, herniography, etc.

## Peritoneography/Herniography

Peritoneography is highly reliable for detecting clinically occult inguinal hernia and has a low complication rate. Peritoneography involves the intraperitoneal injection of nonionic contrast for evaluation of the abdominal parietes. When used selectively for evaluation of the inguinal region and pelvic floor, it is termed herniography.

### *Indications*

1. Inguinal pain (Inguinodynia).
2. Clinically absent inguinal hernia on physical examination.

## Herniography Technique

The technique of herniography is performed as follows: An initial physical examination of the inguinal regions is performed standing and then supine to exclude hernia and to evaluate for other causes of inguinal pain related to the symphysis pubis, adductor musculature, and hip joints. With the patient in the supine position on the radiographic tilt table, the patient is asked to elevate head and shoulders off the table, and the tensed abdomen is examined. The midline region of the supraumbilical linea alba and the linea semilunaris at the lateral margin of the rectus sheath adjacent to the umbilicus are identified and marked where possible, depending on operator preference. An intravenous line is instituted that can be used for conscious sedation (rarely needed) or treatment of vagal reactions (again, rarely needed), reactions to the local anesthetic or the contrast medium. The chosen area is prepared and draped in sterile fashion, and the skin and subcutaneous tissues down to the peritoneum are infiltrated with 1% xylocaine. A small dermatotomy is made and the 7 or 12 cm 21-gauge micropuncture needle (depending on body habitus) from a 10 or 15 cm micropuncture set is inserted in an oblique fashion (not vertically) until the patient's face registers the characteristic grimace and the characteristic pop is felt, indicating passage of the needle tip through the peritoneum. At this time, a small amount of contrast is injected by hand under fluoroscopy. If necessary, the needle is repositioned until the injected contrast shows the characteristic interloop appearance on fluoroscopy, indicating the needle tip is within the peritoneal cavity and not within the parietes, the greater omentum, and the small bowel mesentery or within the bowel lumen. The 0.018-inch-diameter guidewire from the micropuncture set is passed through the needle and the needle is removed. The 4F micropuncture sheath/ dilator is passed over the wire into the peritoneal cavity, the wire and dilator are removed, and then 150 ml nonionic contrast medium (Omnipaque 300), is injected by hand through the sheath into the peritoneal cavity. The sheath is capped off and left *in situ*, covered by a sterile occlusive dressing. The patient is turned into the prone position and the head of the table is elevated 20° to 25° to optimally pool the intraperitoneal contrast over the inguinal regions. Radiographs are then obtained with the patient in prone and prone oblique positions at rest and during provocative maneuvers such as coughing, sniffing, Mueller maneuver (forced inspiration against a closed glottis), and straining or Valsalva maneuver (forced expiration against a closed glottis). In addition, the patient is occasionally asked to elevate up on knees and elbows to relieve compression from obesity on the inguinal regions (a cause of false-negative results). Cross-table lateral radiographs are occasionally used as well. As an important adjunct to the examination, the patient is asked to point with a single index finger or to place a radiographic marker at the site of his or her pain, and a radiograph is obtained for correlation. In male patients, standing images are sometimes useful. In male patients, the scrotum should be briefly evaluated with fluoroscopy after all the provocative maneuvers to see whether any contrast has entered the scrotum. This can indicate hernia when the neck is not apparent or compressed. If there is a teat appearance in the supravesical or medial or lateral inguinal fossae, the patient can be turned supine and the feet elevated 20° to 25° and air or $CO_2$ can be injected through the indwelling sheath. This occasionally detects a hernia, the sac filling with negative contrast. This usually requires abdominal distention with gas.

The entire procedure takes approximately 20 to 30 minutes. When the procedure is complete, the 4F sheath is removed and a sterile dressing is applied.

Herniography has great value in excluding inguinal hernia in patients with chronic symptoms in the groin. It is a useful diagnostic tool for the identification of clinically occult herniae and this investigation can prevent needless surgery and re-exploration in those cases with previous hernia repair. Its principal role is to establish the diagnosis of occult hernia as a cause of obscure pain in the groin.

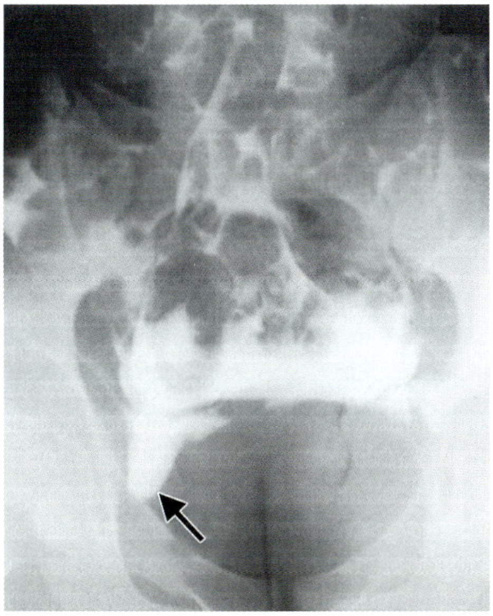

**Fig. 7.10:** X-ray showing right inguinal hernia (arrow)

## Ultrasonography

Sonography has been used in the diagnosis of abdominal wall herniations as well as pathologic conditions affecting the inguinal and femoral regions. It provides a rapid and noninvasive method of imaging the scrotal contents and has enabled differentiation of testicular from extratesticular pathology in most cases.

Ultrasonography can also aid in prenatal diagnosis of hernia in fetus, e.g. hiatus hernia.

*Criteria for prenatal hiatus hernia diagnosis:* The ultrasound criterion for prenatal diagnosis is the presence of a herniated stomach in the posterior mediastinum, sometimes having a dynamic position during examination, with no mediastinal shift associated with normal diaphragm appearance on parasagittal sections of the thorax.

## Inguinal Hernia (Fig. 7.10)

In the obese, distortion of anatomy, the presence of pannus, and the sound-attenuating properties of adipose tissue may make identifying the anatomy more difficult. Initially, examination of the inguinal region is done with the patient supine. It is essential to ask the patient to increase abdominal pressure (Valsalva maneuver) at each of the sonographic steps to identify transient hernias.

The Valsalva maneuver is a critical component of the examination, because in many patients the hernia may be completely reduced at rest. In addition, the characteristic movement of the herniating tissues often clinches the diagnosis. This dynamic capability of sonography is an advantage when compared with other cross-sectional imaging techniques. Re-examination with the patient standing is also recommended if supine evaluation does not reveal herniation. Herniated bowel contents may show peristalsis, and herniated fat will appear hyperechoic. It is also important to evaluate for reducibility and bowel viability identified by peristalsis or mucosal blood flow.

### *Indirect Inguinal Hernia (Fig. 7.11)*

For an indirect inguinal hernia, once the transducer is positioned where the inferior epigastric artery originates from the external iliac artery, it is rotated obliquely so that the medial aspect is inferior, along the long axis of the inguinal ligament. In men, the healthy spermatic cord can be seen in longitudinal and transverse planes as a heterogeneous hyperechoic structure with hypoechoic tubules and vascularity, originating from the internal inguinal ring. This structure should be differentiated from the inguinal ligament, which has a more compact fibrillar appearance, is taut extending from the ilium to the pubis, and is just inferior in relation to the internal inguinal ring. With the transducer positioned longitudinal to the inguinal canal and visualizing the inferior epigastric artery at its origin, an indirect inguinal hernia can be seen protruding anteriorly toward the transducer from its origin lateral to the inferior epigastric artery. The herniated tissue then turns medially anterior to the inferior epigastric artery and extends inferomedially as it traverses and often distends the inguinal canal parallel to the skin surface. An indirect inguinal hernia may reach the pubic tubercle and exit the superficial ring and may enter the scrotum in a man.

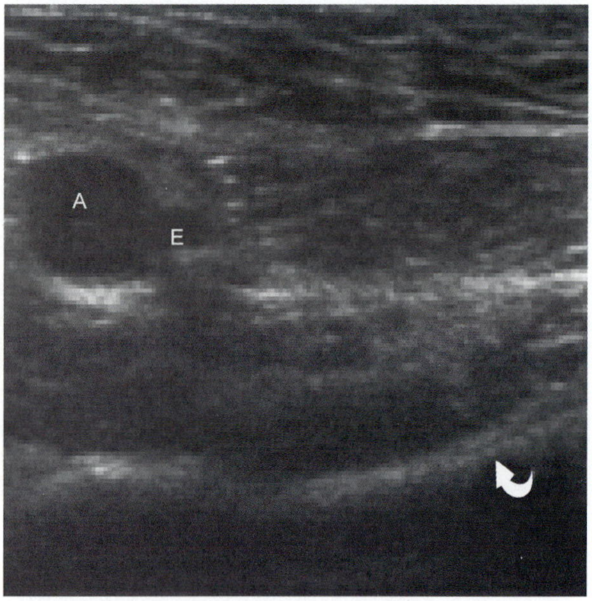


**Fig. 7.11:** Indirect inguinal hernia-right

### *Direct Inguinal Hernia*

Similar to indirect inguinal hernia evaluation, for a direct inguinal hernia the transducer is placed longitudinal to the inguinal canal and anterior to the inferior epigastric artery origin. However, the transducer is moved medially because direct inguinal hernias originate medial to the inferior epigastric artery in Hesselbach's triangle. Imaging superior to the inguinal canal as well as in the orthogonal plane will ensure complete evaluation of Hesselbach's triangle. With the Valsalva maneuver, this hernia will protrude directly anteriorly toward the transducer.

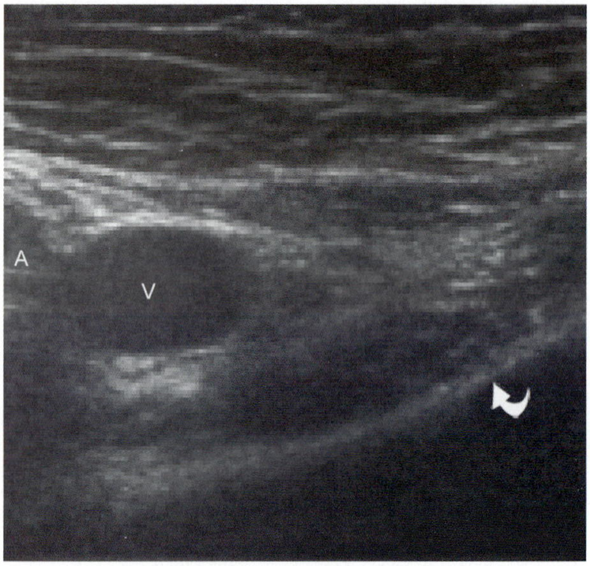


**Fig. 7.12:** Femoral hernia

## Femoral Hernia (Fig. 7.12)

Having evaluated the inguinal region superior to the inguinal ligament, the transducer is moved inferior to the inguinal ligament, and the area medial to the femoral vein is evaluated for femoral hernia. During the Valsalva maneuver, the femoral vein will normally dilate and should be differentiated from a femoral hernia.

## Spigelian Hernia (Fig. 7.13)

The sonography examination for a spigelian hernia should begin at the lateral margin of the rectus abdominis

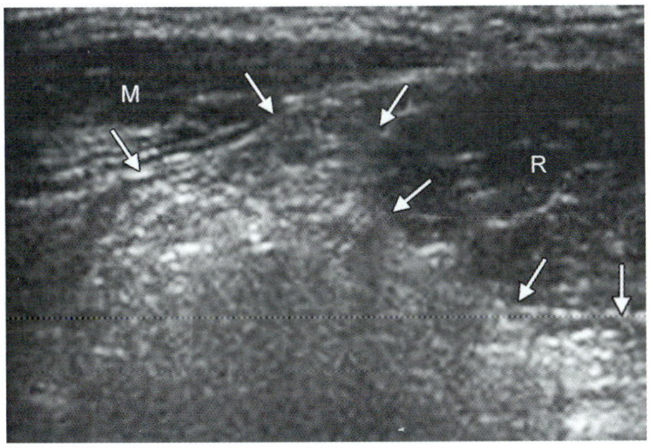


**Fig. 7.13:** Spigelian hernia

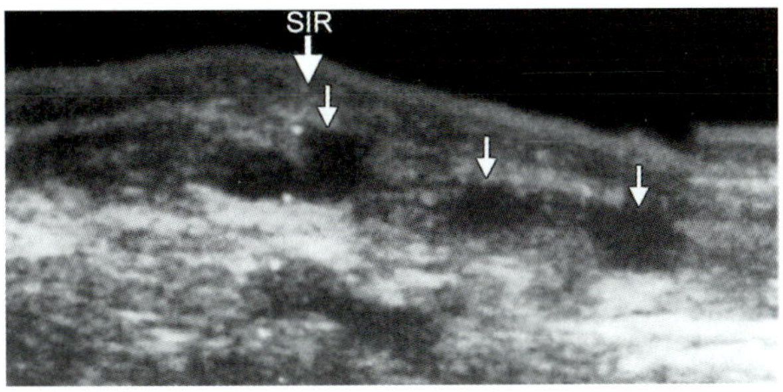


**Fig. 7.14:** Scrotal hernia with bowel loops

(the linea semilunaris) in the transverse plane from the level of the umbilicus. As the transducer is moved inferiorly, the inferior epigastric artery can be identified as it passes deep in relation to the lateral border of the rectus abdominis muscle. Just superior to this location, along the linea semilunaris, is the site where a spigelian hernia may occur. The inferior epigastric artery is then followed inferiorly to the external iliac artery, defining the lateral boundary of Hesselbach's triangle.

### Scrotal Hernias (Fig. 7.14)

Sonography has been used in the diagnosis of abdominal wall herniations as well as pathologic conditions affecting the inguinal and femoral regions. It provides a rapid and noninvasive method of imaging the scrotal contents and has enabled differentiation of testicular from extratesticular pathology in most cases. Scrotal hernia constitutes a secondary extratesticular mass with its origin in the abdomen. The contents of the hernia sac includes small bowel or colon and/or omentum in most cases. If the scrotum alone is scanned, the diagnosis of scrotal hernia containing bowel is based on the recognition of valvulae conniventes on haustrations and on the detection of penistalsis on real-time sonography. In the absence of these features, the diagnosis of scrotal hernia is difficult. Even when these features are present, extratesticular pathology, such as multiloculated hydrocele and hematocele containing fibrous septa, can simulate fluid-filled loops of bowel. In addition, fatty tissue and fat-containing masses can produce high-amplitude echoes similar to a primary scrotal mass containing fat. Due to similarity in their echo amplitude, these masses may be impossible to differentiate from a scrotal hernia containing omentum. For these reasons, scanning along the plane of the inguinal canal and the region of the Hesselbach's triangle should always be performed when evaluating a scrotal mass.

The inferior epigastric artery at its origin is a critical anatomic landmark in differentiating indirect from direct inguinal hernias; a hernia originating lateral to the inferior epigastric artery is indirect, whereas one that is medial is direct.

Femoral hernias characteristically occur medially to the femoral vein and inferiorly in relation to the inguinal ligament.

Spigelian hernias occur at the lateral margin of the rectus abdominis superior to the inferior epigastric artery where it crosses the linea semilunaris.

With an understanding of inguinal region anatomy and knowledge of the variety of hernias found in the inguinal region, sonographic diagnosis can assist the surgeon in managing this common clinical condition.

This technique has sensitivity of 100% and specificity of 97.9%.

## Dynamic Ultrasound Versus a CT or MRI Scan for Diagnosing Hernias

A dynamic ultrasound may be ordered to diagnose a hernia or to characterize the contents of a hernia and determine its reducibility. The ultrasound examination is dynamic because it is performed in real time, showing motion live, and because it can be performed while the patient is lying on his/her back or standing upright. It can also be performed when the patient is breathing quietly or straining vigorously. Finally, ultrasound can be performed while the hernia is being compressed with the ultrasound transducer. Computed tomography (CT) and magnetic resonance (MR) scans, on the other hand, can only be done with the patient lying on his/her back and generally without straining. Because of the ability of ultrasound to show motion during dynamic maneuvers, ultrasound has several advantages over more expensive CT and MR scans in evaluating for groin and anterior abdominal wall hernias.

1. CT and MR can show only nonreducible hernias—those hernias that are "out all the time". Only a minority of hernias are nonreducible. Most hernias are reducible and will fall back into the abdomen when the patient is quietly lying on his/her back on a CT or MR table.
2. Ultrasound, like CT and MR, can show larger nonreducible hernias, but can also smaller show reducible hernias that CT and MR cannot show. Because ultrasound images show real time motion, we can see reducible hernias moving in and out during dynamic maneuvers.
3. During the ultrasound examination, any hernia that is found can be compressed with the ultrasound probe to determine if the hernia is reducible or tender. CT and MR, on the other hand, even when they show a hernia, cannot determine whether the hernia is tender. Tenderness is important, because hernias are so common, that we often find "incidental" small hernias that are not the cause of the patient's pain. If a hernia is tender when compressed by the ultrasound probe, it is far more likely that the hernia is, indeed, the cause of pain, and not merely a common incidental finding.
4. Ultrasound can identify hernias that are completely reducible when the patient is lying down, but become nonreducible and more tender when the patient is standing. CT and MRI cannot.

## Computed Tomography

In the modern era, computed tomography (CT) scans come to help surgeons diagnose hidden, difficult to diagnose hernias. Also occult hernias are well visualized with the help of CT scan modality.

*Aim:* Unlike other diagnostic modalities; the aim of computed tomography (CT) scanning for diagnosis of hernia is to identify the fascial defect rather than visualization of hernia contents. The assessment of defect in the fascia helps surgeon to ascertain the method of repair and plan surgery accordingly.

### Obturator Hernia (Fig. 7.15)

Obturator hernia, although rare, is a well-documented problem. In many elderly, emaciated, debilitated and ill women, symptoms and signs of small bowel obstruction without previous abdominal surgery history and pain along the ipsilateral thigh and knee (Howship-Romberg's sign) probably indicated an incarcerated obturator hernia. CT scan is useful in the early diagnosis. Prompt diagnosis and early surgery can reduce the mortality rate and produce good clinical result.

Plain radiographs often show nonspecific findings of small bowel obstruction and seldom helpful in diagnosing obturator hernia. Noticing gas shadow in the obturator foramen area may be helpful. Barium enema or small bowel series can be helpful if a bowel loop is in the obturator canal, but barium study is more time consuming in diagnosing case of acute abdomen and retained barium in bowel loop may increase the risk of subsequent operation.

Ultrasonography is useful and reliable in diagnosis of obturator hernia, but it is often limited by the relative inaccessibility of this deep region and operator-dependent. The use of CT scan in detecting obturator hernia was first reported by Meziane et al in 1983. The common CT scan finding is low density mass between obturator externus and pectineus muscle. The low density mass may contain air density in some cases and apparently different from

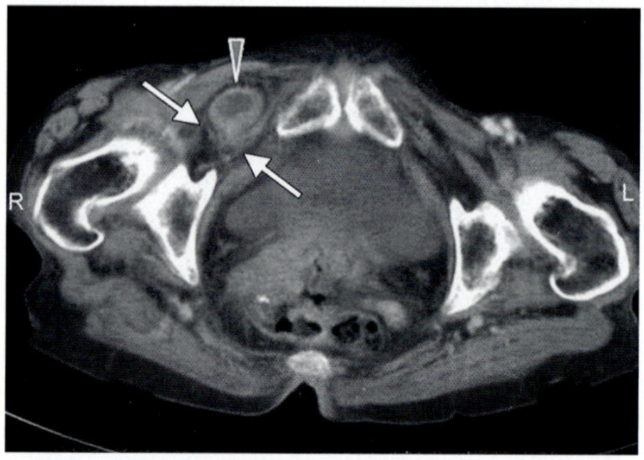


**Fig. 7.15:** Herniated bowel (arrow head) between superior and middle fasciculi of right obturator externus muscle (arrows). Mild wall thickening of herniated bowel with blurring of adjacent fat plane can be found

the opposite side. Associated bowel loop dilatation in the abdomen is common. Since the use of CT scan, pre-operative diagnosis rate was improved from 43 to 90%. CT scan can accurately diagnose not only obturator hernia but also other condition of bowel obstruction.

## Incisional Hernia

Computed tomography (CT) scanning in incisional helps to diagnose the fascial defect, mass of rectus muscles prior to repair.

It also renders information about contents of the sac of hernia, incarceration of bowel/omentum in sac.

- Scan showing transverse colon incarcerated in ventral abdominal wall hernia (incisional).
- Soft tissue stranding in subcutaneous fat around incarcerated hernia.
- Absence of enteric contrast past area of incarceration with collapse of left colon consistent with complete large bowel obstruction (Fig. 7.16).

## Barium Swallow for Hiatus Hernia (Fig. 7.17)

Barium swallow is considered essential in the preoperative assessment of gastroesophageal reflux disease and hiatal hernias.

## Endoscopy for Hiatus Hernia (Fig. 7.18)

- Hiatal hernia is diagnosed easily using upper gastrointestinal endoscopy.
- The diagnosis of a hiatal hernia actually is incidental, and endoscopy is used to diagnose complications such as erosive esophagitis, ulcers in the hiatal hernia, Barrett esophagus or tumor.

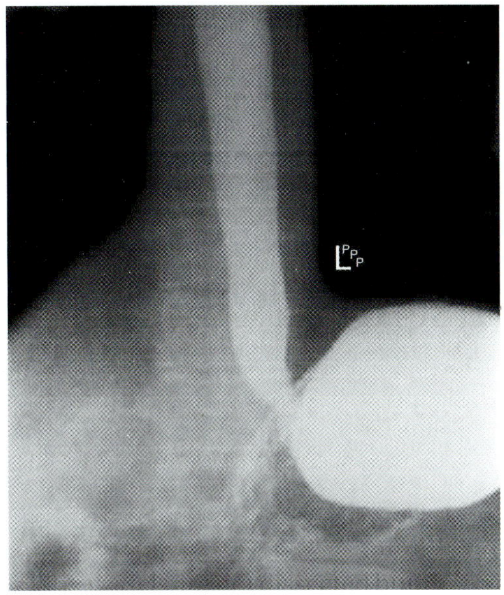

**Fig. 7.17:** X-ray contrast filled in hiatus hernia

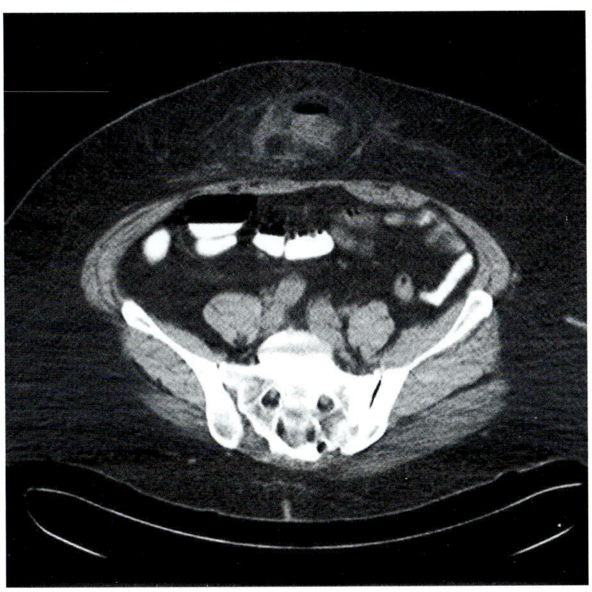

**Fig. 7.16:** Scan showing transverse colon incarcerated in ventral abdominal wall hernia (incisional)

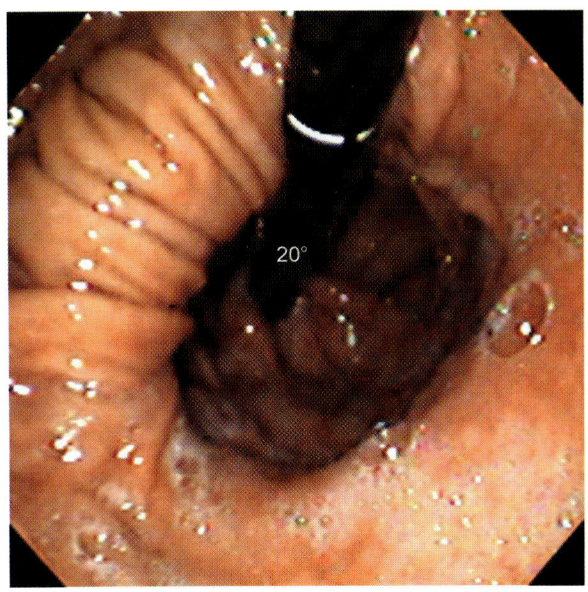


**Fig. 7.18:** Endoscopic view of hiatus hernia

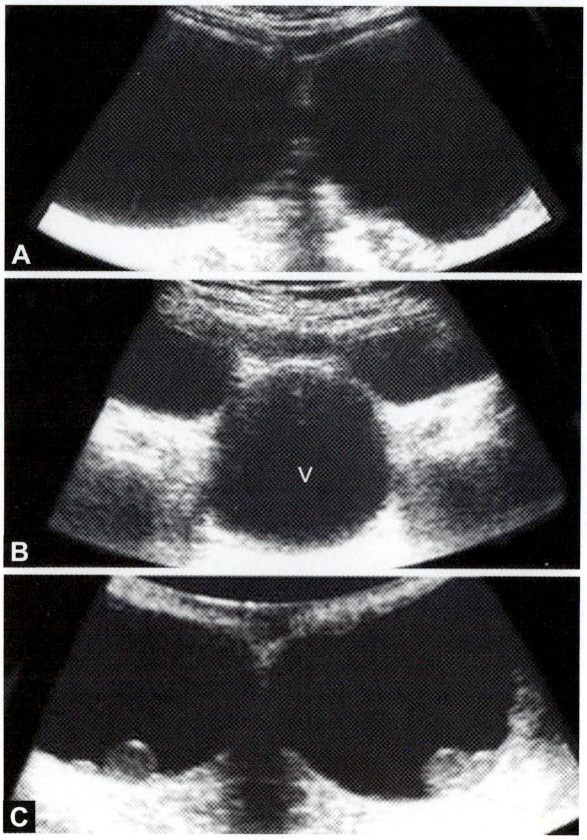


**Figs 7.19A to C:** Supravesical hernia

- A hiatal hernia is confirmed when the endoscope is about to enter the stomach or on retrograde view once inside the stomach. If any doubt remains, the patient may be asked to sniff through the nose, which causes the diaphragmatic crura to approximate, seen as a pinch, closing the lumen.
- Endoscopy also permits biopsy of any abnormal or suspicious area.

## Magnetic Resonance Imaging

In patients with clinically uncertain herniations, magnetic resonance imaging (MRI) is a valid diagnostic tool with a high positive predictive value.

### Indications

1. Clinically uncertain hernias
2. Supravesical hernia (Figs 7.19A to C)
3. Inguinal hernia
4. Osteitis changes in pubic bone after inguinal hernia surgery.
5. Abnormalities in myotendinous structures.

# Chapter 8

# Principles of Hernia Repair

## Current Guidelines in Hernia (Abdominal) Surgery

Following factors are considered mandatory in Principle of Hernia Repairs. These factors are very crucial in successful healing of hernia without any complication. The outcome of the surgery will be positive if these guidelines are followed.

### Hemostasis

Meticulous hemostasis is essential in any hernia surgery. It prevents the formation of hematoma and serum collection in dead space.

Perfect suturing and well approximation of tissues in hernia is priceless. It helps to prevent formation of hematoma. Chances of hematoma formation is more with inguinal hernia operated under local anesthesia.

Suction drains of closed type should be inserted in hernias like incisional, umbilical, epigastric, hiatus which prevents the formation of seroma and hematoma . These surgeries for hernia involve the excessive dissection, so it is wise policy to incorporate use of drains.

### Infection

A strict aseptic procedure should be followed for hernia surgery as the infection is detrimental for the healing of hernia. Infection reduces the healing of hernia and increases chances of recurrence. Infected status of post-operative hernia patient may lead to re-exploration and removal of mesh prosthesis.

While operating any hernia, one should apply adhesive film to abdomen to prevent translocation of micro-organisms.

### Wound Repair

#### *Phases of Wound Healing*

The entire wound healing process is a complex series of events that begins at the moment of injury and can continue for months to years. This overview will help in identifying the various stages of wound healing.

#### *Inflammatory Phase*

- Immediate to 2 to 5 days
- Hemostasis
  - Vasoconstriction
  - Platelet aggregation
  - Thromboplastin makes clot.
- Inflammation
  - Vasodilation
  - Phagocytosis.

#### *Proliferative Phase*

- Two days to three weeks
- Granulation
  - Fibroblasts lay bed of collagen
  - Fills defect and produces new capillaries.
- Contraction
  - Wound edges pull together to reduce defect
- Epithelialization
  - Crosses moist surface
  - Cell travel about 3 cm from point of origin in all directions.

#### *Remodeling Phase*

- Three weeks to two years
- New collagen forms which increases tensile strength to wounds
- Scar tissue is only 80% as strong as original tissue.

## Wound Healing in the Presence of Prosthetic Mesh

Stages in wound healing with mesh implantation:

- Coagulation
- Inflammation
- Angiogenesis
- Epithelialization
- Followed by fibroplasias
- Matrix deposition
- Scar contraction
- Maturation of mesh with scar contraction.

### Causes of Delayed Wound Healing

- Severe protein deficiency
- Vitamin C deficiency
- Prolonged hypovolemia
- Increased blood viscosity
- Intravascular coagulation
- Cold vasoconstriction
- Chronic stress
- Hypoxia
- Irradiation
- Collagen disorders.

### It is Better Practice to Avoid all these Above Listed Causes to Achieve Successful Hernia Repair

The remodeling process of hernia repair takes 6 to 12 months. First 70% repair and remodeling takes place in the first six months and the remaining process is completed in next six months. A total of 80% strength of aponeurosis is achieved at the end of one year from date of hernia surgery ; as long as there are no offending causes of delayed wound healing.

## Suturing Materials

A nonabsorbable, monofilament polypropylene, stainless steel suture is supposed to be the best for hernia repairs and tissue approximation till today.

Absorbable suture materials have risk of losing strength over the period of time and hazards into recurrence of hernia.

The suture material used for reconstruction of anatomy in hernia surgery should be as strong as the tissues to be sutured. The interval for loss of strength of suture material should be longer than the interval of loss of strength of tissue. By the time tissue loses strength and suture material also there should be enough time to strengthen the repair.

## Placement of Prosthetic Mesh

Suggested locations for placing mesh in hernia surgery:

1. Extra-aponeurotic/subcutaneous
2. Subaponeurotic and extraperitoneal
3. Subaponeurotic and intraperitoneal
4. For laparoscopic repair—subaponeurotic plane.

Chapter 9

# Anesthesia in Hernia Surgery

## Anesthesia for Hernia Repairs

There are many choices for anesthesia in hernia surgery today. Surgeon is in position to decide the type of anesthesia for hernia repairs. There are many types of anesthesias used today for different types of hernia. Every hernia in a patient is different so as the anesthesia.

### Anesthesia Used in Hernia Repairs

1. General
2. Spinal
3. Epidural
4. Local
5. Blocks.

Categorywise choice of method of anesthesia is done for safety of the patient, like an epigastric hernia would require a general anesthesia, incisional hernia will require a general anesthesia, strangulated inguinal hernia requires a general anesthesia. While umbilical, femoral, inguinal, spigelian hernias can be performed under local, spinal, epidural anesthesia.

### General, Spinal, Epidural, Local Anesthesia are Best Suited for Hernia Repairs

More and more specialized hernia centers worldwide are employing local anesthesia in hernia surgery which is easy and cost-effective. It reduces the hospitalization time. Here, we will see special local anesthesia technique for hernias amenable to local anesthesia like femoral, inguinal, umbilical, spigelian, etc.

The description about general, regional anesthesia is beyond scope of this book.

## Local Anesthesia for Hernias (Inguinal)

### Introduction

Many practitioners and institutions routinely and successfully employ local anesthesia for inguinal hernia repairs. Although there are certainly other options (including general anesthesia and regional anesthesia such as spinal or epidural), local offers some unique advantages to the patient. As such, here is a short summary about the use of local for these operations including a discusssion of advantages and disadvantages.

Obviously, the choice of anesthesia will be influenced by patient preferences and needs. In addition, to complete any operation successfully under local anesthesia requires a surgeon who is comfortable with the technique and willing to stop surgery and place additional local anesthesia should this become necessary. Interestingly with inguinal hernia repair, it is rarely, if ever, necessary to supplement with additional injections once the initial infiltration is complete. Reported experiences with it have been uniformly positive.

### Advantages of Local Anesthesia

Minimal physiological disturbance which may be an advantage in the patient in whom you wish to avoid a general anesthetic and in whom a regional technique may be contraindicated. This could include patient's with serious cardiac or respiratory diseases which could tolerate other types of anesthesia but would be at reduced risk if given only local anesthesia.

Postoperative pain relief is another benefit injection with a mixture of lidocaine and bupivacaine which gives quick anesthesia but long-lasting pain relief following the operation.

The primary advantage is quick recovery and ambulation allowing a quick discharge of ambulatory surgery patients to home.

## Disadvantages of Local Anesthesia

Surgery on the awake patient must be carried out gently and the surgeon must be willing to adapt both technique and pace to the needs of the patient. Incisional pain is usually blocked. However, some pressure sensation and traction on tissues, particularly the peritoneum, can be uncomfortable for the patient. The patient should be warned about these possibilities and be told that the operation may be slightly uncomfortable at times but should not be painful. Obviously careful patient selection, proper informed consent, and preoperative patient education are very important.

Some sedation during the operation may be required for anxious patients which loses some of the benefits of avoiding other anesthetic techniques in higher risk patients. Again utilize this technique on relatively healthy, ambulatory patients. In this population, the addition of small amounts of sedation, especially with the shorter acting agents available today, does not delay discharge. Patients, who are excessively nervous may not be suitable for surgery with this technique. Almost always, these patients can be identified during pre-operative interview, but always take consent of patients for regional and general techniques as backup anesthetic methods just in case.

## Local Anesthetic Agents

Several anesthetic agents may be used including lignocaine, bupivacaine. Lignocaine acts more quickly than bupivacaine but wears off more rapidly. Careful attention should be paid to the maximum doses of the local anesthetic agent that can be used. Plain lignocaine 0.5% or 1% lignocaine with adrenaline 1:200,000 or plain 0.25% bupivacaine are satisfactory.

## Technique

The patient should be weighed preoperatively and the maximum permissable volume of local anesthetic calculated. Resuscitation equipment must be available in case the patient develops a reaction to the local anesthetic and a cannula inserted into a vein.

Explain to the patient that since the operation will be carried out under a local anesthetic they will not feel pain but that some sensation of touch and perhaps pulling will remain. Reassure the patient that if they experience any discomfort it can easily be remedied by the surgeon injecting some more local anesthetic.

As the skin is being prepared for surgery explain to the patient what is happening as he may be aware of the sensation. If possible, place a surgical towel so that the patient cannot see the operation site.

The patient must be observed throughout the procedure by a trained attendant. The pulse should be monitored and the blood pressure checked regularly. Nervous patients may enjoy talking quietly to a nurse, who will be able to inform the surgeon if the patient is in any discomfort. The surgeon should avoid asking the patient if he can feel anything, but rather ask if he is comfortable.

Local infiltration can be performed on virtually any inguinal hernia, but it is usually reserved for patients of average weight with a primary unilateral hernia. Surgery for recurrent hernias, bilateral hernias, and hernias in obese patients are generally performed with either a subarachnoid or epidural block. The local anesthetic is usually a combination of a rapid-acting anesthetic, such as lidocaine, and a longer-acting agent, such as bupivacaine, which also provides several hours of postoperative pain relief.

Addition of sodium bicarbonate to buffer local instillation decreases the pain at the injection site and accelerates the onset of the anesthetic effect. Addition of epinephrine may provide some hemostasis and prolong the effects of local anesthetics. Many surgeons, however, prefer to observe bleeding points at the time of surgery, rather than risk a postoperative hematoma, when the effects of the epinephrine wear off.

## Anatomy

The nerve supply to inguinal and femoral herniae comes from the anterior branches of the six lower intercostal nerves which continue forward on to the anterior abdominal wall accompanied by the last thoracic (subcostal) nerve. The iliohypogastric and ilioinguinal nerves (T12 and L1) supply the lower abdomen. They are blocked by an injection of local anesthetic between internal and external oblique muscles just medial to the anterior superior iliac spine. The genitofemoral nerve (L1,2) supplies inguinal cord structures and the anterior scrotum via its genital branch and supplies the skin and subcutaneous tissues of the femoral triangle via the femoral branch.

The local anesthesia should:

1. Produce skin anesthesia in the line of the incision. This is best achieved by injecting local anesthetic subcutaneously in the line of the incision.
2. Block the nerve supply to the deeper tissues which are to be dissected and manipulated.
3. Produce anesthesia of the parietal peritoneum of the hernia and especially the neck of the sac which is very sensitive.

## Method—Step-by-Step (Figs 9.1 and 9.2)

1. Identify the anterior superior iliac spine and the pubic tubercle. From a point 2 cm above and medial to the anterior superior iliac spine inject 5 to 10 ml of local anesthetic under the external oblique aponeurosis in a fanwise fashion.
2. You may feel a 'click' as the needle pierces the aponeurosis. Now, inject under the aponeurosis from just lateral to the pubic tubercle, 5 ml towards the umbilicus and 5 ml laterally.
3. Wait a short-time and then infiltrate subcutaneously in the line of the incision. Allow time for the anesthetic to take effect before starting the operation. Keep some local anesthetic ready to inject into the sac when it is exposed, and to supplement any parts which are not adequately anesthetized.
4. Ensure anesthesia of the parietal peritoneum of the hernia and especially of the neck of the sac, which is very sensitive.

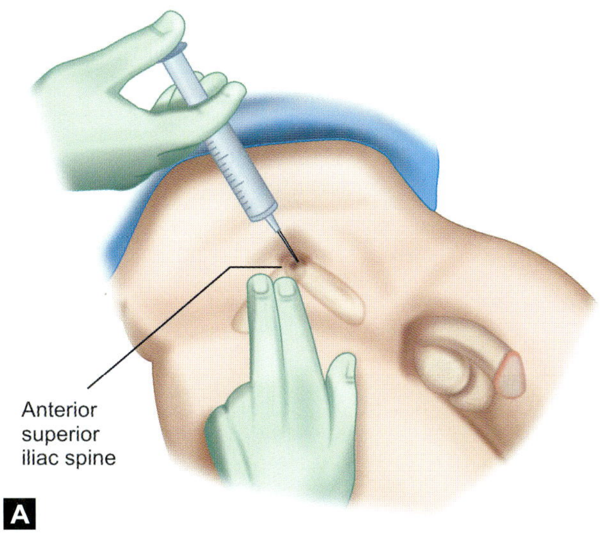


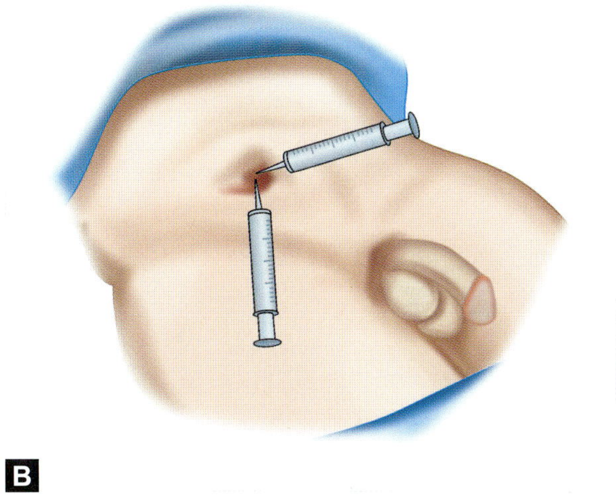


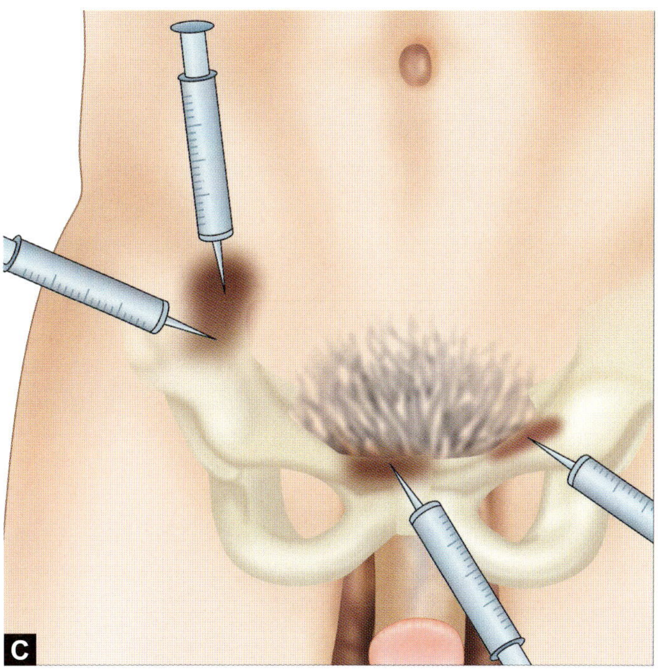


**Figs 9.1A to C:** Local anesthesia to inguinal area

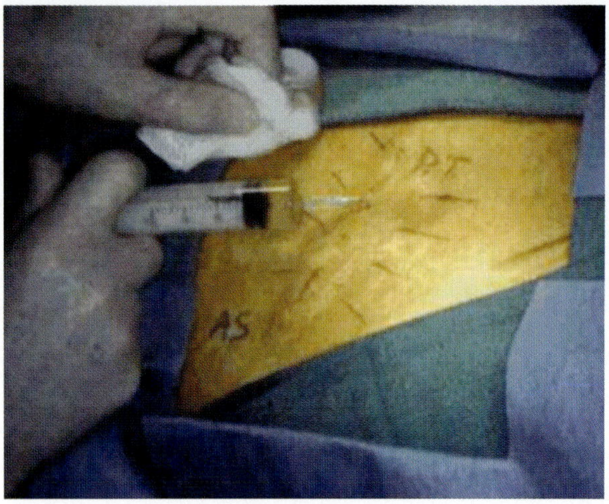

**Fig. 9.2:** Local infiltration anesthesia for inguinal incision in hernia repair

## Complications

These are much more likely to occur if local anesthetic is injected whilst the tip of the needle is in vein. Always, therefore keep the needle tip moving when infiltrating large volumes of local anesthetic.

If the block proves inadequate for surgery consider converting to a general anesthetic. Sometimes sedation with small doses of an intravenous opiate will help.

If traction is applied to the hernial sac without adequate anesthesia, the patient may feel faint and become bradycardic. This is best treated by interrupting the surgery, infiltrating more local anesthetic and giving some intravenous atropine if required.

If bupivacaine is being used, the block will take longer to develop compared with lignocaine. Some surgeons prefer to inject bupivacaine before putting on their gown and gloves and draping the patient. This gives extra time for the block to develop.

## Toxicity of Local Anesthetic Agents

Local anesthetic agents are relatively free from side effects if they are administered in an appropriate dosage and in the correct anatomical location. However, systemic and localized toxic reactions may occur, usually from the accidental intravascular or intrathecal injection, or the administration of an excessive dose of the local anesthetic agent. Systemic reactions to local anesthetics involve primarily the central nervous system (CNS) and the cardiovascular system.

The initial symptoms of CNS toxicity involve feelings of light-headedness, dizziness and circumoral paresthesia which may precede visual and/or auditory disturbances such as difficulty focusing and tinnitus (ringing in the ears). Other subjective CNS symptoms include disorientation and feelings of drowsiness.

Objective signs of CNS toxicity are usually excitatory in nature and include shivering, muscular twitching and tremors initially involving muscles of the face and distal parts of the extremities. Ultimately, generalized convulsions of a tonic-clonic nature occur. If a sufficiently large dose, or rapid intravenous injection of local anesthetic is given, the initial signs of excitation may progress very rapidly to generalized CNS depression and coma. Respiratory depression may result in respiratory arrest.

CNS toxicity is exacerbated by hypercarbia and acidosis.

Cardiovascular toxicity usually occurs at doses and blood concentrations which are higher than those required to produce CNS toxicity. Local anesthetics can exert a direct effect both on the heart and the peripheral blood vessels. Extremely high concentrations of local anesthetics depress spontaneous pacemaker activity in the sinus node resulting in sinus bradycardia and sinus arrest. They also exert a dose-dependent negative inotropic action on isolated cardiac tissue.

**Table 9.1**

**Volumes and doses of local anesthetic which should not be exceeded with different sized patients**

| *Drug* | *Small adult 50-60 kg* | *Medium adult 60-70 kg* | *Large adult 70-100 kg* |
|---|---|---|---|
| 0.5% lignocaine plain | 30 ml (150 mg) | 36 ml (180 mg) | 42 ml (210 mg) |
| 0.5% lignocaine + adrenaline | 70 ml (350 mg) | 84 ml (420 mg) | 98 ml (490 mg) |
| 1% lignocaine + adrenaline | 35 ml (350 mg) | 42 ml (420 mg) | 49 ml (490 mg) |
| 0.25% bupivacaine | 40 ml (100 mg) | 48 ml (120 mg) | 56 ml (140 mg) |

The more potent local anesthetics depress cardiac contractility at lower concentrations than the less potent drugs.

Local anesthetic agents appear to exert a biphasic effect on peripheral vascular smooth muscle (Table 9.1). In lower doses they may increase peripheral vascular resistance, and in higher doses, reduce it. Cocaine is the only anesthetic that causes vasoconstriction consistently because of its ability to inhibit the reuptake of noradrenaline by storage granules at the synapse. The excess concentration of free circulating noradrenaline is responsible for the vasoconstriction associated with the use of cocaine. In general, a direct relationship exists between the anesthetic potency and cardiovascular depressant potential of the various agents. The more potent drugs, e.g. bupivacaine and etidocaine, have been reported to cause rapid and profound cardiovascular depression in some patients following accidental intravascular injection.

**The Clinical Advantage**

The clinical advantages of local anesthesia include the decreased blood ooze when local anesthetic solution with adrenaline is employed, the prolonged analgesia provided without any central effects, enhanced definition of tissue planes afforded by the hydrodynamic dissection by local anesthetic distending the tissues, and lastly the patient cooperation possible in testing and identifying anatomic defects, particularly in inguinal hernioplasty. The patient is saved the anxiety of general anesthesia and the hangover effect of recovery.

Severe cardiac arrhythmias such as resistant ventricular fibrillation may occur.

Local anesthesia has considerable advantages over regional or general anesthesia in the repair of groin hernia.

# Chapter 10

# Open Anterior Repair of Inguinal Hernia in Adult

## Techniques of Open Anterior Inguinal Hernia Repair

### Techniques of Hernia Repair

- Anterior rrhaphies or plasty
- Posterior rrhaphies or plasty.

#### *Anterior Rrhaphies*

1. Lytle's and Marcy repair
2. Bassini repair
3. Shouldice repair
4. McVay/Lotheissen repair
5. Iliopubic tract repair.

#### *Anterior Plasties*

1. Lichtenstein's repair (Prosthetic mesh repair)
2. Mesh plug repair (Rutkow and Robbins).

#### *Posterior Rrhaphies*

Nyhus posterior preperitoneal approach.

#### *Posterior Plasty*

Stoppas giant prosthetic reinforcement of the visceral sac (GPRVS).

#### *Laparoscopic Hernia Repair*

1. Transabdominal preperitoneal repair (TAPP)
2. Total extraperitoneal repair (TEP)
3. Intraperitoneal onlay mesh
4. Double buttress laparoscopic herniorrhaphy.

## Details of Procedure

### Lytle and Marcy Repair

When the internal ring is weak and stretched and TF is bulging the repair should include Lytle's method of repairing and narrowing ring by the lateral displacement of cord. The internal ring should be narrowed to admit the tip of the little finger.

*Marcy repair*: Narrowing of the internal ring by plication of TF

*Lytle's repair*: Narrowing of the internal ring by placation of conjoint tendon.

### Bassini Repair (Fig. 10.2)

The greatest contribution to hernia surgery was that of Italian Surgeon Edorado Bassini. He is considered to be the father of modern herniorrhaphy. He performed his first operation in 1884. Next 100 years most inguinal hernia are repaired by his technique or variation of it.

#### *The Incision*

The skin incision is placed 1 cm above and parallel to the inguinal ligament. It should extend from the pubic tubercle medially to about 1 cm lateral to the deep ring (Fig. 10.1).

The procedure consist of strengthening posterior wall of inguinal canal by stitching the lower border of the conjoint muscle and tendon to the inguinal ligament.

Bassini stressed the importance of dividing the fascia transversalis and reconstructing the posterior wall of the canal by suturing the fascia transversalis and transverses muscle to the upturned, deep edge of inguinal ligament.

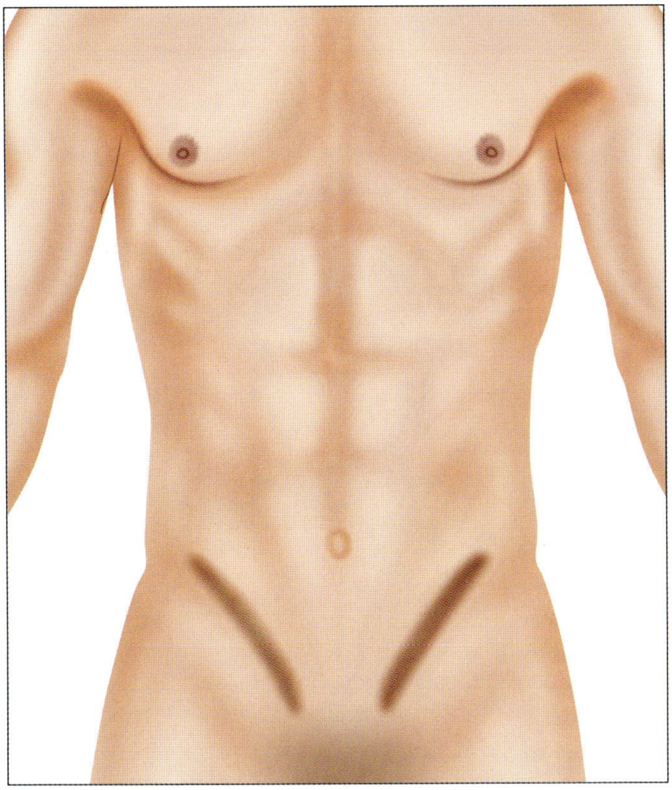

**Fig. 10.1:** Lines of incision for Bassini's repair of inguinal hernia

In this repair, Bassini included the lower arching fibers of the internal oblique muscle where they form the conjoint tendon with the transverses muscle.

Bassini's operation epitomized the essential steps for an ideal tissue repair. He opened the external oblique aponeurosis through the external ring, then resected the cremasteric fascia to expose the spermatic cord. He then divided the canal's posterior wall to expose the preperitoneal space and did a high dissection and ligation of the peritoneal sac in the iliac fossa. Bassini then reconstructed the canal's posterior wall in 3 layers. He approximated the medial tissues, including the internal oblique muscle, transversus abdominus muscle and transversalis fascia to the shelving edge of the inguinal ligament with interrupted sutures (Fig. 10.3). He then placed the cord against that newly constructed wall and closed the external oblique aponeurosis over it, thereby restoring the step-down effect of the canal and reforming the external inguinal ring.

*Modified Bassini:* Bassini's original repair yielded outstanding results for a pure tissue technique, but, as noted above, problems occurred when surgeons failed to open the posterior wall. This operation became known as the "modified" or "North American" Bassini. By not opening the posterior wall, the wall tissue was damaged in its most medial portion by sutures placed under

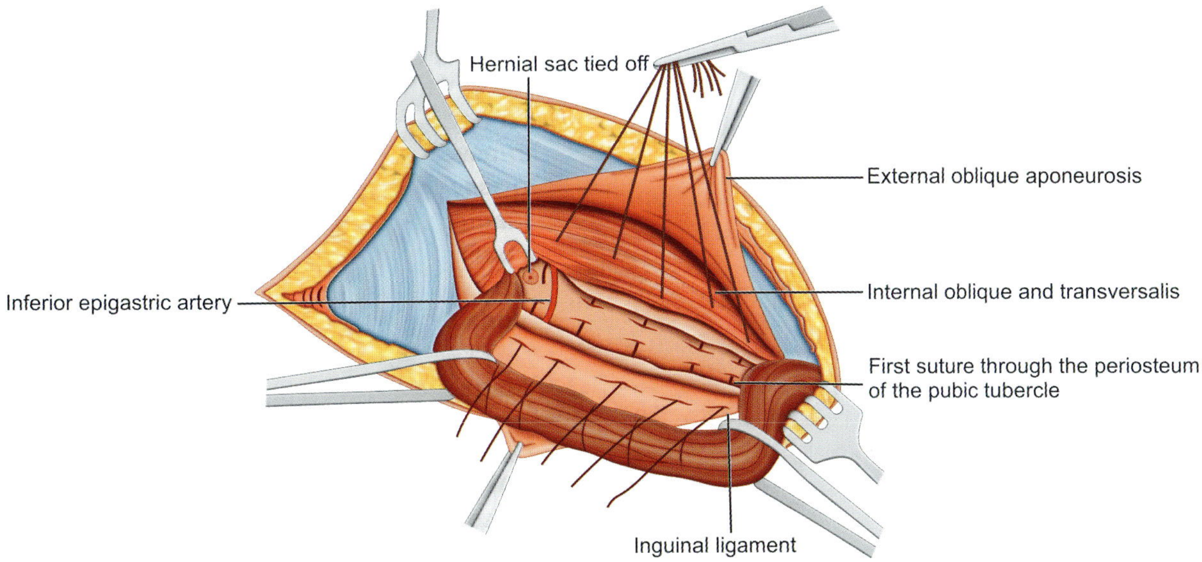


**Fig. 10.2:** Bassini repair

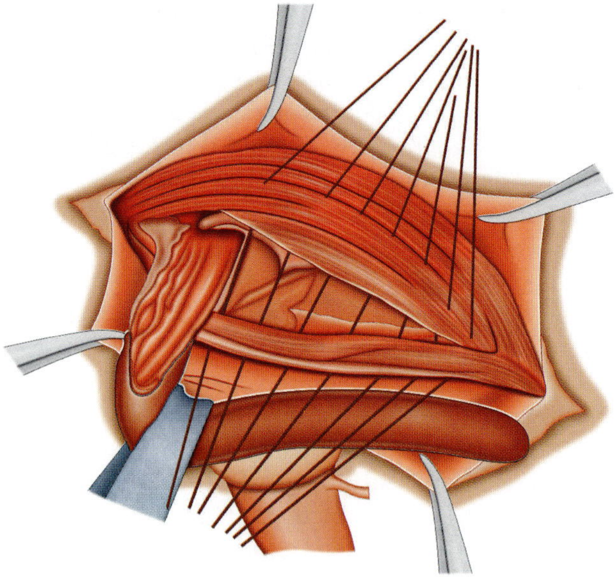

**Fig. 10.3:** Original Bassini operation. The canal's posterior wall is opened and the deep epigastric vessels are exposed

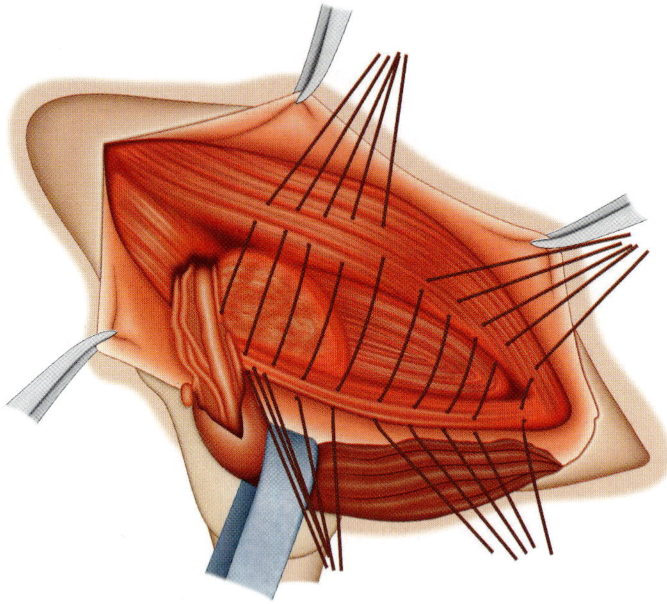

**Fig. 10.4:** Modified Bassini. The posterior wall is not opened. Sutures placed between the transversus arch and the inguinal ligament create tension on the tissues approximated

tension, and recurrences resulted, primarily in the pubic tubercle area. Thus, the failure of this operation in its first year was more likely due to an overlooked second hernia or to poor surgical technique, rather than a metabolic or tissue defect that might predispose to recurrent hernia (Fig. 10.4).

There have been numerous modifications of Bassini's original technique, although many of the less detailed renditions have yielded poor results. Those that avoided opening the posterior wall, e.g. resulted in suture-line tension between tissues at the most medial part of the inguinal canal just cephalad to the pubic bone. Some help was afforded the Bassini technique and other tissue repairs by the introduction of relaxing incisions by surgeons such as Wolfer, Halsted, Tanner, and McVay.

## Shouldice Repair

It is basically a Bassini repair. It is a pure tissue repair. The essential steps in this method of repair are:

1. Double breasting the TF (Two layers)
2. Approximation of conjoint tendon to inguinal ligament in two layers.

The operation depends on removal of cremasteric muscle from that portion of spermatic cord which lies with in the inguinal canal. This is the optimum method of repair (Fig. 10.6).

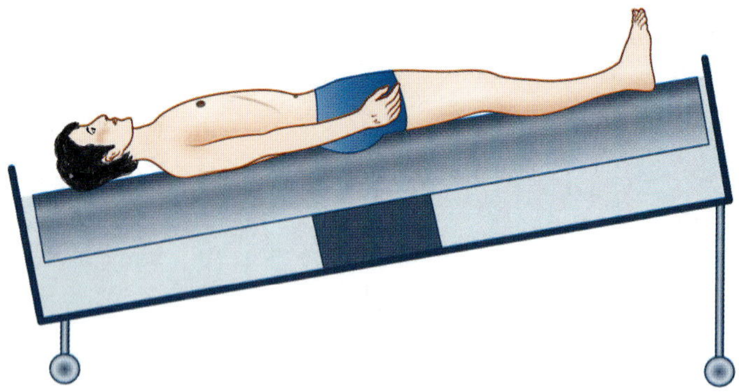

**Fig. 10.5:** Trendelenburg position

The Shouldice technique for the treatment of inguinal hernia.

# Inguinal Dissection

A comprehensive intraoperative examination of the inguinal region is performed in all cases. This is integral to attaining a very low recurrence rate. The frequency of secondary hernias found at the time of surgery is 15.4%. The assessment should include the direct, indirect, interstitial and femoral spaces.

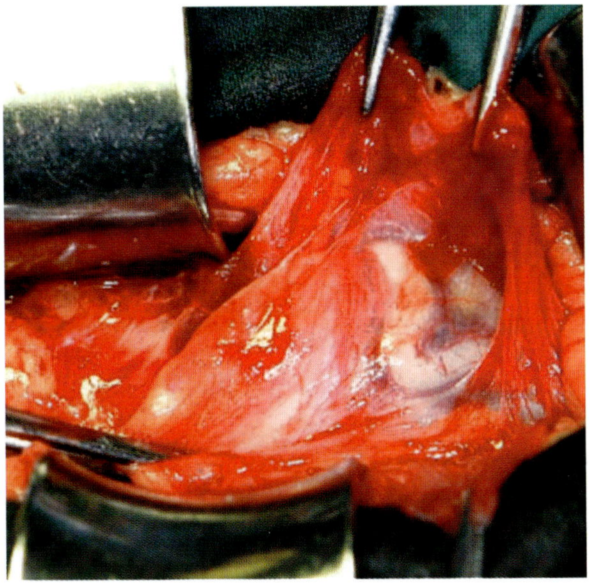

**Fig. 10.6:** Right inguinal hernia repair: dissection of cremasteric muscle. Mobilization of the spermatic cord through the cremasteric muscle and creation of medial and lateral flaps for transection

The incision is made from 2 cm inferiomedial to the ASIS to the pubic tubercle, parallel to the inguinal ligament. This allows generous exposure to both inguinal canal and femoral space. Trendelenburg's position (Fig. 10.5) may be used to reduce intra-abdominal pressure, facilitating the repair.

Dissection is deepened to expose the external oblique fascia and superficial inguinal ring. Local anesthesia is required at this point prior to opening the canal. Care is required to identify and avoid injury to the ilioinguinal and iliohypogastric nerves. Their course usually runs deep to the external oblique, superior to the deep ring and superficial to the cord structures. Infiltration of the internal oblique muscle superior to the canal can provide anesthesia for the internal oblique and peritoneum used later in the reconstruction. If the nerves are traumatized at any point, do not hesitate to resect the damaged segments to avoid neuropathy postoperatively. The resultant numbness after nerve resection is not usually of any clinical significance.

The spermatic cord is isolated by a longitudinal anterior opening in the cremasteric muscle fibers at the midpoint of the canal extended medially to the pubic tubercle, creating two flaps of muscle medial and lateral to the cord.

This maneuver allows a complete examination of the posterior floor, in particular the medial aspect. The larger lateral cremasteric flap, which includes the genital branch, is infiltrated with local anesthetic, as is the internal ring. If a lipoma is present, this is dissected from the cord towards the internal ring and excised. This facilitates identification of the indirect sac in its typical anteromedial position. An indirect sac should be isolated from the cord and internal ring and excised. The stump should retract naturally into the peritoneal cavity. Some surgeons choose only to reduce the sac to avoid peritoneal irritation and discomfort. Care should be taken if the sac is thicker, contains more fat than usual or is broad based, as this may be an indication of a sliding hernia. These are reduced and not opened. If a sac is not identified, the dissection of the cord at the internal ring must identify a peritoneal protrusion, which can be aided by gentle traction on the cord. The identification of this structure, which is in its normal anatomic position, assures the surgeon that the indirect hernia has not been missed. After complete dissection of the cord, both flaps of the cremasteric muscle are divided sharply and ligated. These stumps are used to support the repair at a later point in the procedure.

The posterior wall of the inguinal canal is examined for a direct hernia then opened beginning at the internal ring in parallel to the internal oblique muscle fibers. Care should be taken not to injure the inferior epigastric vessels found medial to the internal ring. The lateral flap should be wide enough, at least 1 cm, to reach the edge of the rectus sheath in the first layer of the repair. Any redundant transversalis fascia of a direct hernia should be excised. Preperitoneal examination of the internal oblique muscle and fascia cephalad to the internal ring and the inguinal canal, should confirm the presence of an interstitial hernia. If present, the internal ring can be incised laterally to include an interstitial defect. The internal ring would then be displaced laterally after reconstruction. Dissection below the inguinal ligament should identify Cooper's ligament and thus confirm the presence or absence of a femoral hernia (Figs 10.7A and B).

The superficial thigh fascia or cribiformis fascia candal to the inguinal ligament should be incised to examine the femoral space from Figure 10.7. In addition, this mobilizes the inguinal ligament and external oblique for use in the reconstruction.

## Reconstruction

A continuous repair with 32 to 34 gauge stainless steel wire is used for the reconstruction. This may be

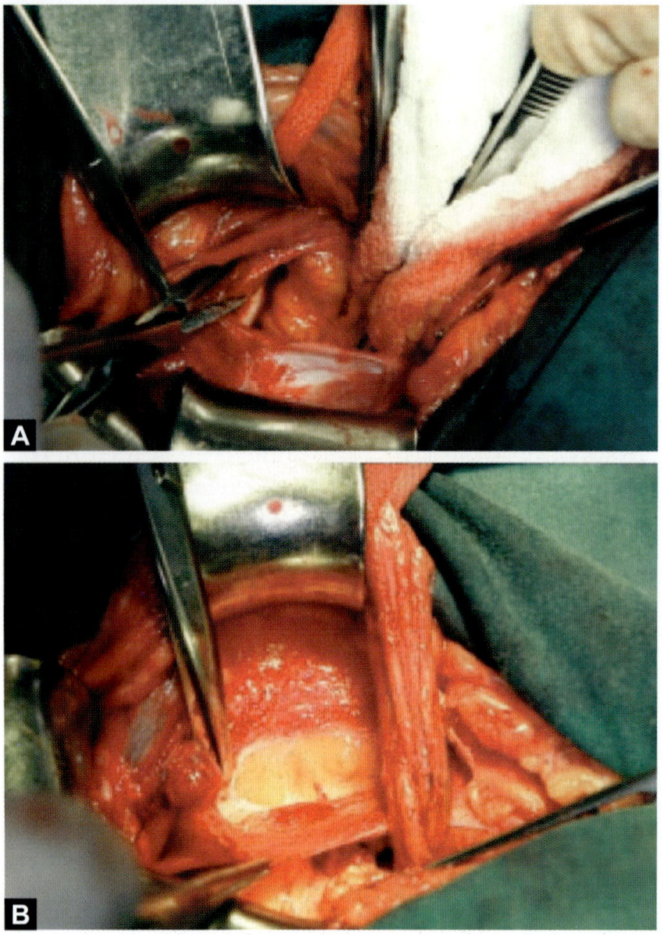


**Figs 10.7A and B:** Dissection of femoral space. (A) Cooper's ligament seen through the preperitoneal space, deep to the tips of the clamp; and (B) Incision of the cribiformis ligament below the inguinal ligament

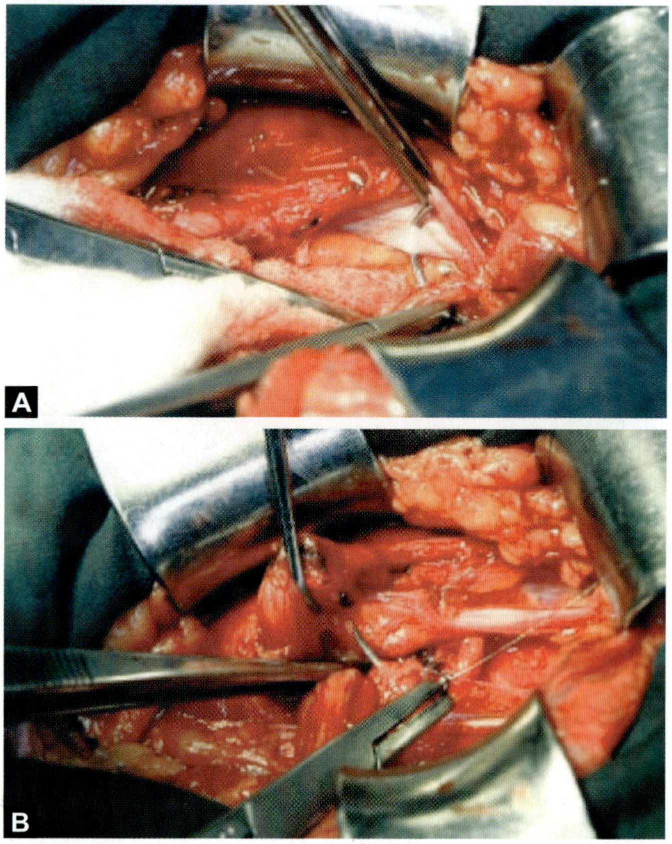


**Figs 10.8A and B:** Reconstruction: the first layer. (A) Starting at the pubic tubercle, the lateral flap of transversalis fascia is taken to the edge of rectus sheath underneath the medial flap; and (B) The layer is completed with the reconstruction of internal ring. The lateral stump of cremasteric muscle is taken with the bite of transversalis to buttress its medial edge of the new internal ring, prior to emerging with a full thickness bite of internal oblique

substituted with a 3-0 polypropylene suture. It is a four-layer tissue reconstruction using two separate sutures. A continuous technique distributes the strength of the repair evenly and should be without tension. A relaxing incision is rarely required.

The first two layers represent an overlapped reconstruction. It begins medially, anchoring over the pubic tubercle, leaving a sufficient end to tie the returning suture after the second layer. The inferolateral flap of transversalis fascia is sutured to the lateral edge of the rectus sheath by reaching underneath the superior-medial flap.

The reconstruction then moves laterally to the aponeurosis of the transversus abdominis and the edge of the internal oblique muscle. The lateral extent of this layer redefines the internal ring and should include the superior stump of the divided lateral flap of cremasteric muscle (Figs 10.8A and B). This buttresses the internal ring and helps prevent an indirect recurrence. The suturing is then reversed to begin the second layer. The superior flap of transversalis fascia is sutured to the shelving portion of the inguinal ligament then tied at the pubic tubercle. The periosteum should not be included in any bite as this can result in a painful osteitis.

The next stage of reconstruction creates a two-layered imbrication to provide reinforcement. The layer is begun superior and slightly lateral to deep ring, anchoring the suture to the internal oblique fascia. The inferior flap of

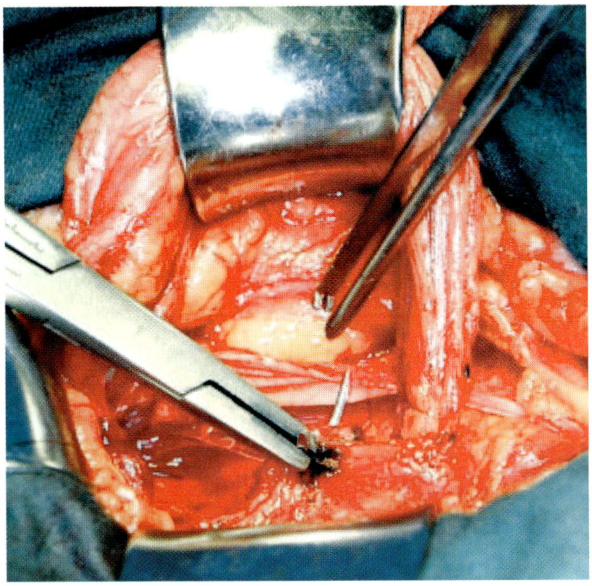

**Fig. 10.9:** Reconstruction: the second layer using the same suture, it is continued from the internal ring back, taking the medial flap of transversalis fascia to the shelving portion of the inguinal ligament. Overlapping layers are created

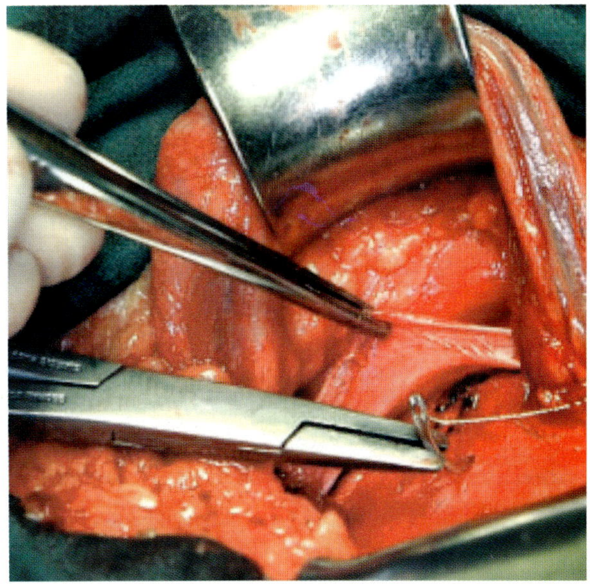

**Fig. 10.10:** Reconstruction: the third layer. Starting at the medial side of the internal ring, the external and internal oblique are used to imbricate the first two layers. Small bites of external oblique are taken just above the inguinal ligament

the external oblique, millimeters above and parallel to the inguinal ligament, is tacked to the edge of the internal oblique and transversus muscles (Figs 10.9 to 10.11).

In addition, only a small bite of the internal oblique is required, no more than 5 mm. Excessively large bites will create tension. At the pubic tubercle, the direction is reversed for the fourth layer and taken back to the internal ring and affixed.

The importance of mobilizing the inferior flap of external oblique by previously incising the superficial thigh fascia is realized here. The additional mobility allows the external oblique to be used in the third and fourth layers to cover the medial portion of the repair that is susceptible to recurrence. The inguinal canal is reconstructed by re-approximating the remaining external oblique fascia, returning the cord to its anatomical position. The inferior stump of the medial flap of cremasteric muscle is included in the first suture medially to stabilize the position of the testes to the abdominal wall and prevent drooping.

## Postoperative Course

In the postoperative care, oral narcotic analgesia is usually required during the first 48 hours. Ambulation is encouraged the evening after the operation and light exercises commence the first postoperative day. Upon discharge, heavy lifting can be resumed at 4 weeks.

Lichtenstein technique first described about 18 years ago. It is every simple effective and associated with very low recurrence rate (ranging from 0 to 2%).

The concept is based on two important facts:

1. Inguinal hernias are caused by a metabolic disorder, which leads to a progressive destruction of the fibroconnective tissue of the groin, making the tissue unsuitable for being used in hernia repair.
2. The fact that traditional tissue repairs are associated with undue tension at the suture line, which leads to more postoperative pain, longer recovery time, and higher rate of recurrence.

A tension-free repair is performed under local anesthesia and consists of reinforcement of the inguinal floor using polypropylene mesh. The prosthesis is approximately 8 × 16 cm to provide sufficient tissue-mesh interface beyond the floor of the inguinal canal. As a result, the entire inguinal floor is completely and permanently protected from all future mechanical and degenerative adverse effects. Therefore, the procedure is both therapeutic and prophylactic.

Skin, subcutaneous tissues are incised as usual up to the external oblique; the anterior wall of the inguinal canal. Inguinal canal is opened by splitting the external

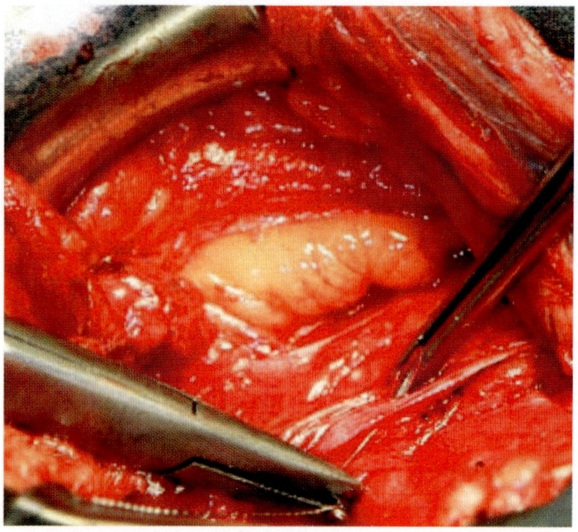

**Fig. 10.11:** Reconstruction: the fourth layer. The second layer of imbrication using the external and internal oblique. The benefit of incising the cribiformis fascia and the mobilization of the lateral flap of external oblique is realized as a small flap of external oblique remains after the four layers. This small flap is used to reconstruct the inguinal canal and restore the natural anatomic position of the cord structures

oblique along the direction of its fiber, the spermatic cord with its cremasteric covering is elevated with a Penrose drain. Care must be taken to include the external spermatic vessels when elevating and dissecting the spermatic cord from the floor of the inguinal femoral canal. This assures that the genital branch of the genito nerve, which is always in close contact with the external spermatic vessels is preserved.

Next cremasteric fiber are transversely incised at the level of the deep inguinal ring to thin out the cord. Indirect hernia sacs are dissected free up to the neck marked by collar of extraperitoneal fat and than opened for digital examination of the femoral ring. The sac was transfixed at the neck using 1/0 vicryl and excised. A prolene mesh 7.6 × 15 cm size used is trimmed to accommodate the varying sizes of the inguinal floor. The medial end of the mesh is rounded to the shape of medial corner of the inguinal canal. With cord retracted upward a running suture of 3/0 proline used to fix the mesh. The rounded corner is sutured first to the aponeurotic tissue over the pubic bone by 1.5 to 2 cm (this is a crucial step in the repair, since failure to overlap this bone may result in recurrence). The periosteum of 8 the bone is avoided. Then, the suture continue to attach the lower edge of the mesh to the shelving margin of the inguinal ligament to a point just lateral to the internal ring.

A slit is made in the lateral end of the mesh creating two tails, the wider on (2/3) above, the narrow one (1/3) below. The upper wide tail is grasped with a hemostat and passed underneath the spermatic cord. This maneuver positions the cord between the two tails. The wider upper tail is then placed over the narrower one and held in a hemostat with the cord retracted downward, the upper edge of the mesh is sutured to the internal oblique aponeurosis or muscle using a few intercepted 3/0 prolene suture. During the placement of these sutures the external oblique aponeurosis is retracted upward when the retraction is released, the mesh buckles slightly. This is desirable and 'looseness' assures tension free repair and will flatten out when the patient strains or resumes an upright position. The lower edges of the two tails are fixed to the shelving margin of the inguinal ligament. This creates a new internal ring made up of mesh. The tails are trimmed leaving approximately 3 to 4 cm of mesh beyond the internal ring. After meticulous hemostasis a closed suction drain is placed beneath the external oblique aponeurosis specially in large inguinal hernias, when an extensive dissection was performed during the plastic reconstruction. The aponeurosis of the external oblique is then closed using absorbable suture (Vicryl 1/0) skin closed by subcuticular proline (3/0).

## The Repair Technique (Other Way Around)

A 5 to 6 cm transverse incision is made within a Langer's line, beginning from the pubic tubercle. The external oblique aponeurosis is opened. As it is shown in Figure 10.12, the spermatic cord with its cremasteric covering, external spermatic vessels, and the genital nerve are freed from the inguinal floor and lifted with a Penrose drain. An easily visible landmark for the genital nerve is the external spermatic vein. Usually, referred to this as "the blue line." If the blue line is kept with the spermatic cord, the surgeon can be sure that the genital branch of the genitofemoral nerve, which is always adjacent to this vein, is completely protected. The spermatic cord is also dissected free from the pubic bone area for approximately 2 cm medial to the pubic tubercle in order to make room for extending the mesh beyond the pubic tubercle. This dissection is easy because the space between the cremasteric sheath and the pubic bone area is avascular. This is a critical part of any mesh repair because if the pubic tubercle area is not overlapped, the stage is set for

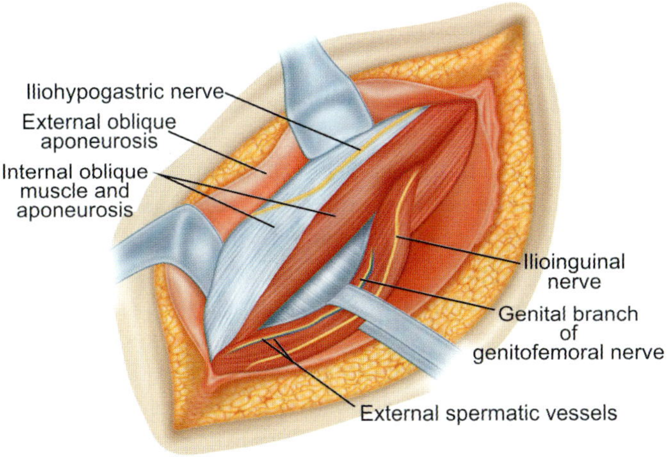


**Fig. 10.12:** The external oblique aponeurosis is opened. The spermatic cord with its cremasteric covering,external spermatic vessels, and the genital nerve are freed from the inguinal floor and lifted with a Penrose drain

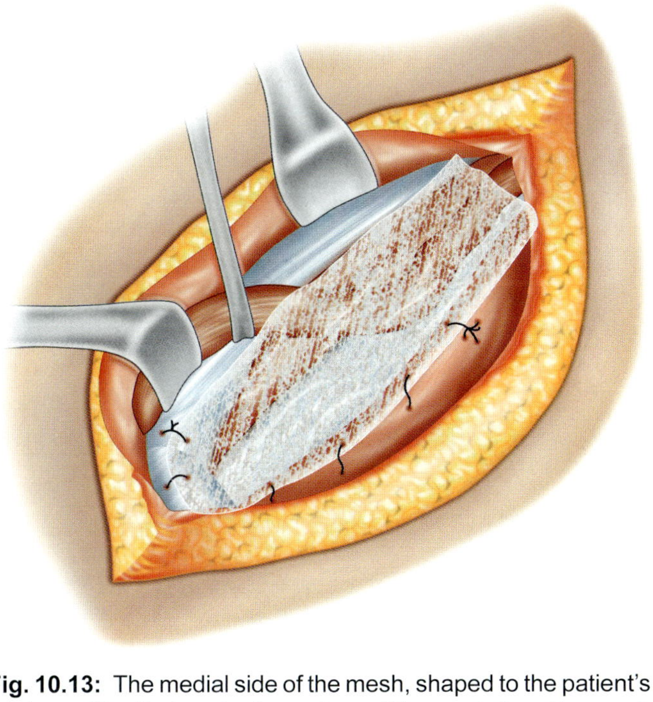

**Fig. 10.13:** The medial side of the mesh, shaped to the patient's anatomy. The first anchoring suture of the mesh fixes the mesh to the anterior rectus sheath where it inserts into the pubic bone

one of the most common causes of recurrence after any mesh repair, open or laparoscopic.

Next, the external oblique aponeurosis is dissected from the underlying internal oblique muscle and aponeurosis high enough to make room for a prosthesis that is 6 to 7 cm in height. The iliohypogastric nerve comes into the view during this part of the dissection. Identification of this nerve protects it from incorporation during suturing of the mesh.

For indirect inguinal hernias, the cremasteric sheath is incised longitudinally for approximately 3 cm. Removal of the cremasteric muscle is unnecessary. Approximately, 15% of the time, the ilioinguinal nerve is within the cremasteric muscle and, therefore, removal of the muscle can injure the nerve as well as injuring the pampiniform plexus.

The sac is then dissected from the cord beyond its neck and inverted into the properitoneal space without ligation or excision. If the sac is very large, as in a scrotal hernia, the sac is divided at the midpoint of the inguinal canal. The proximal end is closed, dissected away from the cord structures, and inverted into the preperitoneal space. The distal end is left behind in order to reduce the possibility of testicular complication. Of course, if the hernia is a sliding type, this cannot be achieved.

No special preparation is needed for direct inguinal hernias if it is not too large. When the direct hernia bulge is large, it is inverted utilizing a purse-string or a continuous suture on the transversalis fascia without incorporating the iliopubic tract or the inguinal ligament. This is only to make the floor of the inguinal canal flat in order to facilitate placement of the mesh. It adds no strength to the repair.

The medial side of the mesh, as seen in Figure 10.13, is shaped to the patient's anatomy. The first anchoring suture of the mesh fixes the mesh to the anterior rectus sheath where it inserts into the pubic bone. This suture is placed approximately 2 cm medial to the pubic tubercle in order to be sure that area is covered by the mesh. While doing this, care must be taken not to pass the needle through the periosteum of the bone or through the pubic tubercle because this is one of the most common causes of chronic postoperative pain. The lower edge of the mesh is sutured to the inguinal ligament using the same suture in a continuous fashion with not more than 4 passages. This suture ends at the lateral border of the internal ring.

At this point, a slit is made on the lateral end of the mesh, as seen in Figure 10.14, creating 2 tails—2/3 above and 1/3 below. The upper tail is then passed under the cord and pulled toward the head of the patient, placing the spermatic cord in between the 2 tails.

The upper tail is then crossed over the lower one and held with a pair of hemostat as seen in Figure 10.15. The tails are later sutured together and tucked under the

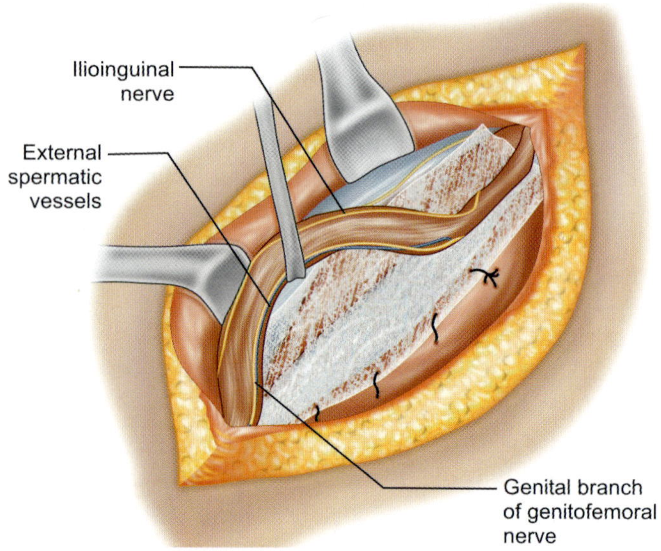


**Fig. 10.14:** At this point, a slit is made on the lateral end of the mesh, creating 2 tails—2/3 above and 1/3 below. The upper tail is then passed under the cord and pulled toward the head of the patient, placing the spermatic cord in between the 2 tails

external oblique aponeurosis, leaving 5 to 6 cm of mesh lateral to the internal ring. Leaving this much of mesh lateral to the internal ring is very important because if the tails are too short, there is a possibility of recurrence in that area. Also, failure to cross the 2 tails of the mesh is another source of internal ring recurrence. And, in fact, this is the subject of a recent article from Spain, showing that if the edges of the tails are simply sutured together without having overlap or without being crossed, then an indirect recurrent hernia can occur at internal ring.

While the upper edge of the mesh is fixed in place, care is taken to keep the mesh slightly relaxed. This laxity produces a dome-like ripple in the mesh to compensate for increased intra-abdominal pressure when the patient stands up from his or her recumbent position during the operation. It is particularly important to have this convexity to compensate for the inevitable future shrinkage of the mesh, which, according to our study reported 6 or 7 years ago during one of the American College of Surgeon meetings, is approximately 20%. If the mesh is kept completely flat, it becomes subject to tension when the patient stands up. We can see this pulling effect on the mesh and the tissue, when the mesh is kept flat in

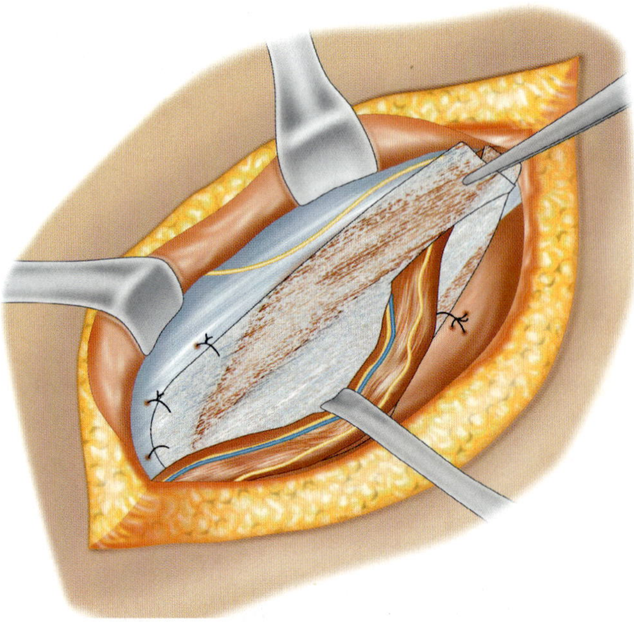

**Fig. 10.15**

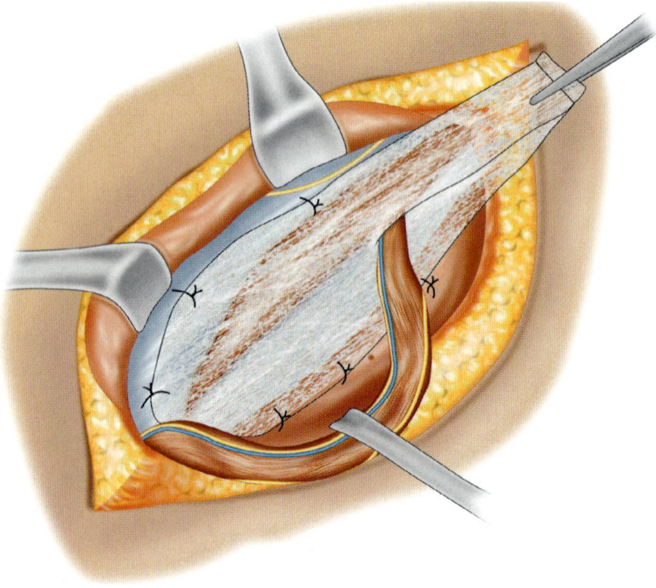

**Fig. 10.16**

**Figs 10.15 and 10.16:** Pulling effect on the mesh and the tissue, when the mesh is kept flat in Figure 10.16. The mesh becomes subject to even more tension after shrinkage of the mesh is completed. Failure to keep the mesh slightly convex is the second most common cause of recurrence after mesh repair

Figure 10.16. The mesh becomes subject to even more tension after shrinkage of the mesh is completed. Failure to keep the mesh slightly convex is the second most common cause of recurrence after mesh repair.

## Advantages and Disadvantages

The Lichtenstein operation, including the administration of local anesthesia, takes between 20 and 40 minutes, depending on the complexity of the hernia. Patients are discharged after 1 or 2 hours postoperatively, and no restriction of activity is imposed on them. Postoperative pain is minimal, and, in fact, according to a meta-analysis of all reported randomized studies, is equally comparable with the postoperative pain after laparoscopic repair. Based on more than 150 articles in the surgical literature, the recurrence rate is consistently less than 1%, ranging between 0% and 0.7%.

The complications of the procedure are not life threatening and include less than a 2% rate of infection, hematoma, or seroma. Using mesh does not increase the risk of infection, provided that the mesh is monofilament and microporous. If the wound gets infected for other reasons, such a mesh does not have to be removed. The most significant complications after Lichtenstein repair are testicular atrophy and chronic neuralgia with a reported rate of less than 1%. To summarize, the operation is simple, can be performed under local anesthesia, is easy to learn, and is economical.

### Currently Used Other Tension-Free Techniques

At recent times the special mesh instrument called as prolene hernia system (PHS) or ultrapro hernia system (UHS) are used increasingly. These instruments provide a strong support to the inguinal tissues and prevents the recurrence (Fig. 10.16).

The prolene hernia system (PHS, Fig. 10.16) is an innovative method of treating hernias. The mesh is made up of three elements. There is an underlay mesh, which slips behind the muscle, an onlay mesh which lays on top of the muscle, and a cylinder which connects the two layers. The cylinder fits through the hernia defect, and it is held in place primarily by its shape. Stitches may be used to hold it in position, but usually only a few are necessary and they do not have as much tension on them as stitches in the older types of repair. This means less pain in the postoperative period.

The PHS bilayer patch device has a combined onlay graft (like a Lichtenstein repair) and underlay graft (like a Stoppa or Kugel patch); these are held together by a connector (like a plug) (Figs 10.18 and 10.19).

### Equipment

- Standard operating room anesthesia equipment, outfitted for possible conversion to general anesthesia and endotracheal intubation, is required.
- A standard open surgical tray, including self-retaining retractors, a Penrose drain, and different size meshes, should be available on standby.
- *Mesh*: The mesh must be a permanent material large enough to produce a wide overlap beyond the defects edges. A polypropylene or polyester mesh (5 × 10–7 × 15 cm) is generally used. Recently, manufacturers have shifted toward lighter, more porous constructions that maintain the strength of the repair but putatively reduce the inflammatory response. Different mesh configurations may be chosen, primarily based on surgeon preference and training. None have been shown to be better at preventing recurrence (Fig. 10.17).
- The question of absorbable versus permanent sutures to secure the mesh is based on surgeon preference; to date, no evidence supports one over the other. A theoretical advantage of absorbable suture is that, if nerve impingement is inadvertently caused, the suture material disappears with time. The authors

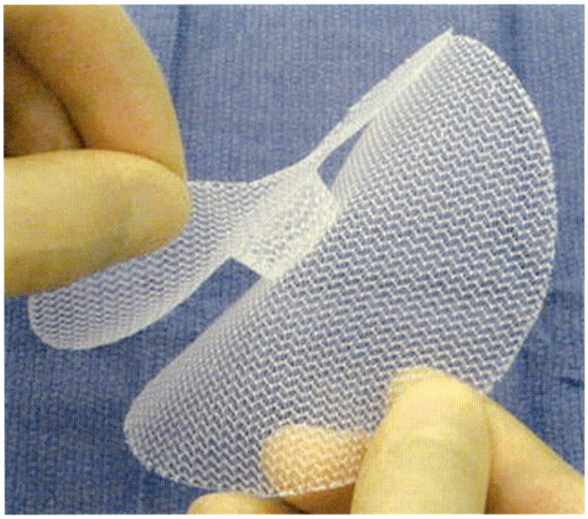

**Fig. 10.17:** Polypropylene hernia system–I

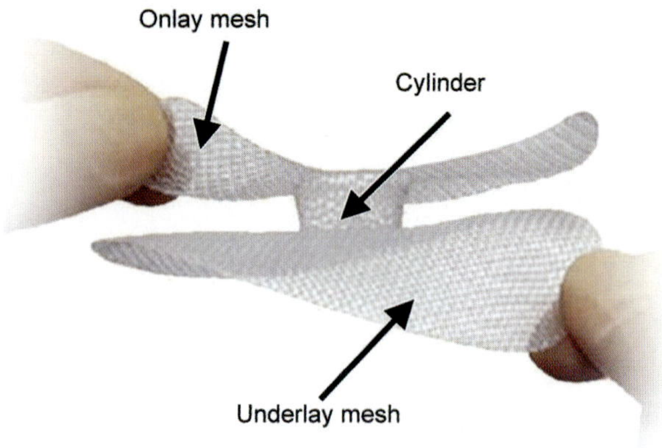


**Fig. 10.18:** Polypropylene hernia system–II

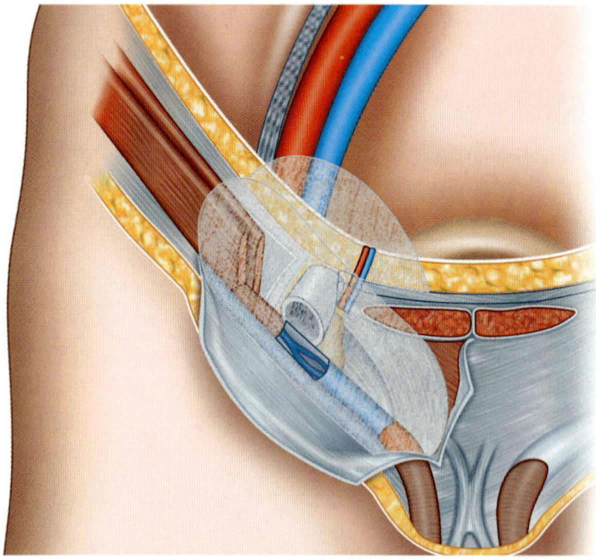

**Fig. 10.19:** The PHS repair gains its strength from the patients tissues healing into the patch

prefer to use absorbable (2-0 polyglactin) suture for mesh fixation.

## Positioning

- Confirm and mark the correct surgical site preoperatively in the holding area.
- Position the patient supine, comfortably securing the upper extremities.
- For large defects, slight Trendelenburg positioning may help exposure by reducing the visceral contents into the abdomen.
- Shave the surgical site with electric clippers.
- Prepare and drape the surgical site in standard surgical fashion, exposing only the intended operative groin site.

## Technique

After final verification of the correct side of surgery and the infiltration of local anesthesia, make an oblique skin incision (or along the Langer lines) approximately 2 finger breadths (2 cm) superior to and parallel to the thigh crease (Fig. 10.20), and extend it 5 cm toward the anterior superior iliac spine, starting from just lateral to the pubic tubercle. In thin patients, the external ring can actually be palpated just lateral and slightly above the pubic tubercle and should be the medial starting point of incision.

- Continue the dissection deeper through the subcutaneous tissue until the aponeurosis of the external oblique is identified. During dissection, take note of the superficial vessels that can be ligated and divided when encountered.
- Identify the external oblique aponeurosis. The following three landmarks must also be identified before incising the external oblique:
  1. Firstly, the Scarpa fascia can mimic the external oblique, as it is well developed and thickened in some patients. Avoiding this mistake, especially in patients who are overweight, can be accomplished if the fibers of the external oblique aponeurosis (Fig. 10.21) are always visualized, since the Scarpa fascia does not have these fibers.
  2. Secondly, the inguinal canal should be entered at its apex. To correctly identify the apex of the canal, identify the lower wall of the canal, which is where the external oblique aponeurosis disappears into the fat of the thigh. Approximately one finger breadth above this point is a good entry site into the canal.
  3. Thirdly, the external ring must be identified. This is important because the external ring is ultimately the end point of the division to be made in the external oblique aponeurosis and defines the orientation of this cut.

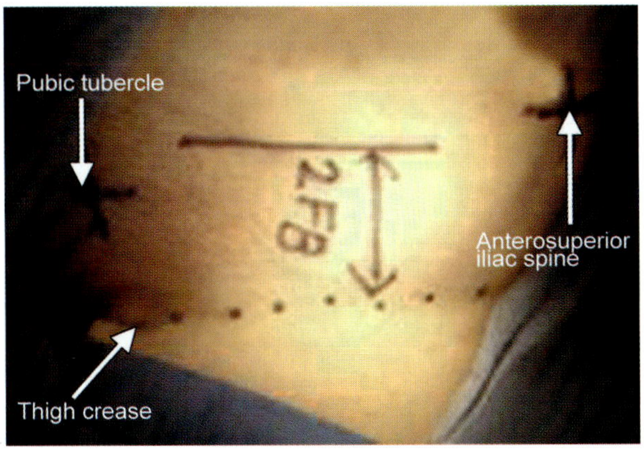


**Fig. 10.20:** Skin incision

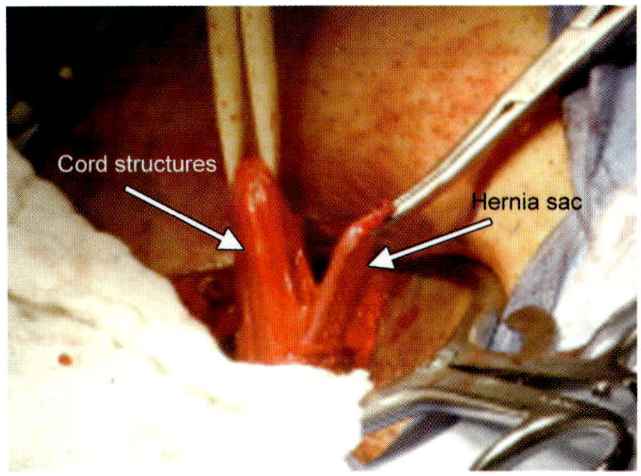


**Fig. 10.23:** Hernia sac separated from the cord structures

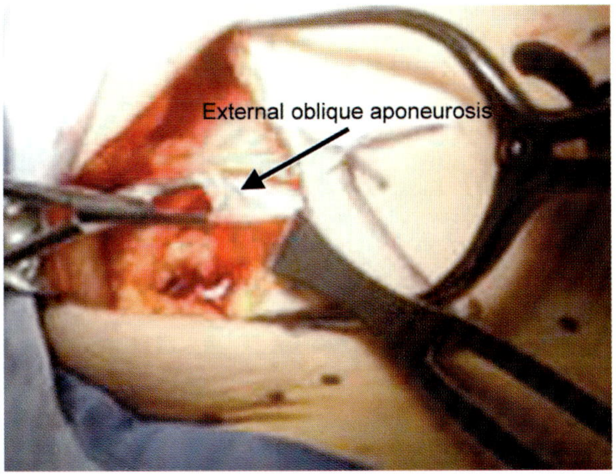


**Fig. 10.21:** Division of the external oblique aponeurosis

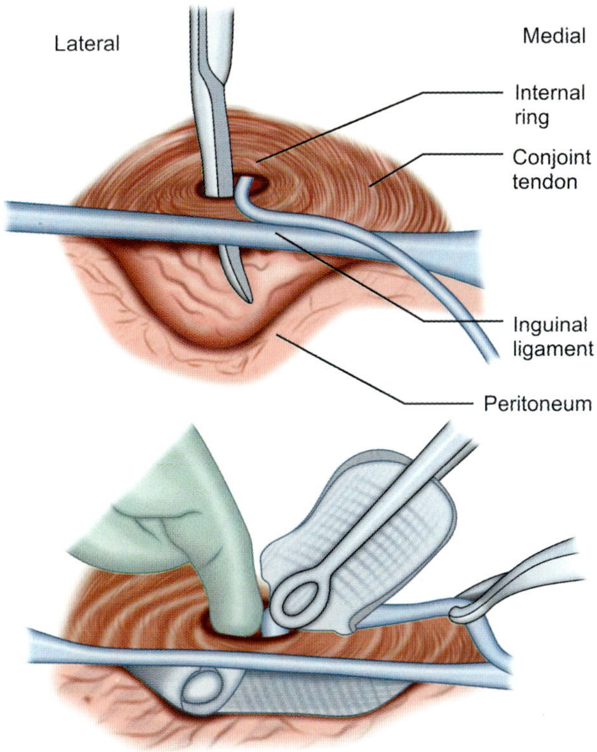


**Fig. 10.24:** Development of the preperitoneal space

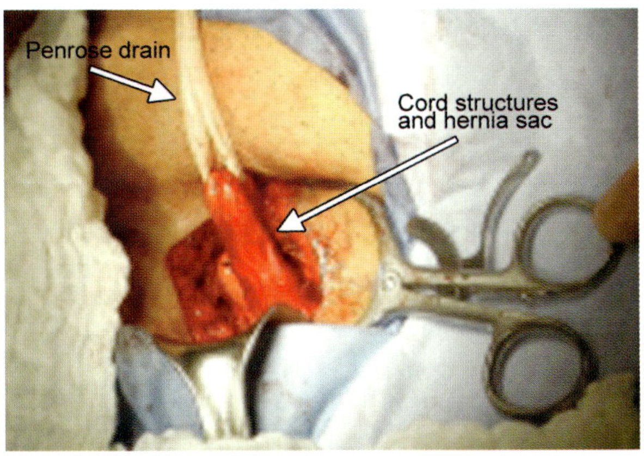


**Fig. 10.22:** Cord structures and hernia sac encircled by a Penrose drain

- Once the external oblique aponeurosis is identified, thoroughly expose it and make a gentle stab incision in its mid-portion along the orientation of its fibers. Extend this incision superiorly, and medially downward, through the superficial ring, thus exposing the inguinal canal and the cord structures.

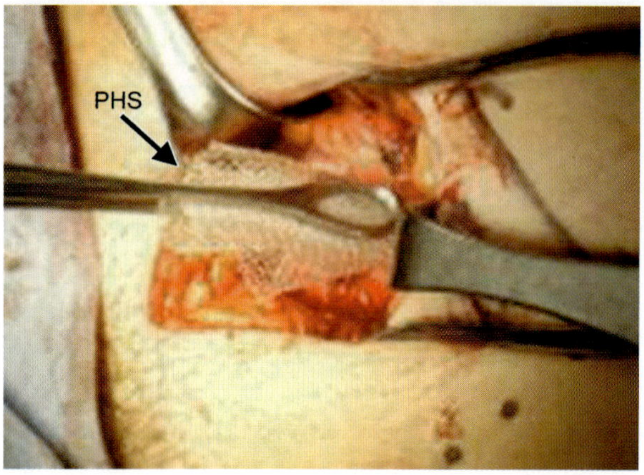


**Fig. 10.25:** Deployment of the prolene hernia system (PHS)

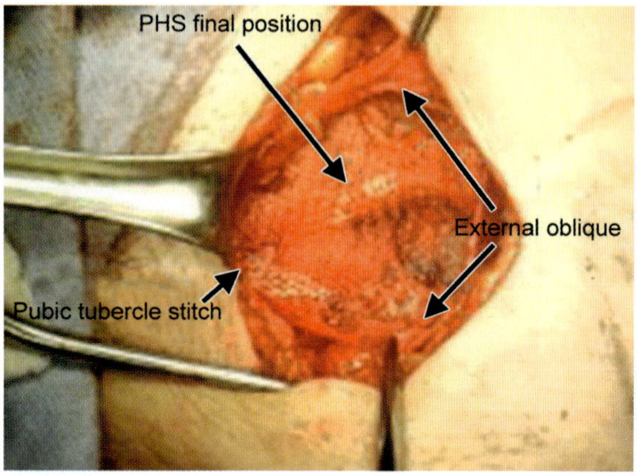


**Fig. 10.26:** Final position of the prolene hernia system mesh

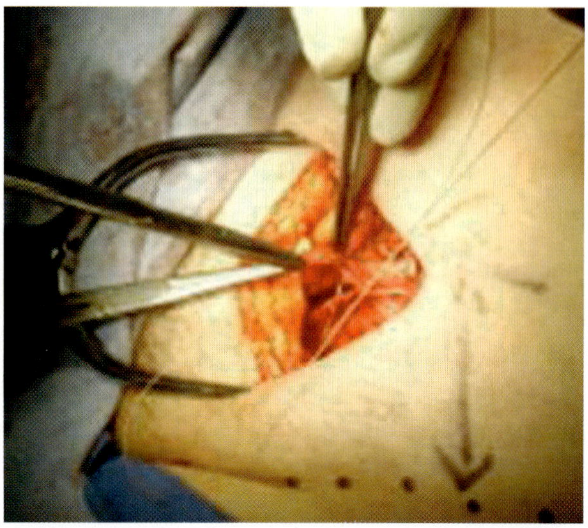

**Fig. 10.27:** Closure of the external oblique aponeurosis

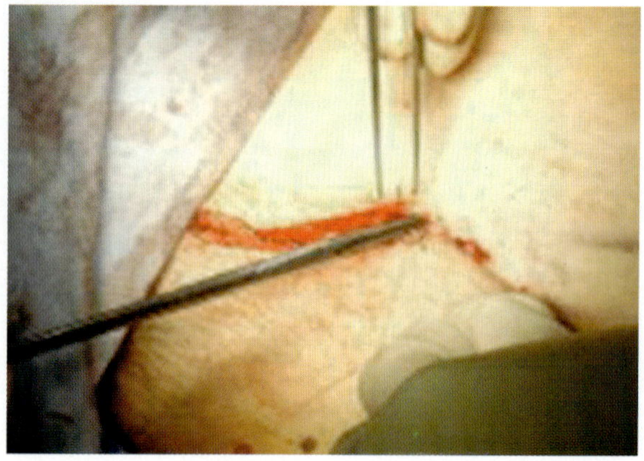

**Fig. 10.28:** Skin closure

- Circumferentially mobilize the cord structures off the floor of the canal by working on the pubic tubercle as a fulcrum. With blunt dissection of the index finger in a sweeping and medially encircling fashion, the cord is sufficiently freed, so that the cord structures can be surrounded by a Penrose drain for convenient retraction. This allows exposure of the inguinal floor and protects the cord structures (Fig. 10.22).
- Next, examine the anteromedial aspect of the cord for an indirect component of the hernia. Separating the cremasteric muscle along its fibers often facilitates this. The cremasteric muscle fibers must be dissected carefully with slow electrocautery coagulation, as the cut muscle fibers tend to bleed (Fig. 10.23).
- If an indirect hernia is present, dissect the sac off the cord structures, down toward its base at the internal inguinal ring (Fig. 10.24), until it is comfortably invaginated into the preperitoneal space. This is preferably achieved without division of the sac. However, if necessary, as with certain large hernias, the sac can be entered carefully and examined for visceral contents, and then divided with a high ligation (i.e. proximal)
- Direct hernias, which protrude through the inguinal floor at the Hesselbach triangle, are similarly dissected away from the cord structures toward their base and then inverted below the transversalis fascia.
- Closure of the defect and buttressing of the inguinal canal floor can now be performed. This can be done using a prosthesis.
  - *Prolene hernia system (PHS) (Fig. 10.25)*: This system consists of an anterior oval polypropylene mesh connected to a circular posterior component.

a. The posterior component is deployed in a bluntly created preperitoneal space.
b. The anterior portion is then laid out with a cut made to recreate the internal ring.
c. The anterior portion is then sutured above to the conjoined tendon and below to the shelving edge of the inguinal ligament and is tucked behind the external oblique (Fig. 10.26).

- Reapproximate the external oblique aponeurosis with a running 3-0 polyglactin suture; be mindful of the underlying ilioinguinal nerve (Fig. 10.27).
- Follow this with reapproximation of the Scarpa fascia with interrupted 3-0 polyglactin suture and then a running subcuticular closure of the skin with 3-0 poliglecaprone suture (Fig. 10.28).
- Clean the operative site and apply sterile dressing.

**Important Tips**

- Injury to the ilioinguinal, iliohypogastric, or genital nerves is a common cause of chronic postherniorrhaphy pain (defined as pain persisting more than 3 months postherniorrhaphy, after the process of wound healing is complete). This can be minimized by the identification and careful dissection of the nerves.
- The ilioinguinal nerve, which runs anterior to the spermatic cord, can be protected by its gentle dissection and by isolating it behind a leaf of the incised external oblique aponeurosis with use of a straight hemostat clamp.
- When dissecting the hernia sac, awareness of the posteriorly located vas deferens must always be at the forefront of the surgeon's mind, to protect the vas deferens from injury. In adults, the rate of vas deferens injury is estimated at 0.3%.
- Another cause of significant postherniorrhaphy pain is the placement of a stitch into the periosteum. This is often the point of maximal postoperative tenderness and, therefore, mandates mindful maneuvering when anchoring the pubic tubercle bite.
- Vascular injury is a less common but reported and potentially disastrous pitfall. This can be avoided by respecting the proximity of the femoral vessels, particularly when suturing the mesh to the inguinal ligament. Hematoma formation can be due to injury of the inferior epigastric vessels or failure to ligate the superficial subcutaneous veins.
- In male patients, always remember to gently pull the testes back down to their normal scrotal position after the procedure is completed.

# Chapter 11

# Laparoscopic Inguinal Hernia Repairs

## Introduction

The surgical history of inguinal hernias dates back to ancient Egypt. From Bassini's heralding of the modern era to today's mesh-based open and laparoscopic repairs, this history parallels closely the evolution in anatomical understanding and development of the techniques of general surgery.

Today, the minimally invasive technique of laparoscopic surgery can be used to repair the most common types of hernias. Although both traditional and laparoscopic hernia surgery are performed on an outpatient basis, patients treated laparoscopically seem to experience more rapid healing and far less pain during recovery. They can return to normal activity, including work, after only a few days, while recovery from traditional hernia repair can be a three- to five week process.

The laparoscopic repair of inguinofemoral hernias has had a tumultuous beginning in the surgical arena. Laparoscopic repairs have had to compete with the current gold standard for anterior or conventional inguinal hernia repairs. Initially, some of these laparoscopic repairs, such as the "plug and patch" (PAP) and "on lay technique" (IPOM), failed to demonstrate good results and were abandoned. Only two laparoscopic repairs have proven to be viable with early results comparable or superior to the Liechtenstein repair. These repairs are the extraperitoneal laparoscopic repair (TEP) and the trans-abdominal preperitoneal repair (TAPP). Some authors are now claiming newer and simpler open laparoscopic inguinal hernia repairs such as "Plug" or "Klug" repair are effectively competing with the laparoscopic inguinal hernia repairs without the increased cost.

Currently, the two most popular laparoscopic techniques are the TAPP and the TEP. The most ardent critique of the TAPP procedure is that it is an intra-abdominal procedure with significant potential morbidity. On the other hand, the TEP procedure avoids intra-abdominal access. In our studies, the morbidity rate of both these laparoscopic repairs was minimal and/or similar to other open repairs with comparable early recurrence rates. The most persuasive argument for using this procedure is the same argument favoring all laparoscopic procedures: the postoperative benefits to the patients, i.e., less postoperative pain, decreased disability and small incisions. However, it continues to be a procedure with limited long-term follow-up and analysis. We strongly believe surgeons performing laparoscopic inguinal hernia repair should be familiar with the TEP and TAPP Repair.

Accounting for 75% of all abdominal wall hernias, and with a lifetime risk of 27% in men and 3% in women, inguinal hernia repair is one of the most commonly performed surgeries in the world. Most randomized studies comparing laparoscopy to open repair have confirmed the following findings:

- Pros
  - Reduced postoperative pain
  - Earlier return to work
- Cons
  - Increased cost
  - Lengthier operation
  - Steeper learning curve
  - Higher recurrence and complication rates early in a surgeon's experience.

Although open, mesh-based, tension-free repair remains the criterion standard, laparoscopic herniorrhaphy, in the hands of adequately trained surgeons, produces excellent results comparable to those of open repair.

## Definitions

Laparoscopic inguinal herniorrhaphy can refer to any of the following three techniques:

- Totally extraperitoneal (TEP) repair
- *Transabdominal preperitoneal (TAPP) repair:* The abdomen is accessed and pneumoperitoneum is achieved using standard laparoscopic techniques. The preperitoneal space is then exposed transabdominally by sharply incising and bluntly stripping the peritoneum that overlies the inguinal anatomy. A mesh is then deployed and fixed in place as with the TEP technique and the peritoneum returned to its anatomical position.
- *Intraperitoneal onlay mesh (IPOM) repair:* A dual-layer mesh is placed over the myopectineal orifice transabdominally and fixed in place. The preperitoneal space is not entered and minimal dissection is carried out.
- The most commonly performed laparoscopic techniques are the TEP and TAPP repairs.

### Anatomy-Understanding

Poor familiarity with the complex anatomy of the posterior inguinal view is an important contributor to the steepness of the laparoscopic inguinal herniorrhaphy learning curve (Fig. 11.1).

The preperitoneal space is contained between the transversalis fascia and the parietal peritoneum. It contains areolar and adipose tissue and the inferior epigastric artery and vein.

Transabdominal laparoscopic landmarks useful when performing the TAPP repair are the obliterated fetal remnants, which divide the posterior surface of the anterior abdominal wall into three fossae.

- The median umbilical ligament is a remnant of the embryonic urachus. It forms the center divide by arising in the midline from the apex of the bladder toward the umbilicus.
- Laterally, the paired medial umbilical ligaments, vestiges of the fetal umbilical arteries, arise from the superior vesicle arteries toward the umbilicus.
- Between the median and medial ligaments lie the supravesical fossae, where external supravesical hernias occur.

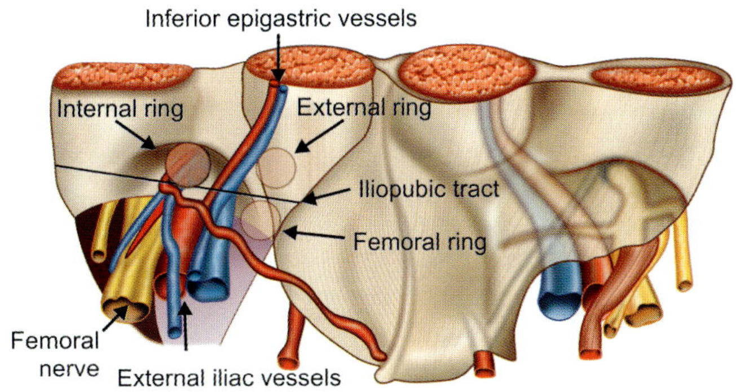


**Fig. 11.1:** Inguinal anatomy from the laparoscopic viewpoint

- Most lateral are the paired lateral umbilical ligaments, which contain the inferior epigastric arteries. Between them and the medial ligaments lies the medial fossa, which contains the Hesselbach triangle, the zone of direct hernias. Lateral to the inferior epigastric arteries is the lateral fossa, which is the site of indirect hernias. Thus, the lateral umbilical ligaments separate the lateral and medial fossae, and delineate between indirect and direct hernias, respectively.

The following three landmarks found in the preperitoneal space are constant in their presence and location. They are a good starting point to get one's bearings in this difficult region. They are also helpful in cases of large hernias or recurrences.

- *The inferior epigastric artery and vein complex:* This complex lies on the rectus muscles bilaterally.
  - Medial to these vessels but above the iliopubic tract is the external ring, which is not visible in patients without a direct hernia.
  - The internal ring is lateral to the inferior epigastric artery and vein but is often obscured by them, even when a hernia is present. The location of the internal ring can be approximated by locating the junction of these vessels and the cord structures.
  - The femoral ring is inferior and lateral to the external ring and lies below the iliopubic tract just medial to the external iliac vessels (The external iliac vessels change their name to the common femoral vessels after they pass beyond the inguinal ligament. Since preperitoneal hernia repair is performed dorsal to the inguinal ligament, these vessels still retain their intra-abdominal name)

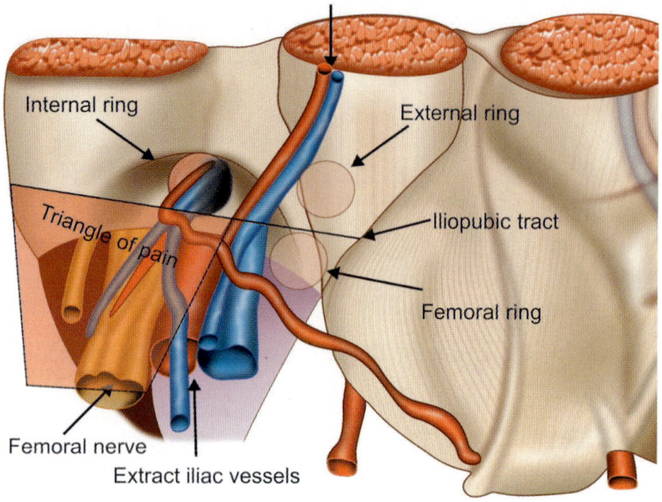


**Fig. 11.2:** Triangle of pain

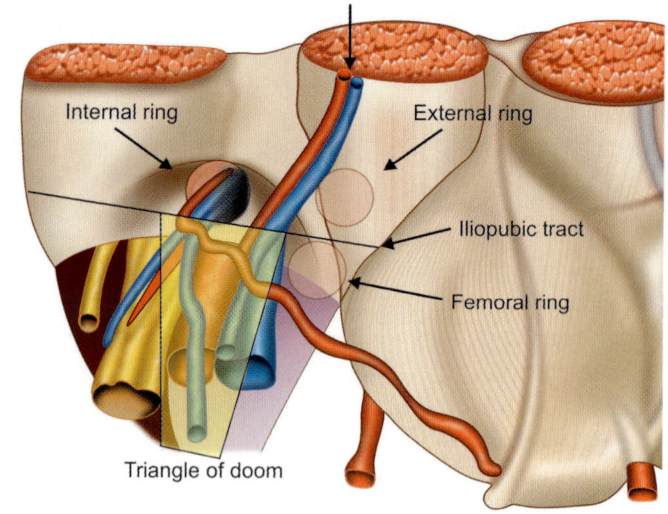


**Fig. 11.3:** Triangle of doom

- *Cooper ligament:* This is the name given to the periosteum of the superior pubic ramus. The pubic ramus can be easily palpated with a blunt grasper and is an excellent starting point for dissection.
- *Iliopubic tract:* Another fundamental structure that deserves careful recognition is the iliopubic tract (commonly referred to as the shelving edge of the inguinal ligament in open surgery)
  - This aponeurotic stretch of tissue is located posterior to the inguinal ligament and extends from the anterosuperior iliac spine to the superior pubic ramus. As a continuation of the transverse abdominus aponeurosis and fascia at the upper border of the femoral sheath, it passes medially to form the inferior border of the internal inguinal ring, crossing over the femoral vessels.
  - Importantly, the iliopubic tract forms the superolateral border of the so-called "triangle of pain (Fig. 11.2)," an area bounded medially by the spermatic vessels. In this area, tacking of the mesh is to be avoided because of the risk of injury to the femoral branch of the genitofemoral nerve or the lateral femoral cutaneous nerve.

Another anatomical zone that requires the surgeon's awareness is the so-called "triangle of doom (Fig. 11.3)," bordered medially by the ductus deferens, laterally by the spermatic vessels, and with its apex at the deep inguinal ring. This area contains the external iliac artery and vein; thus, tacking of the mesh must be avoided within its boundaries.

## Laparoscopic Inguinal Anatomy

The anatomy of the inguinofemoral region viewed via a telescope placed in intra-abdominal position differs radically from the anatomy observed via an open or anterior approach (Fig. 11.4). The laparoscopic surgeon needs to become familiar with the anatomical structure of this region. As all anatomical landmarks are covered

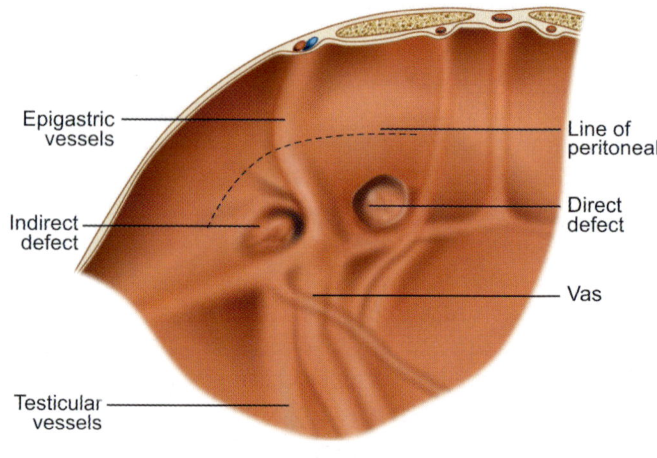


**Fig. 11.4:** Anatomy with and without peritoneal coverage

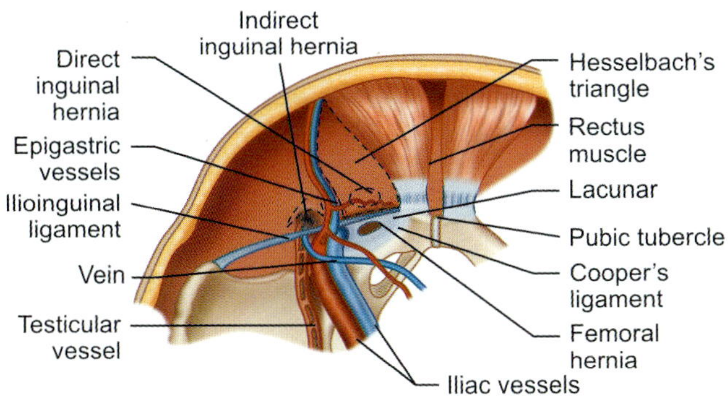


**Fig. 11.5:** Actual views—TAPP repair

with peritoneum, in the TAPP technique (Fig. 11.5) the peritoneum has to be first incised and a lower flap developed in order to expose the region adequately. In the TEP repair (Figs 11.6A and B), the anatomical landmarks need to be meticulously exposed with blunt dissection.

Our guidelines for the performance of a safe and secure laparoscopic inguinal hernia repair, mandate the following structures should be clearly and unequivocally identified:

- Cooper's ligament
- The epigastric vessels
- The spermatic cord or the round ligament
- The femoral canal and the iliac vessels
- In addition, the laparoscopic anatomical distinction between direct, indirect inguinal and femoral hernias should be well understood. Before a surgeon attempts to perform a laparoscopic inguinal or femoral hernia repair, he should memorize and be very familiar with the diagrams.

## Indications

- The general indications for laparoscopic inguinal hernia repair versus watchful waiting are the same as for open inguinal hernia repair.
- Classically, the existence of an inguinal hernia has been reason enough for operative intervention. However, recent studies have shown that the presence of a reducible hernia is not, in itself, an indication for surgery and that the risk of incarceration is less than 1%.
- Symptomatic patients (with pain or discomfort) should undergo repair; however, up to one-third of patients with inguinal hernias are asymptomatic.

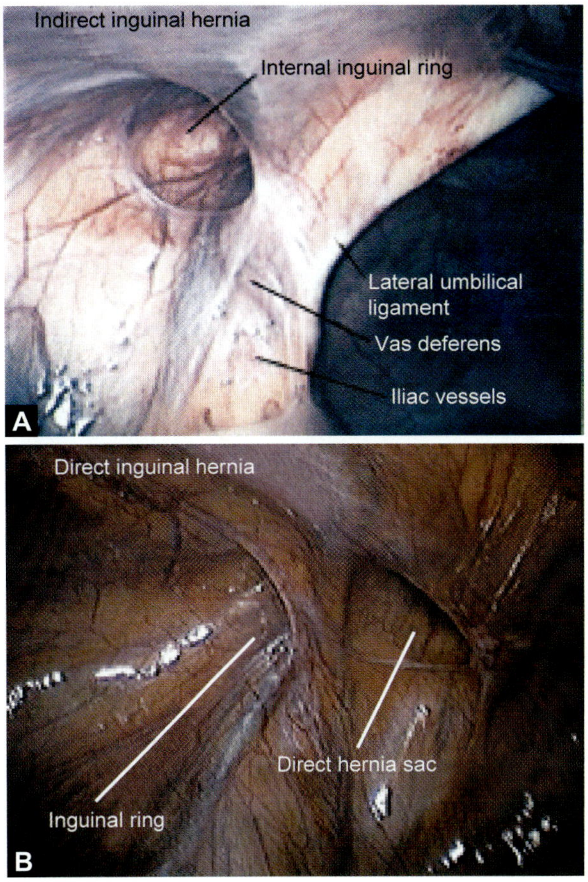


**Figs 11.6A and B:** Actual views—TEP repair

- Some reports have listed specific indications for laparoscopy over open repair, including recurrent hernias, bilateral hernias, and the need for earlier return to full activities (Figs 11.7A to F).
- Patient's preference plays perhaps the greatest role in choosing one type of repair over another.
- Surgical expertise also plays a role in selecting the appropriate type of repair. Data show that the recurrence rate drops significantly with increased surgeon experience with the laparoscopic technique. Some studies suggest that the learning curve for totally extraperitoneal (TEP) laparoscopic herniorrhaphy may be as high as 250 cases (as opposed to 25 for open repair). Transabdominal preperitoneal (TAPP) repair has a learning curve closer to that of the open technique. A large randomized controlled trial comparing laparoscopic to open repair found that, with adequate training, laparoscopic repair produced equivalent recurrence

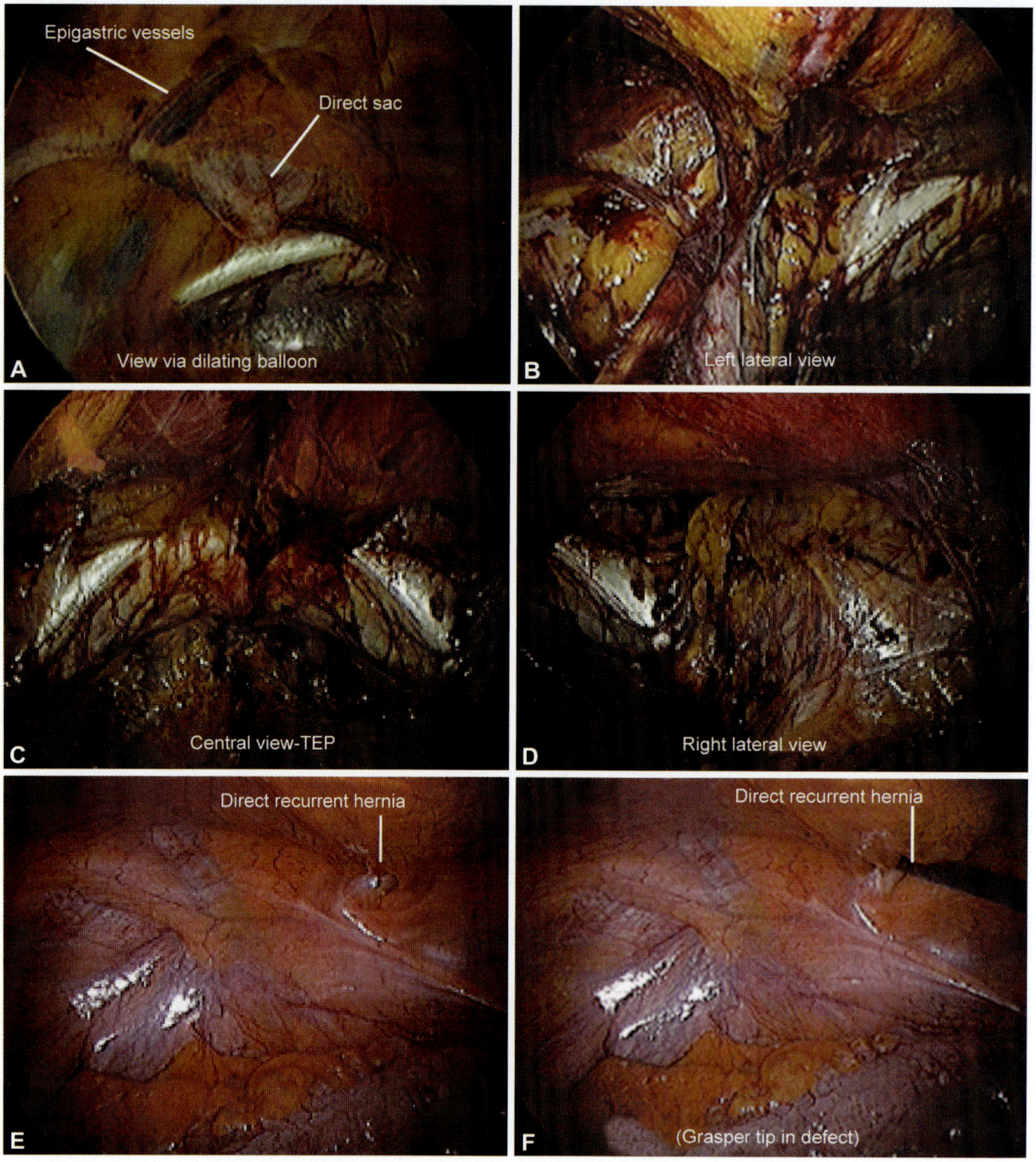


**Figs 11.7A to F:** Recurrent inguinal hernia from an open repair

rates but reduced postoperative pain and allowed earlier return to work.

- A Cochrane database meta-analysis comparing TEP to TAPP found no significant difference in recurrence but did find that TAPP was associated with a higher risk of intra-abdominal injury. The author concluded that further randomized controlled trials are needed to definitively compare these two techniques.
- The intraperitoneal onlay mesh (IPOM) technique has fallen out of favor because of reports of unacceptably high rates of organ injury, nerve injury, and hernia recurrence.

- Conclusions regarding inguinal hernias in female patients are difficult to draw because the most of the inguinal hernia literature involves male patients. In fact, Koch et al found that recurrence rates were higher in women and that recurrence in women was 10 times more likely to be of the femoral variety than in men. This has led some to the conclusion that repairs that provide coverage of the femoral space (e.g. laparoscopic repair) at the time of initial operation are better suited for women as a primary repair. A well-designed randomized controlled trial comparing laparoscopic to open herniorrhaphy has yet to be completed.
- The actual hospital costs of laparoscopic repairs are higher than those of open repairs but may be offset by the societal benefits of earlier return to full activities.

We use these techniques in the following settings:

- Incarcerated inguinofemoral hernia: TAPP repair
- Inguinofemoral hernia/patients with previous major lower abdominal surgery: TEP repair
- *Massive inguinal hernias with scrotal extension:* TEP repair or anterior repair
- *Bilateral inguinal hernias:* TAPP or TEP repair.

## Contraindications

- General contraindications for laparoscopic herniorrhaphy parallel those of open repair.
- Inguinal hernia repair has no absolute contraindications. Just as in any other elective surgical procedure, the patient must be medically optimized. Any medical issues, whether acute (e.g. upper respiratory tract or skin infection) or exacerbations of underlying medical conditions (e.g. poorly controlled diabetes mellitus), should be fully addressed and the surgery delayed accordingly.
- Contraindications specific to the laparoscopic technique include a lower midline incision, previous preperitoneal surgery (e.g. prostatectomy), irreducible hernia, and inability to tolerate general anesthesia.

## Anesthesia

- General anesthesia is preferred for laparoscopic inguinal hernia repairs.
- Although the totally extraperitoneal (TEP) technique can be performed with epidural anesthesia, the author routinely use general anesthesia for the occasional development of pneumoperitoneum due to an inadvertent peritoneal rent.
- Elective inguinal hernia repair is considered a clean procedure and, as such, should carry a < 2% surgical site infection rate. Typically, a cephalosporin antibiotic is administered by the anesthesiologist as a single dose prior to the skin incision.

### Equipment (Fig. 11.8, Table 11.1)

- All methods of laparoscopic hernia repair require the following standard laparoscopic equipment:
  - Blunt graspers
  - Hook electrocautery
  - A 30° laparoscope
  - A tacking device or fibrin glue applicator system
- A laparoscopic clip applier and suction irrigator should be available on standby.
- *Foley catheter:* The author routinely place a Foley catheter to decompress the bladder and maximize the preperitoneal space. Patients undergoing unilateral hernias and with no history of urinary retention can probably avoid a Foley catheter if they void immediately prior to the operation.
- *Balloon dissector and trocars:* The author finds that a balloon dissector saves time but does add cost to the totally extraperitoneal (TEP) technique. Simple blunt dissection with the laparoscope can be used instead to create the preperitoneal space. The author routinely uses an integrated trocar/dissector balloon system for the infraumbilical port. In addition, the author use a 5-mm trocar and an 11-mm trocar. The TAPP technique requires an umbilical Hasson 12 mm trocar and 25 mm trocars placed at the midclavicular lines bilaterally.
- *Mesh:* The mesh must be a permanent material large enough to produce a wide overlap beyond the defect's edges. Although some surgeons prefer anatomical mesh configurations, a polypropylene or polyester flat sheet of mesh (5 × 10 cm to 7 × 15 cm) works just as well and is more cost-effective.
- *Tacks:* The author routinely uses nonabsorbable tacks for mesh fixation and exercise extreme caution to avoid the danger zones. Laparoscopic absorbable tackers are now available, which may add an extra layer of security. The potential benefit is that even if a nerve is inadvertently impinged, the tack will be resorbed with time. This benefit has not been critically evaluated.

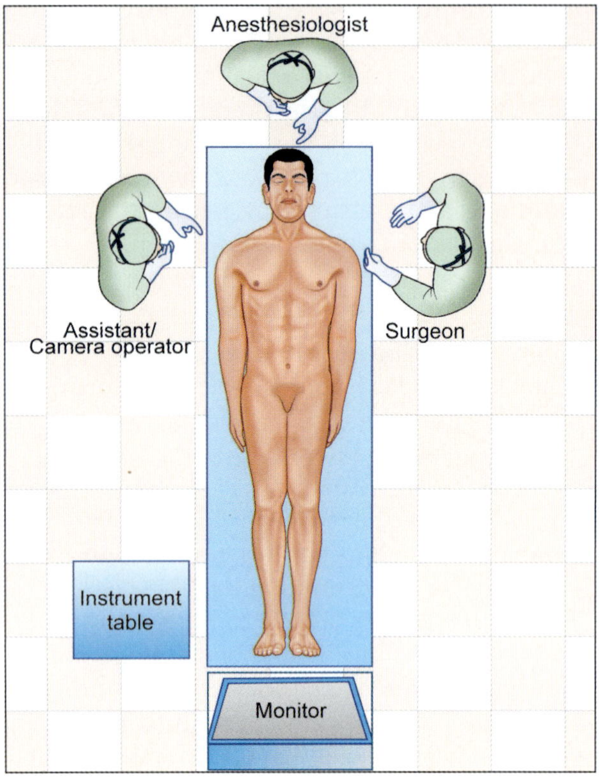


**Fig. 11.8:** Scheme of operation theater trolley and operating staff

**Table 11.1**

| Operating room setup | |
|---|---|
| Operating room table | Electric |
| Patient position | Supine—arms tucked at the sides |
| Surgeon position | Opposite side of the hernia |
| Assistant position | No dedicated assistant needed |
| Nurse position | Side of the hernia—sitting down while holding the camera |
| Pneumatic stockings | YES |
| Foley | No (Patient to urinate immediately prior to surgery) |
| CVP | No |
| Monitors | 1—at the feet of the patient |
| Monitors height | 5 feet minimum |
| Mayo stand | By left foot of the patient |
| Surgery Robot | Not standard—optional |

- Some authors have reported on the use of fibrin glue for mesh fixation with excellent results.
- Still others use no fixation at all but instead rely on peritoneal pressure to maintain the mesh in proper position (Fig. 11.9).

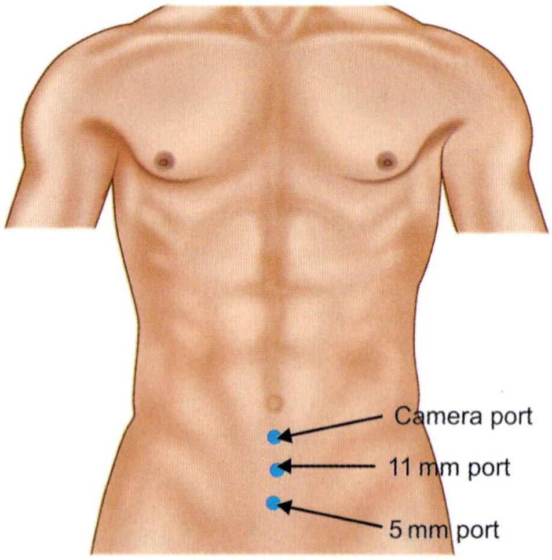


**Fig. 11.9:** Locations of port placement

## Positioning

- Confirm and mark the correct surgical site preoperatively in the holding area.
- Position the patient supine, comfortably securing the upper extremities at the patient's sides.
- For large defects, slight Trendelenburg positioning may help exposure by reducing the visceral contents into the abdomen.
- Shave the surgical site with electric clippers.
- Prepared and drape the surgical site in standard surgical fashion, exposing an area from above the umbilicus to below the pubis. The prepared area should be wide enough to allow for conversion to an open technique if this becomes necessary.
- The author places a single monitor at the foot of the bed. The operating surgeon stands on the side opposite the hernia. The assistant stands on the same side as the hernia.

## Technique TEP—Total Extraperitoneal Repair

- Make a longitudinal 10 mm infraumbilical incision and deepen it to expose the anterior rectus sheath.

- Incise the anterior rectus sheath longitudinally slightly off the midline (thus avoiding entering the peritoneal space in the midline, where the anterior and posterior rectus sheaths merge). Grasp the midline raphe with a Kelly clamp and retract the underlying rectus muscle fibers laterally, revealing the posterior rectus sheath.
- Using the posterior rectus sheath as a guide, introduce a dissecting balloon and slip it along the rectus sheath. Advance the balloon past the arcuate line and into the preperitoneal space down to the pubic symphysis. Then, inflate the dissection balloon under direct laparoscopic vision to dissect the preperitoneal space.

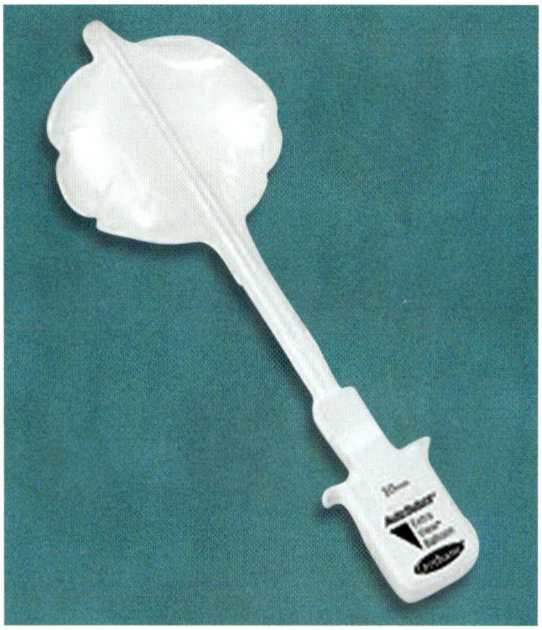

**Fig. 11.10:** Baloon for making properitoneal space

## Balloon Dissection (Fig. 11.10)

- Once adequate dissection is attained, deflate and remove the dissector balloon.
- Insufflate the preperitoneal space with $CO_2$ to a pressure of 12 mm Hg.
- Insert a 5-mm trocar 2 finger breadths above the pubis. Place an 11-mm trocar midway between the 5 mm trocar and the umbilical port.

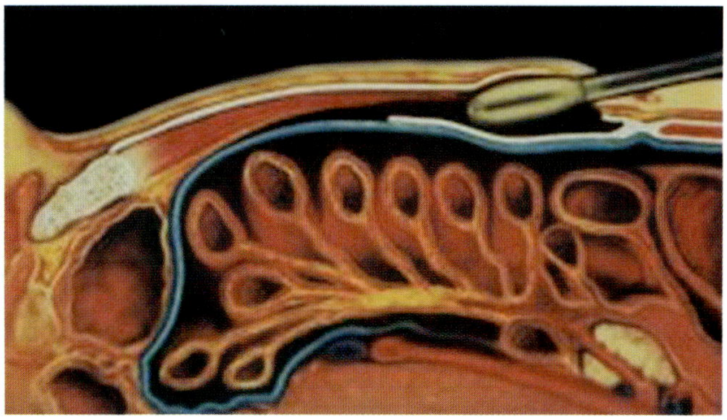

**Fig. 11.11:** Trocar placement in preperitoneal space

## Trocar Placement (Fig. 11.11)

- Insert a 30°-angled laparoscope at the umbilical port. This provides the best visualization of the inguinal region in the tight preperitoneal space.
- The author always begin the dissection with exposure of the Cooper ligament and the pubic tubercle. This is most easily performed using a 2-handed technique, whereby two blunt graspers are placed against the bone at a single point, then gently spread apart. Carry out continued gentle dissection with meticulous hemostasis to expose the direct space and the femoral space by clearing the Cooper ligament down to the iliac vessels.

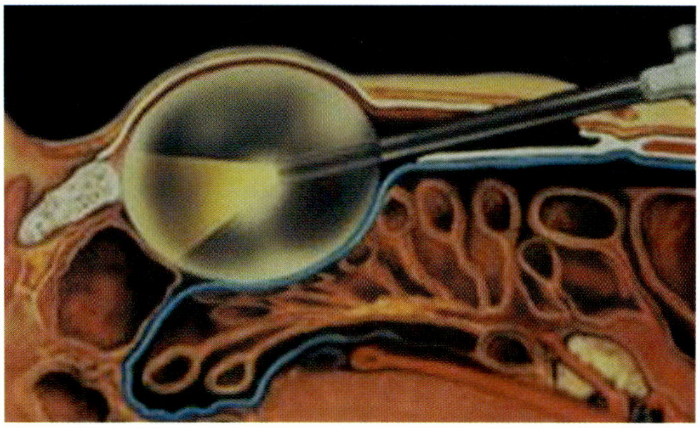

**Fig. 11.12:** Space dissection

## Direct Space Dissection (Fig. 11.12)

- A direct hernia often reduces spontaneously with pneumopreperitoneum but may require careful gentle traction and freeing of fibrous bands to get a complete reduction. Clearing the Cooper ligament in its entirety ensures that a direct hernia is fully reduced (*See* Fig. 11.7A)
- It is essential for the surgeon to get familiar with the actual properitoneal view as seen in Figure 11.13.

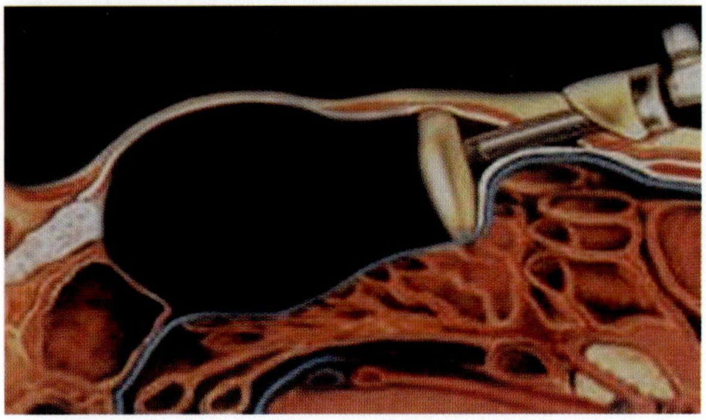

**Fig. 11.13:** Creating propneumoperitoneum

- Great care must be exercised as one approaches the iliac vessels. In addition, obturator vessels often cross the dissection planes and may need to be clipped and divided.
- Carry out the dissection of the preperitoneal space superolaterally toward the anterior superior iliac spine by gently pushing the peritoneum away from the ventral abdominal wall (*See* Figs 11.7B to D). Care must be exercised when separating the peritoneum from the muscle layers of the abdominal wall. The peritoneum is often very thin and may be tightly adhesed. Attempting to disconnect these structures may result in a peritoneal rent. This is especially evident cephalad. Inferolaterally, the abdominal wall must be cleared to below the iliopubic tract.

## Lateral Abdominal Wall Dissection

- Next, attention is shifted to the internal ring to identify an indirect hernia sac. Perform careful gentle separation of the cord structures from the sac by elevating the cord/sac bundle then delicately stripping the areolar tissue downward until a window is found between the sac and cord structures.

## Indirect Sac Isolation

- If possible, the sac should then be reduced back into the peritoneal cavity. If this is not possible, ligate the sac proximally and leave it open to drain distally to prevent formation of a hydrocele. The simplest way to do this in a wide mouth sac is to fire a vascular 30-mm linear stapler across the sac and then divide the sac distal to the staple line. Other techniques for sac ligation include Endoclips or an Endoloop.
- Be careful to avoid injury to any intra-abdominal sac contents or slider component.
- Once the dissection is complete, introduce a mesh under direct vision via the 11 mm trocar and drag it as lateral as possible toward the anterosuperior iliac spine (ASIS). Then flatten out the mesh across the myopectineal orifice and drape it over the cord structures. Place a single tack at the pubic tubercle. This serves as a fixation point that allows for easy arrangement of the mesh in the tight preperitoneal space.

## Mesh Deployment and Fixation

- Manipulate the mesh so its upper border lies above a line from the pubic symphysis to the ASIS. Then place the remaining tacks down the Cooper ligament, up the midline, and along the upper border of the mesh.
- Each fire of the tacker beyond the inferior epigastric artery and vein complex must be above a line from the pubic symphysis to the ASIS. This ensures that no tacks are placed in proximity to nerve structures or iliac vessels (the triangle of pain and triangle of doom). This can be further verified by carefully palpating the tacker head through the abdominal wall and comparing its relationship to this line prior to each fire. No more than 1 to 2 tacks are needed in this hazardous location.
- Anchoring the mesh has been subject to most controversy. Early on in the history of this laparoscopic technique, some surgical teams claimed the anchoring or stapling of the mesh has been responsible for a significant rate of postoperative neuropathy. Compression of branches of the genitofemoral and lateral cutaneous nerve by staples or tacks on the lateral aspect of the inguinal ring may have been the cause for this postoperative complication. For these reasons, author has developed numerous techniques, i.e. "no anchor-staple technique" or no lateral fixation of the mesh. Experience is somewhat different. A recent analysis of 2300 laparoscopic inguinal hernia repair (with lateral fixation of the mesh) demonstrated that patients may develop a transient neuropathy without any reported permanent neuropathy. In addition, we firmly believe that stapling or anchoring the mesh is responsible for reported low recurrence rate.
- Attention is now turned to the contralateral side if the patient has bilateral pathology. Close the larger

trocar site fascial defects with a figure-of-eight 0-absorbable suture, approximate the skin, and remove the Foley catheter.

## Important Tips

- *Warning:* Extreme care must be exercised when placing the mesh fixation tacks. This point cannot be overstated. A nerve injury caused by an errant tack can be truly debilitating, and treating these injuries can be very challenging. Tacks should be placed only above the iliopubic tract. The author routinely draws a line from the pubic tubercle to the anterosuperior iliac spine (ASIS) at the start of the procedure. Prior to firing each tack, carefully palpate the tacker head through the abdominal wall to ensure that it is above this line.
- Violation of the peritoneum during totally extraperitoneal (TEP) repair causes loss of insufflation from the preperitoneal space into the peritoneal cavity. The preperitoneal space then collapses to some degree, which may make completing the procedure difficult. In addition, it puts intra-abdominal organs at risk for injury and may lead to adhesion formation. Tearing the peritoneum should, therefore, be avoided, if possible. If the rent is small, Endoclips can be placed to close the defect and minimize the leak. Otherwise, conversion to transabdominal preperitoneal (TAPP) or open hernia repair may be necessary. Another option is to place a Veress needle through a stab incision into the abdominal cavity to drain the $CO_2$.
- Trocar placement should always be done under direct vision. To prevent bleeding and hematoma formation, the trocars should be placed exactly in the midline so as to avoid tearing the rectus muscle fibers.
- During preperitoneal dissection, the inferior epigastric artery and vein sometimes become separated from the abdominal wall. They then hang down into the operative field. The author prefer to clip and divide these vessels early in the case rather than struggle and, invariably, injure them anyway.
- Placing the mesh in such a way as to help with its flush deployment is very helpful. The authors' technique is to fold the mesh in half lengthwise, grasp the mesh by the fold, and advance the mesh through the trocar toward the ASIS. When the grasper is released, the natural memory of the mesh causes it to spring open in a properly oriented position without the need for time-consuming manipulation.
- At the completion of the operation but prior to desufflation, the author likes to spray the preperitoneal space with 20 ml of 0.5% bupivacaine with epinephrine for long-acting local analgesia and improved hemostasis.
- A blunt grasper should be placed against the lower corner of the mesh just lateral to the cord structures while the preperitoneal space is desufflated under direct vision. This prevents the mesh from rolling upward and exposing the lateral aspect of the internal ring to recurrence.

### Desufflation

- Rather than pumping the dissector balloon to a preset number of pumps, (manufacturer recommendation is 30–40), the author prefer to pump under direct vision until no further movement of the tissues is visible, indicating no benefit from further dissection.
- Vascular injury is a less common but potentially disastrous pitfall. This can be avoided by respecting the proximity of the femoral vessels, particularly when tacking the mesh to the Cooper ligament.
- The use of an ample-sized mesh is the key to minimizing recurrences. It must be large enough to extend 2 cm medial to the pubic tubercle, 3 to 4 cm above the Hesselbach triangle, and 5 to 6 cm lateral to the internal ring.
- In male patients, always remember to gently pull the testes back down to their normal scrotal position at the end of the case.

## Complications

- *Hematoma or seroma formation*: This is usually self-limited because of the tamponade effect of the peritoneum. On rare occasions, this complication may require surgical intervention.
- *Nerve injury*: Great care must be exercised when securing the mesh with tacks. Nerve injury is usually self-limited but may require steroid injections or, if persistent, neurectomy.
- *Intra-abdominal injury*: This is uncommon with totally extraperitoneal (TEP) repair but may occur if the peritoneum is torn and the abdominal cavity is entered. Take extra care with wide-neck hernia sacs that contain abdominal organs. A final intraperitoneal evaluation may be helpful at the completion of the case if an injury is suspected.

- *Adhesion formation*: This is very uncommon with TEP repair but has been reported with large peritoneal rents. Closure of this defect may be warranted and can be performed laparoscopically with Endoclips or an Endoloop.
- Ischemic orchitis leading to atrophic testicle or even necrosis is a catastrophic but known complication of inguinal herniorrhaphy. The exact cause of this vascular injury is unclear, but it is thought to be secondary to venous thrombosis rather than arterial injury. Although rare, a high index of suspicion for this complication and emergency testicular ultrasonography may help avoid orchiectomy. Symptoms include painful testicular swelling and fever commencing 2 to 3 days after surgery.

## Transabdominal Preperitoneal Hernia Repair (Figs 11.14A to F)

Among all inguinal hernia repair techniques that utilize a preperitoneal placement of mesh, the advantage of laparoscopic hernioplasty (TAPP) is based on the fact that any type of groin hernia can be treated safely and effectively in a standardized way. Diagnostic laparoscopy allows an immediate evaluation of the type of hernia on both the sides. In case of difficult preparation of a large hernial sac, it is possible to observe the sac and its content continuously. A disadvantage of the TAPP is that the placement of the mesh cannot be checked while deflating the pneumoperitoneum. The mesh needs to be placed without any wrinkles, with a wide overlap of the hernia defect (> 3–5 cm), whereas the parietalization plays the most important role.

The degree of difficulty of TAPP is not only determined by pathologic-anatomic substrate of hernia (type, size, cicatrization, associated lipoma) but also by physical attributes of the patient (size; weight; pelvic width; local obesity; strength of musculature of the abdominal wall; thickness and distensibility of the abdominal wall; abdominal previous surgery, e.g. appendectomy).

To perform a first TAPP, the ideal patient is older than 60 years, has a flabby abdominal wall, has a poor muscular tone, has a wide pelvis, is slightly obese, has a small direct hernia and has had no previous abdominal surgery.

### Patient Selection

In the initial part of the learning curve, patient selection is important. Indirect hernial sacs are closely applied to the cord structures and are more often complete, making

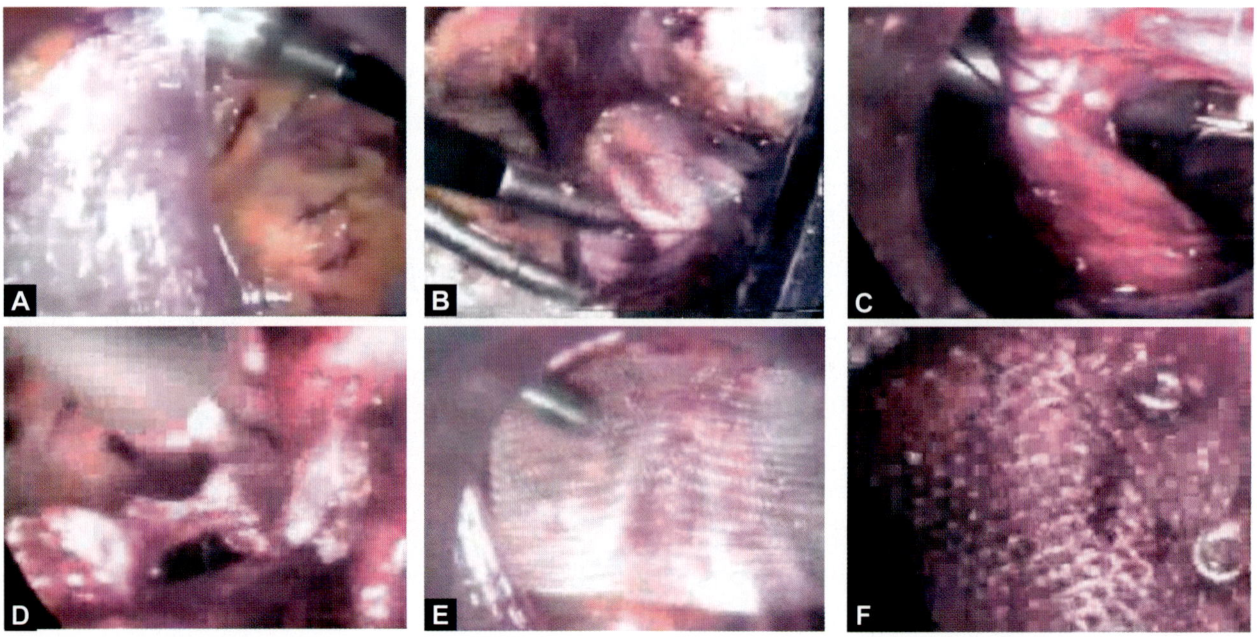

**Figs 11.14A to F:** The totally extraperitoneal hernia repair. (A) Trocar insertion into the extraperitoneal space; (B) Separation of the hernial sac from the vas deferens and spermatic veins; (C) Hernial sac ligation; (D) Division of the sac and leave the distal sac *in situ*; (E) Covering with a mesh; (F) Mesh fixation

dissection difficult. Left sided hernias are more difficult to dissect than the right sided ones. Bilateral hernia repair during the learning curve may significantly increase the operating time. Recurrent hernias and irreducible hernias should be repaired only after expertise is gained in repair of simple hernias. Direct or small indirect primary hernias in lean and thin subjects are the best. Indirect, left sided hernias, large, irreducible or complicated hernias in obese patients are best avoided during the learning curve. Laparoscopic inguinal hernia repair is an advanced laparoscopic procedure. The dissection is performed in the vicinity of major vessels (iliac vein and artery) and the potential for injury to adjoining viscera (urinary bladder) is high. It is, therefore, required that the surgeon planning to undertake the repair should have experience in laparoscopic surgery. Laparoscopic anatomy of the inguinal area is totally different from what is seen during the anterior approach. The surgeon has to learn this anatomy. Familiarization with this anatomy by working in a unit performing laparoscopic hernia repair regularly is very helpful for proper orientation.

## Anesthesia

Laparoscopic TAPP hernia repair is performed under general anesthesia. In elderly subjects, a detailed cardio-respiratory work up should be done prior to surgery for safe general anesthesia and pneumoperitoneum. The patient is asked to pass urine just before shifting to the operation theater. If the patient is more than sixty years of age, has symptoms of prostatic enlargement or post-void residual volume is more than 50 ml, it is advisable to place a Foley's indwelling catheter prior to surgery. This may be removed 24 hours after the surgery. Perioperative prophylactic antibiotics are administered. After induction of anesthesia, irreducible hernia contents, if any, are reduced before painting and draping is commenced.

Steps of TAPP repair:

- *Step 1:* Entering the intra-abdominal cavity
- *Step 2:* Creating the peritoneal flap
- *Step 3:* Identifying the anatomical landmarks
- *Step 4:* Dissecting the hernia sac
- *Step 5:* Deploying and anchoring the mesh
- *Step 6:* Testing the fixation of the mesh
- *Step 7:* Closing the peritoneum.

## Standard Technique of Transabdominal Preperitoneal Hernia Repair (Fig. 11.15)

*Operation theater layout:* It is customary to perform a diagnostic laparoscopy to inspect the upper abdomen, including the liver. To expose the inguinal area, the patient needs to be positioned as mentioned above. The surgeon should stand on the opposite side of the hernia. The camera operator is required to sit on the hernia side. The video tower is placed at the feet of the patient, whereas the scrub nurse stays on the left side.

*Positioning:* The patient lies supine and flat on the operating table with both arms placed by the side. After obtaining the pneumoperitoneum, the patient needs to be placed in a Trendelenburg position and turned at an angle of 10 to 20° towards the surgeon, so that the surgeon can approach the inguinal region without the hindrance of the intestinal loops (Fig. 11.16).

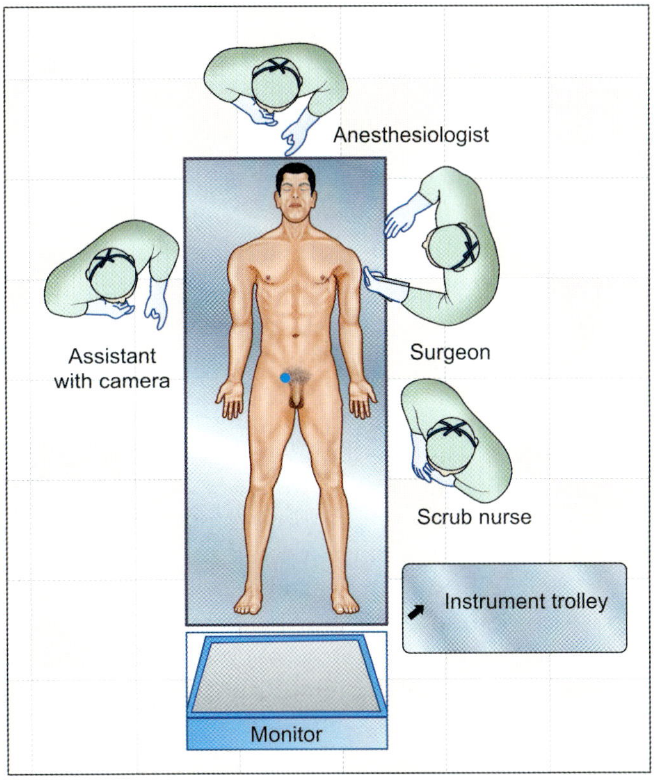


**Fig. 11.15:** Standard technique of transabdominal preperitoneal hernia repair

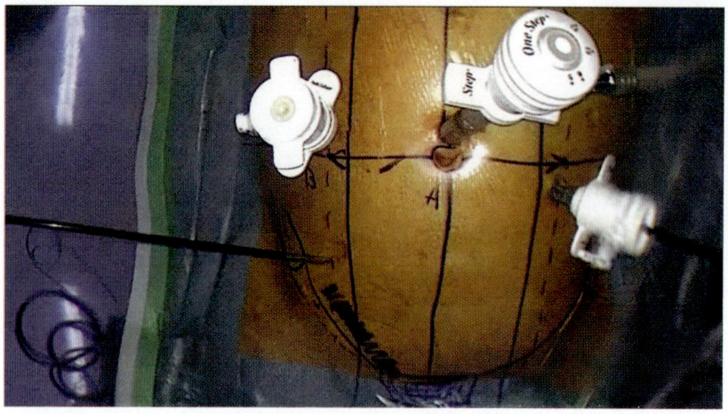

Fig. 11.16: Trocar positioning

*Incision:* To place the optical trocar, an incision of 1 cm needs to be made longitudinally superior of the umbilicus down to the umbilical base. The opposite wound edges are grasped using strong Backhaus clamps to lift up the abdominal wall. Thus, Veress needle can be positioned to induce a pneumoperitoneum.

*Insufflation:* Semm's safety tests are always performed to ensure correct intraperitoneal position of the needle. During insufflation, the intra-abdominal pressure and the gas flow need to be observed. To ensure correct position of the tip of the Veress-needle in the abdominal cavity, the pressure should be low (about 0 mm Hg), whereas the flow is required to be adequately high (about 2 l/min). Then insufflation can be continued until a maximal pressure of 12 mm Hg is reached. The Veress needle is used to create pneumoperitoneum. Patency of the needle and spring function must be checked before insertion. The preferred site of needle insertion is the supraumbilical fold. The springmechanism gives a click sound immediately on penetrating the parietal peritoneum. Insuffulation is commenced with a set pressure of 12 mm Hg. A pressure reading of less than 7 mm Hg suggests that tip position in the cavity. A higher pressure indicates the tip position to be extra-peritoneal or obstruction to the flow by the omentum. All quadrants of the abdomen are inspected and percussed to check for uniform pneumoperitoneum. Insufflation is continued until a pressure of 12 mm Hg is reached, which requires about 2.5 to 3 liters of gas. After satisfactory pneumoperitoneum (Fig. 11.18), the Veress needle is removed and a 10 mm port is placed through the supraumbilical incision. During insertion, the abdominal wall is lifted up and stabilized with the left hand and the trocar is directed towards the hollow of the pelvis. A 300 telescope attached to the camera, is introduced and the groin area is visualized. Two 5 mm ports are placed as working ports for the right and left hand of the surgeon, one on each side, at the level of umbilicus in the midclavicular line. These ports should be placed under vision to prevent injury to the inferior epigastric vessels and underlying bowel (Fig. 11.17).

### *Step 1: Entering the Intra-abdominal Cavity*

The optical trocar is then placed. Again, the abdominal wall should be held tense by using Backhaus clamps. The optical trocar is screwed into the abdominal cavity softly, and the optic can be inserted. Usually we use a 30° angle optic (Figs 11.19 and 11.20).

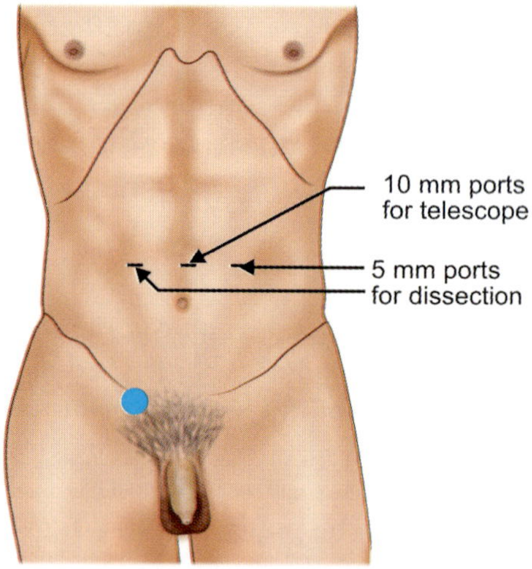


Fig. 11.17: Port positions

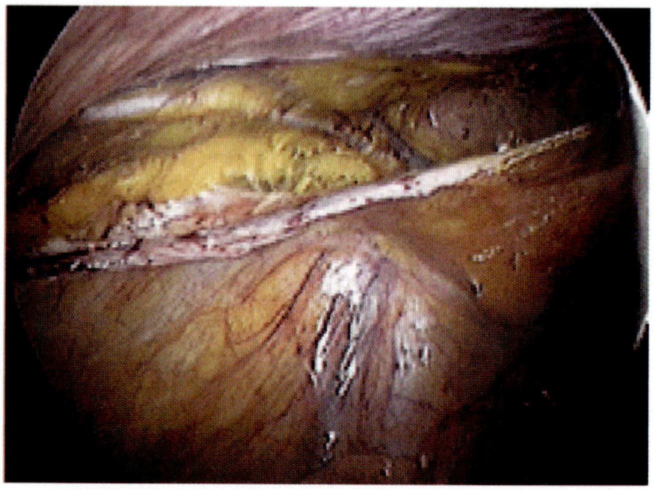

Fig. 11.18: Pneumoperitoneum in TAPP

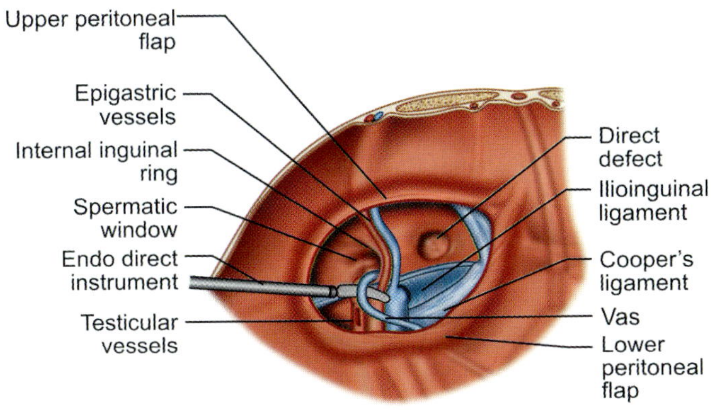


**Fig. 11.19:** TAPP view

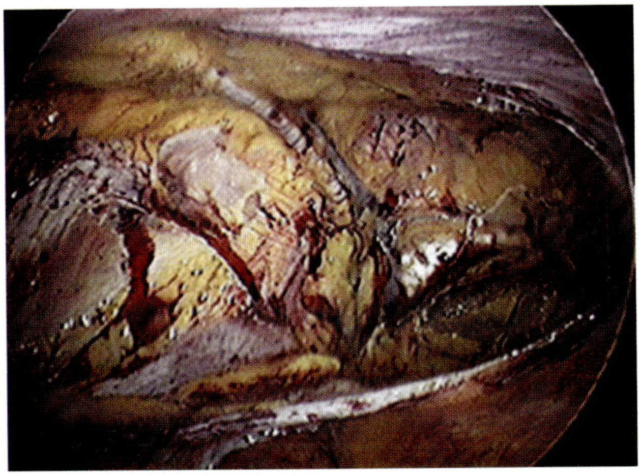

**Fig. 11.20:** TAPP view after opening peritoneum

In case of bilateral hernia, all the trocars are placed at the umbilical and midclavicular levels (right 12 mm, left 5 mm). In case of a unilateral hernia, one trocar can be positioned above the umbilicus at the hernia side, whereas the contralateral trocar may be placed below the umbilicus to avoid collision with the optical trocar.

In order to avoid any injury to intra-abdominal organs, trocars should always be inserted under vision. Without exception, blunt and reusable trocars with expanding and nonincisive cone-shaped tips are used (Karl Storz GmbH, Germany). Consequently, injuries of epigastric vessels causing bleeding complications as well as major tissue trauma, followed by late postoperative hernia formation, can be avoided completely.

### *Step 2: Creating the Peritoneal Flap*

*Opening peritoneum*: The dissection of the right inguinal area begins with a curved and a spacious opening of the peritoneum, starting in the region of the anterosuperior iliac spine, going to the myopectinal orifice and ending at the medial umbilical ligament. In case of a prominent fatty ligament which obscures the access to the inguinal region, it should not be cut (caveat: bleeding from a nonobliterated umbilical artery may ensue), but the incision of the peritoneum should be enlarged towards the cranium in a 'J' shape. The repair is initiated. The laparoscope is pointed toward the afflicted inguinal canal. The peritoneal defect or hernia is identified. The *lateral umbilical ligament* is located as well as the *inferior epigastric artery and vein*. The incision is extended from the lateral aspect of the inguinal region to the *lateral umbilical ligament.*

For obese patients, this ligament may have to be transected in order to obtain additional exposure. The operator should be meticulous in making this incision as high as possible to maximize the exposure of the region.

### *Step 3: Identifying the Anatomical Landmarks*

With blunt dissection, *Cooper's ligament* is exposed as well as the *inferior epigastric vessels* and the *spermatic cord*. The iliac vessels are not dissected but their positions is clearly identified. It is essential to expose the uncovered abdominal wall meticulously (without peritoneum) and remove all fatty layers.

### *Step 4: Dissecting the Hernia Sac*

The dissection of the right inguinal area begins with a curved and a spacious opening of the peritoneum, starting in the region of the anterosuperior iliac spine, going to the myopectinal orifice and ending at the medial umbilical ligament. In case of a prominent fatty ligament which obscures the access to the inguinal region, it should not be cut (note: bleeding from a nonobliterated umbilical artery may ensue), but the incision of the peritoneum should be enlarged towards the cranium in a 'J' shape.

The dissection of the inguinal region is done in accordance with a strict concept. Before dissecting the myopectinal orifice with the hernial sac, a preparation of the lateral and medial compartments is required, particularly in an obese patient. It is advantageous to identify important landmarks—such as the rectus muscle and symphysis, as well as testicular vessels laterally. Consequently, risk of injury to the spermatic cord, iliac vessels, nerves and urinary bladder can be eliminated. Dissection of the hernial sac should not be performed before demonstrating both the compartments clearly. An early identification of the epigastric vessels is recommended. In addition, it is advisable to free the epigastric vessels of fat so as to uncover the inner inguinal ring exactly. In case of a lipoma at the entry into the inguinal canal, dissection is required to identify to the hernial sac.

By following a so-called 'cobweb-like nonvascular zone,' the space of Retzius (medial compartment) as well as the Bogros' space (lateral compartment) can be dissected in a blunt manner. The left hand is used to pull firmly on the leaf-like opened peritoneum, while the right hand performs either a blunt or a sharp dissection with a Metzenbaum scissors, which is connected to unipolar diathermy. As a matter of principle, accurate hemostasis is required to identify landmarks and obtain excellent exposure.

*Dissecting a direct hernia is a simple process (Figs 11.25A to F)*: Immediately after dissecting the medial compartment a preperitoneal lipomatous tissue is observed at the direct hernial orifice. By placing the peritoneum as well as the lipomatous tissue on tension, the transversalis fascia (which forms the hernial sac) becomes visible and appears to be a white circular structure. Stepwise, the lipomatous tissue gets separated from the transverse fascia without penetrating it. Furthermore, a thorough hemostasis with the use of monopolar diathermy as well as a meticulous dissection of the hernial sac play an important role in reducing postoperative formation of serohematoma. It has been observed that as the dissection progresses medial, corona mortis is observed to occur in 20% of patients. Again, careful attention is required to avoid bleeding.

The femoral hernial orifice is located in an angle formed by the Cooper's ligament (iliopubic tract inserting into the pubic os) and the iliac vein. Thus, the femoral hernial orifice can be exposed. Due to the proximity to the femoral vein, the dissection needs to be performed very carefully.

*Caution:* Be attentive not to injure the vas deferens.

Dissection of the indirect hernial sac is much more difficult as compared to the direct hernia, especially when the sac is long and contains scar formation near the cremaster encircling the spermatic cord. Proceeding systematically, at first the testicular vessels, located caudal and lateral, should be dissected. Afterwards, the hernial sac is separated off the adhesions to the above-mentioned structures by starting from caudal lateral and then going to cranial medial. Under careful hemostasis, dissection is achieved partly bluntly and partly sharply. Especially in large hernias, the double-instrument-rope-ladder method should be used, which means that the scissors in the right hand are replaced by a second forceps. Now, the hernial sac can be dissected step-by-step off the inguinal canal by adopting the rope-ladder principle. To release and separate the hernial sac off the spermatic cord, a fine and superficial coagulation of the adhesions normally suffices.

Quite often, strong adhesions can be found at the entrance of the inguinal canal between the hernial sac and cremaster muscle, as well as the medial edge of the epigastric vessels. Again, superficial coagulation suffices to bluntly peel off the hernial sac. A stepwise progress under permanent view of the vessels of the spermatic cord permits the surgeon to reach the tip of the hernial sac. The following procedure is simple and only the freeing up of the vas deferens is left. Once again, the procedure is similar to the one used for the testicular vessels. This time, the dissection goes from cranial lateral to caudal medial. The usage of scissors combined with monopolar diathermy allows even firm adhesions to be dissected free.

(*Note:* Dissect a safe distance away from the vas deferens!)

*Parietalization:* The final step of dissecting the groin includes parietalization, at which peritoneum is dissected off the spermatic cord and the spermatic fascia beyond the middle region of the psoas muscle. In doing so, even the flimsiest of the connections between the peritoneum and the retroperitoneal space and spermatic fascia and spermatic cord respectively should be disconnected. The purpose of parietalization is to prevent the mesh (placed over the hernial orifices) from being lifted up by the remaining connective tissue during peritoneal closure; this may especially occur laterally. Thus, a later recurrence of the hernia from caudal and lateral caused by shifting of the fatty tissue is prevented. One should be able to lift the peritoneum without causing movement of the mesh. Now the preparation of the groin is completed.

### *Step 5: Deploying and Anchoring the Mesh (Figs 11.21A and B)*

Hemostasis should be secured before the mesh is placed and any blood/serum sucked out. If a prominent vein is seen coursing horizontally over the Cooper's ligament, it should be cauterized, else it may be a source of troublesome bleeding when the mesh is being fixed to the Cooper's ligament with stapler. A polypropylene mesh of 15 cm (transverse) × 12 cm (vertical) is used for repair on each side. Three corners of the mesh are rounded off except the lower lateral corner for orientation. Upper half of the mesh is rolled and secured in that position with 2 to 0 vicryl suture in the center. The mesh is now rolled completely and introduced into the operating field through the 10 mm umbilical port by removing the telescope. The telescope is then reinserted. The mesh is taken to the area of dissection and the lower part of the mesh is unrolled. The lower medial part of the mesh is positioned against the Cooper's ligament. The medial border of the mesh should reach the midline and in direct hernia must cross over to the opposite side for a wide overlap. See through property of the prolene mesh, by virtue of its large pore size, is very helpful in proper positioning of the mesh. The mesh is fixed to the Cooper's ligament at two points with stapler. The anchoring suture is now cut away and the remaining half of the mesh is unrolled. It is spread over the anterior abdominal wall, to cover the defect widely. Staples are applied over the medial and upper border of the mesh to anchor it to the underlying muscles. Generally 3 to 4 staples are sufficient; one on the medial border and two on the upper border (one on each side of the EIV). No staple should be applied on the lower and lateral parts of the mesh below the iliopubic tract to avoid injury to the nerves (triangle of pain). In case of bilateral hernia repair, the meshes should overlap each other in the midline and are fixed to each other with stapler so that they function as one mesh .

### *Step 6: Testing the Fixation of the Mesh (Fig. 11.22)*

The operator should check the mesh is well anchored to the surrounding structures. Using a closed grasper, pressure is applied with the end or tip of the grasper directly at the center of the covered direct and indirect defect. The mesh should not migrate and remain in place.

### *Step 7: Closing the Peritoneum*

The peritoneum is closed meticulously and no defect between the peritoneum and the abdominal wall should be left open. In addition, it should cover the entire mesh.

The closure should be initiated on the lateral aspect of the repair. The peritoneal flap is held by a grasper and pulled over the upper peritoneal layer. Tacks are used to close the peritoneal flap. The epigastric vessels should be meticulously visualized prior to stapling around them.

*Caution:* Be attentive not to place staples or tacks over the epigastric vessels.

The trocars are removed under direct vision. The fascia of the subumbilical trocar site is closed as needed.

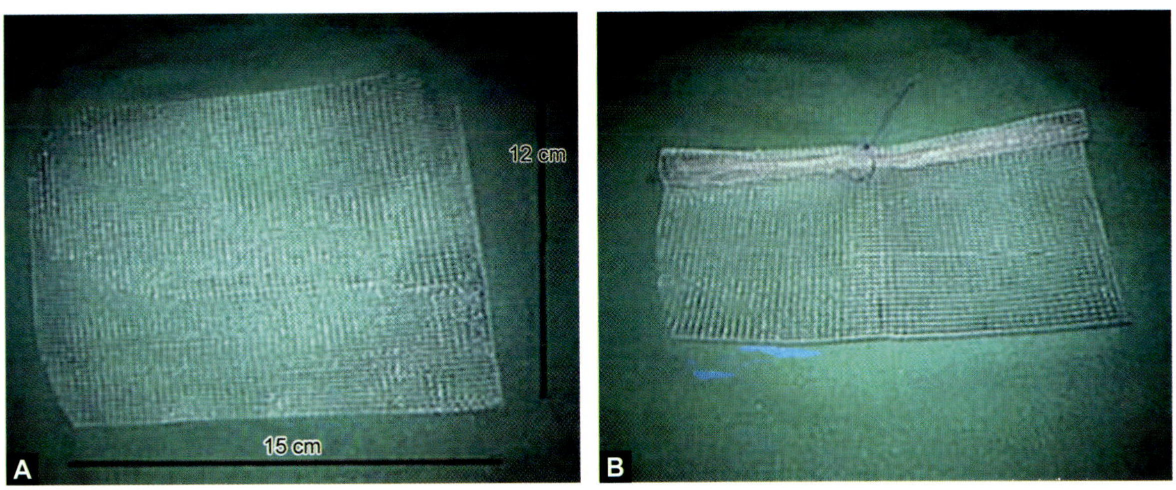


**Figs 11.21A and B:** Mesh and folding of mesh

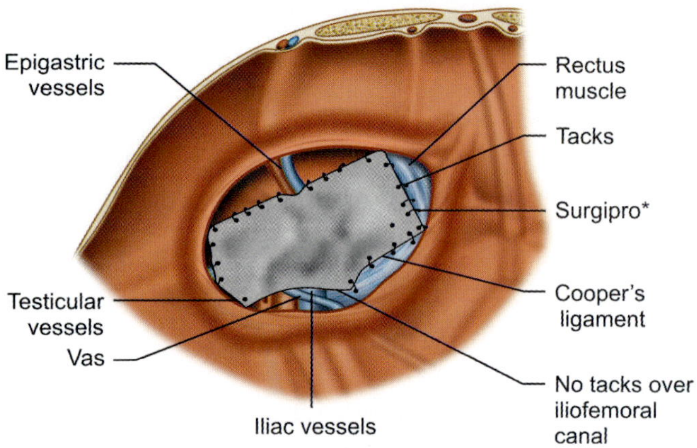


**Fig. 11.22:** Placement of mesh and fixation

*Or else:* As soon as the mesh is placed in position, the peritoneal incision should be approximated using an absorbable, industrially manufactured suture, whose ends get fixed with absorbable clips. At the time of suturing the peritoneum, the intra-abdominal pressure is reduced to 6 to 8 mm Hg, thereby allowing a tension-free peritoneal closure. An alternative is to close the peritoneum with a simple continuous suture with intracorporeal knotting.

The procedure is terminated by removing all trocars under vision. In case, bleeding is observed from the port sites, it is possible to control it by electrocoagulating the area with a grasper from the contralateral port. Finally, after deflating the abdominal cavity, the optical trocar needs to be removed. Therefore, an accurate closure of the fascia with a strong suture is required; because in contrast to the lateral working trocars, the fascial opening at the optical trocar is not covered by muscles (Figs 11.23 and 11.24).

## Intraoperative Complications

The urinary bladder should be emptied before surgery either by self-voiding or by catheterization. A full bladder can create lot of difficulties during medial dissection and also becomes prone to injury. The bladder may sometimes become full intra-operatively if the anesthetist infuses fluid rapidly or the procedure becomes prolonged. In such a situation, it is preferable to insert a catheter intraoperatively than to struggle with a full bladder.

*Bowel injury*: The patient should be in a head low position to move the bowels away from the operating field. During TAPP repair, as in all pelvic surgeries, possibility of thermal injury to the bowel exists. The insulation of the instruments should be checked, use of electrical energy should be kept to minimum and while moving the hand instrument, the foot should be off the cautery pedal to prevent accidental thermal injury to intraperitoneal structures (Figs 11.25A to F).

*Bleeding*: Inferior epigastric or gonadal vessels can cause bleeding during dissection. Gentle careful

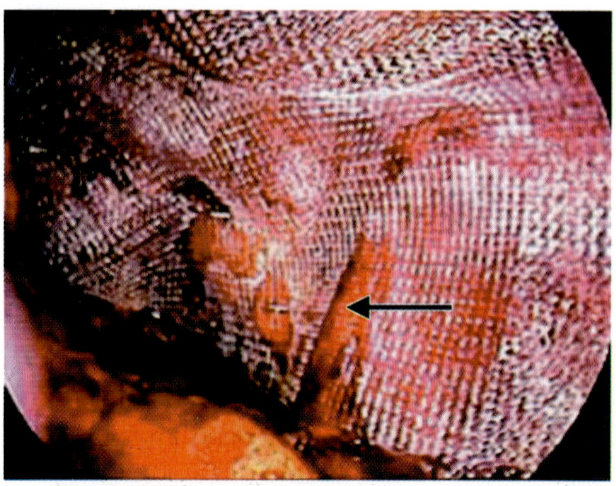

**Fig. 11.23:** Spreading placed mesh

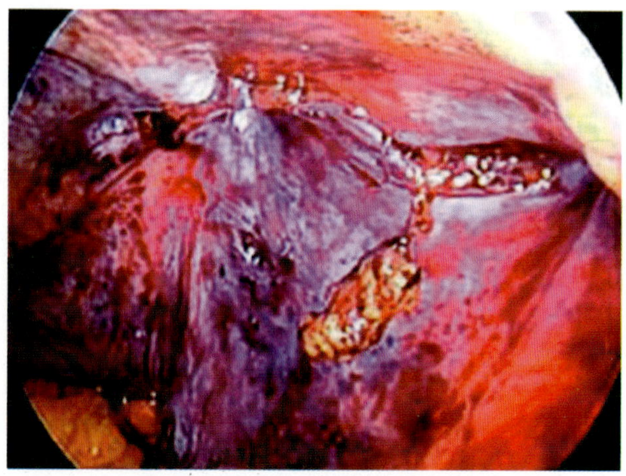

**Fig. 11.24:** Suturing peritoneum

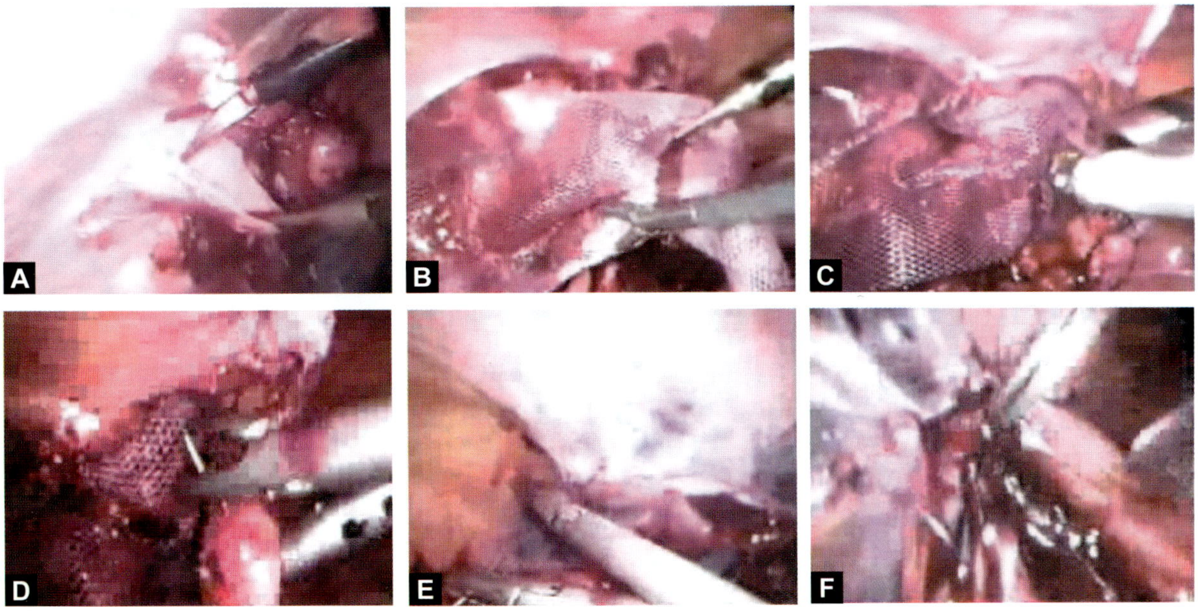

**Figs 11.25A to F:** The transabdominal preperitoneal approach. (A) Open the preperitoneal space and the hernial sac was left in place; (B) Covering with a mesh; (C) Fixation the mesh with staples; (D) Suture closure the peritoneum; (E) Continuous suture; (F) Operation is completed

dissection will avoid bleeding. Mostly, bleeding may be controlled with monopolar cautery or clips. The most disastrous of all is the iliac vessel injury (in the triangle of Doom), which requires an emergency conversion.

A few keys points should always be remembered to keep the recurrence rate close to zero. The peritoneum should be stripped from the midline the medially to the anterosuperior iliac spine laterally. Proximally, the peritoneum should be stripped off the cord structures for a distance to prevent indirect recurrence. In direct hernia, the dissection should cross the midline. Mesh of 15 × 12 cm is recommended, so that the entire myopectineal orifice is covered with wide overlap.

- The mesh should lie in the preperitoneal space without any folds, particularly at the corners. If the mesh is getting folded, the preperitoneal space should be dissected further.
- For bilateral repair, the mesh of both sides should overlap in the center.
- The mesh should be fixed over the Cooper's ligament with minimum two staples. The polypropylene material has memory and after it is unrolled inside, it may again roll back and leave the defect uncovered. Fixing the upper margin of the mesh further decreases the chances of the mesh rolling back and can help in obtaining a zero recurrence.

## Final Word

Laparoscopic hernia repair by the TAPP technique is an excellent operation for treatment of inguinal hernias.

Precondition for excellent results is the strict application of a standardized technique. In experienced hands, all types of hernias, including large scrotal hernias and recurrent hernias after previous preperitoneal repair, can be operated with low morbidity and recurrence rates.

# Chapter 12

# Female Inguinal Hernia

## Anatomy and Surgery Techniques

### Anatomy (Table 12.1)

#### *Site*

The inguinal canal is situated just above the medial half of the inguinal ligament.

#### *Length*

Approximately 4 cm (1.57 inches).

#### *Direction*

It is oblique directed inferiorly, anteriorly and medially.

#### *Boundaries*

A first-order approximation is to visualize the canal as a cylinder, stretching from the deep inguinal ring to the superficial inguinal ring.

To help define the boundaries, the canal is often further approximated as a box with six sides. Not including the two rings, the remaining four sides are usually called the "anterior wall", "posterior wall", "roof", and "floor". These consist of the following:

One way to remember these structures is with the mnemonic "MALT", starting at the top and going counterclockwise:

M–Muscles

A–Aponeuroses (The A in MALT coincides with the position of the wall-anterior. Hence, it is impossible to mix up whether the direction of the mnemonic is clockwise or anticlockwise)

L–Ligaments

T–Transversalis/tendon.

## Contents

- *In males*: The spermatic cord and its coverings + the ilioinguinal nerve.
- *In females*: The round ligament of the uterus + the ilioinguinal nerve.

Table 12.1

| Anatomy of female inguinal canal | | |
|---|---|---|
| | *Superior wall (roof)*: internal oblique transversus abdominis | |
| *Anterior wall*: Aponeurosis of external oblique aponeurosis of internal oblique (lateral third of canal only) superficial inguinal ring (medial third of canal only) | (inguinal canal) | *Posterior wall*: Transversalis fascia conjoint tendon (medial third of canal only) deep inguinal ring (lateral third of canal only) |
| | *Inferior wall (floor)*: Inguinal ligament lacunar ligament (medial third of canal only) iliopubic tract (lateral third of canal only) | |

- The round ligament of the uterus originates at the uterine horns, in the parametrium.
- It leaves the pelvis via the deep inguinal ring, passes through the inguinal canal and continues on to the labia majora where its fibers spread and mix with the tissue of the mons pubis.

## Female Inguinal Hernia (Fig. 12.1)

### In Females

In the female, groin hernias are only 4% as common as in males. Indirect inguinal hernia is still the most common groin hernia for females. If a woman has an indirect inguinal hernia, her internal inguinal ring is patent, which is abnormal for females. The protrusion of peritoneum is not called "processus vaginalis" in women, as this structure is related to the migration of the testicle to the scrotum. It is simply a hernia sac. The eventual destination of the hernia contents for a woman is the labium majoris on the same side, and hernias can enlarge one labium dramatically if they are allowed to progress.

#### *Symptoms*

The most frequent symptom of female inguinal hernia is a nontender, reducible bulging mass located above the labia major, where the canal of Nuck terminates. Such a bulging mass may not be painful, and the patient's attention may not be drawn to the situation; consequently, inguinal hernia often remains untreated. When patients undergo laparoscopy for other gynecological conditions, the vulvar mass bulges under pneumoperitoneal pressure, revealing unexpectedly a patent canal of Nuck and an inguinal hernia that requires surgical correction.

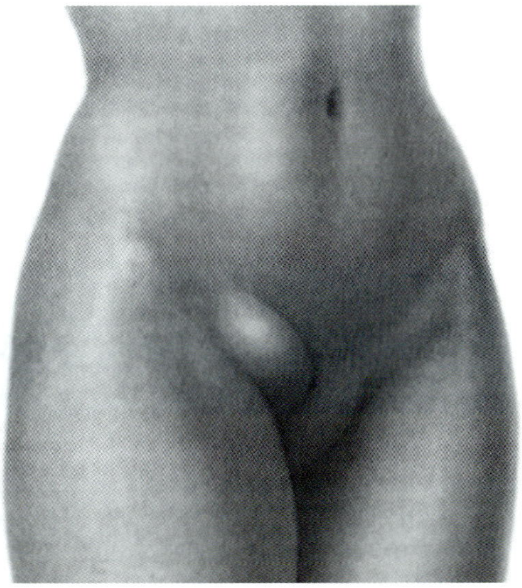

**Fig. 12.1:** Female inguinal hernia

#### *Formation*

Although less common than in males, inguinal hernias may occur in females. During fetal development, the *inguinal* canal is formed by the processus vaginalis, an evagination of peritoneum, and descends on each side of the abdomen to the labio sacral swellings. In female fetuses, however, the processus vaginalis usually occludes and disappears long before birth. If the closure fails, a persistent process—called the 'canal of Nuck'—offers a pathway from the pelvic cavity to the labia major. This opening may sometimes be seen at laparoscopy, but few gynecologists notice that the patent canal might elicit the occurrence of inguinal hernia.

An untreated reducible hernia has the potential to develop into an incarcerated hernia; therefore most surgeons suggest that the hernia is best repaired as soon as a reducible mass is noticed. With the conventional anterior herniorrhaphic method, not only is a larger skin incision required but the postoperative recovery is also lengthy and painful, owing to the delicacy of the tissues manipulated during surgery and the anatomic tension created by the repair. The current techniques of laparoscopic hernia repair are usually carried out with a mesh prosthesis in order to cover the defect in a tension-free manner, to prevent recurrence of tissue attenuation of the repair, and to reduce postoperative pain. The most popular laparoscopic herniorrhaphic procedures include an intraperitoneal onlay mesh (IPOM) technique, a transabdominal preperitoneal (TAPP) approach, and a totally extraperitoneal (TEP) approach (Fitzgibbons et al. 1995; Liem and van Vroonhoven, 1996). A randomized, multicenter trial has been performed which concluded that patients who underwent the TEP technique recovered more rapidly and had fewer recurrences (Liem et al. 1997). However, the mesh prosthesis is a material which evokes a marked tissue reaction and may induce severe pelvic adhesion; the mesh may also, on occasion, migrate across the peritoneum. Complications caused by mesh, including bowel obstruction (McDonald and Chung, 1997), mesh infections (Avtan et al. 1997) and mesh migration into bladder (Hume and Bour, 1996) have been reported when using the TAPP approach. Bowel obstruction has also been reported in TEP (Eugene et al. 1998).

In the past, these hernia repair procedures have been designed mainly for use in male patients, and earlier reports of male inguinal hernia have emphasized the different, albeit stronger, *inguinal* anatomy of females (Glassow, 1973; Spangen, 1995). During development of the female fetus, the processus vaginalis has no testes through which to pass, and contains no spermatic cord except for the gubernaculum, which later becomes the round ligament of the uterus. Thus, most female inguinal canals have fewer weak points, and hence inguinal hernias are of a milder form than those found in males. It is doubtful whether it is necessary to use such complicated and invasive methods to repair a mild female indirect inguinal hernia, especially when the hernia (though symptomatic) has usually been neglected by the patient herself. However, concomitant simple closure of the inguinal canal is a quick and simple way to deal with the problem during the same laparoscopic operation, and disappearance of the bulging mass under pneumoperitoneal pressure offers a good test to confirm complete occlusion of the patent hernial canal. In comparison with traditional anterior herniorrhaphy, the laparoscopic simple closure method provides better results and less postoperative pain. This is because it offers the highest ligation of the hernia sac by using an intraperitoneal approach, as well as a less invasive access, since the surgeon has no need to section a thick layer of fat and muscle. Unlike the laparoscopic mesh hernioplastic method, the simple closure method reported here does not require dissection of the extraperitoneal space, and also eliminates the possibility of mesh infection and severe adhesion or bowel obstruction which may be caused by mesh migrating into the abdominal cavity.

In short, the previously neglected female indirect inguinal hernia with open canal of Nuck may be revealed unexpectedly during laparoscopy for diagnostic work-up of infertility or other gynecological conditions. The hernia may be cured by simple closure of the internal inguinal ring during the same laparoscopic surgery. Disappearance of the vulvar bulging mass under pneumoperitoneal pressure confirms complete closure of the patent canal of Nuck. Overall, the technique involves straightforward surgery, a minimal degree of invasiveness, and virtually no postoperative discomfort. The outcome of this approach has been satisfactory over a 2-year follow-up period.

## Operative Technique

Inguinal hernias are approached by a 6 to 7 cm incision extending horizontally from the pubic tubercle and placed within the hair line. After opening the external oblique the sac is identified. In the female the round ligament which replaces the spermatic cord is excised with the sac if it is seen. No attempt is made to preserve the ilioinguinal or genitofemoral nerves if they traversed the operative area.

Direct sacs are treated by imbrication of the posterior wall of the canal. The repair of all inguinal hernias is then completed with an onlay of polypropylene mesh as in a standard Lichtenstein repair except that the mesh is not split laterally as there is no spermatic cord to accommodate (Fig. 12.2).

All inguinal incisions are closed with absorbable sutures; patients are discharged the same day and encouraged to return to normal activities as early as comfort allowed.

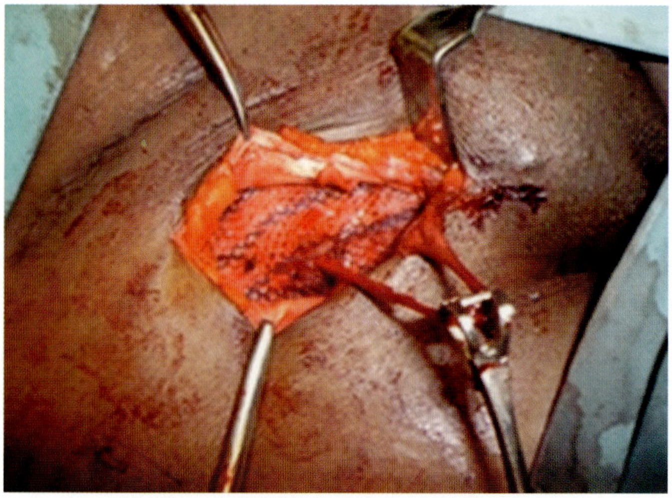

**Fig. 12.2:** Technique of hernia repair

# Chapter 13

# Pediatric Inguinal Hernia

## Inguinal Hernia in Children

### Introduction

Today, inguinal hernia repair is one of the most common pediatric operations performed. Inguinal hernia is a type of ventral hernia that occurs when an intra-abdominal structure, such as bowel or omentum, protrudes through a defect in the abdominal wall. Most hernias that are present at birth or in childhood are indirect inguinal hernias. Other less common types of ventral hernias include umbilical, epigastric, and incisional hernias (Figs 13.1A to D).

### Pathophysiology

The processus vaginalis is an outpouching of peritoneum attached to the testicle that trails behind as it descends

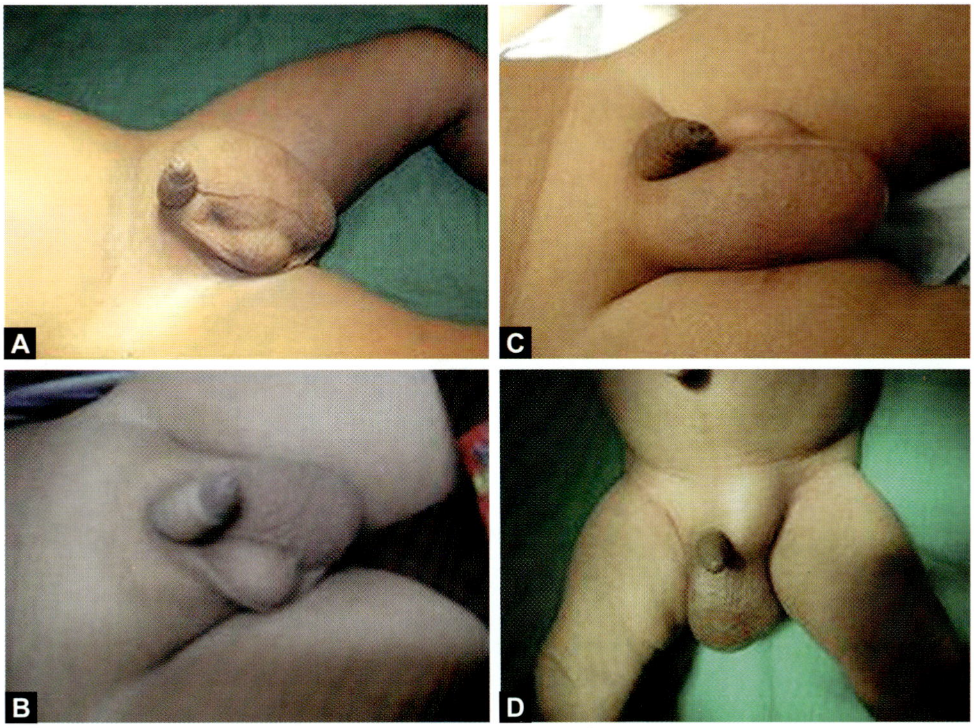

**Figs 13.1A to D:** Pediatric inguinal hernias

retroperitoneally into the scrotum. When obliteration of the processus vaginalis fails to occur, inguinal hernia results. A review of embryonic development of the inguinal region is important to understanding the pathophysiology and surgical management of inguinal hernias.

Although the sex of the embryo is determined at fertilization, the gonads do not begin to differentiate until 7 weeks' gestation. Primordial germ cells migrate along the dorsal mesentery of the gut. They arrive at the primitive gonads early in the fifth week of development and, during the sixth week, invade the genital ridges, which lie on the medial aspect of the mesonephros. The coelomic epithelium proliferates, and the underlying mesenchyme condenses, forming the primitive sex cords.

Under the influence of the Y chromosome, the cords in the male embryo proliferate to form the testes. Near the end of the second month, the testis and mesonephros are attached by the urogenital mesentery to the posterior abdominal wall. As the mesonephros degenerates, only the testis remains suspended. At its caudal end, the attachment is ligamentous and is known as the caudal genital ligament. The gubernaculum, a mesenchymal structure rich in extracellular matrices, also extends from the caudal pole of the testis. This structure attaches in the inguinal region between the differentiating internal and external oblique muscles prior to descent of the testes. As the testes begin to descend at about 28 weeks' gestation, an outgrowth of gubernaculum from the inguinal region grows toward the scrotal area, and as the testis passes through the inguinal canal, this portion of the gubernaculum comes in contact with the scrotal floor.

During this time, the peritoneum of the coelomic cavity is forming an evagination on each side of the midline into the ventral abdominal wall. This evagination, known as the processus vaginalis, follows the path of the gubernaculum testis into the scrotal swellings and forms, along with the muscle and fascia, the inguinal canal. The descent of the testes through the inguinal canal is thought to be regulated by both androgenic hormones produced by the fetal testis and mechanical factors resulting from increased abdominal pressure.

As each testis descends, the layers of the abdominal wall contribute to the layers of the spermatic cord. The internal spermatic fascia is a reflection of the transversalis fascia, the internal oblique muscle helps form the cremaster muscle, and the external spermatic fascia results from the external oblique aponeurosis. In addition, a reflected fold of the processus vaginalis covers each testis and becomes known as the visceral and parietal layers of the tunica vaginalis.

In the female embryo, the ovaries descend into the pelvis but do not leave the abdominal cavity. The upper portion of the gubernaculum becomes the ovarian ligament, and the lower portion becomes the round ligament, which travels through the inguinal ring into the labium majus. If the processus vaginalis remains patent, it extends into the labium majus and is known as the canal of Nuck.

Before birth, the layers of the processus vaginalis normally fuse, closing off the entrance into the inguinal canal from the abdominal cavity. In some individuals, the processus vaginalis remains patent through infancy, into childhood, and possibly even into adulthood. The precise cause of the obliteration of the processus vaginalis is unknown, but some studies indicate that calcitonin gene-related peptide (CGRP), released from the genitofemoral nerve, may have a role in the fusion.

When luminal obliteration fails to occur, a readymade sac is present where abdominal contents may herniate. Even when the processus vaginalis is patent, the entrance may be adequately covered by the internal oblique and transverse abdominal muscles, preventing escape of abdominal contents for many years. Failure of fusion can result not only in an inguinal hernia, but also in a communicating or noncommunicating hydrocele.

In infants, the most common type of hydrocele is the communicating type. A communicating hydrocele results when the proximal portion of the processus vaginalis remains patent, allowing fluid from the abdominal cavity to freely enter the scrotal sac. When closure is present proximally but fluid remains trapped within the tunica distally, a noncommunicating hydrocele results.

## Some Statistics

About 3 to 5% of healthy, full-term babies may be born with an inguinal hernia and one-third of hernias of infancy and childhood appear in the first 6 months of life. In premature infants the incidence of inguinal hernia is substantially increased, up to 30%. In just over 10% of cases, other members of the family have also had a hernia at birth or in infancy.

Right side hernias are more common than left. The figures are as follows:

| | |
|---|---|
| Right | 60% |
| Left | 25% |
| Both sides | 15% |

The occurrence of an inguinal hernia in boys is related to the development and descent of the testes. The testes develop within the abdomen and at around the seventh month of pregnancy they descend into the scrotum. On their way through the abdominal wall, they pass through the inguinal canal. After they reach the scrotum, the opening behind should close. Failure to close adequately results in a hernia with an opening remaining in the abdominal wall at this point.

## Mortality/Morbidity

An incarcerated or strangulated inguinal hernia can result in severe complications and even death. An incarcerated or strangulated inguinal and/or femoral hernia may also result in significant sequela, depending on which visceral structure is involved in the hernia sac. Such sequela can range from life-threatening complications to gonadal dysfunction, including intestinal necrosis and perforation, intestinal obstruction, intestinal stricture, testicular necrosis, testicular atrophy, ovarian necrosis, ovarian atrophy, and tubal stricture.

### Sex

Inguinal hernias are much more common in males than in females. The male-to-female ratio is estimated to be 4-8:1.

### Age

Premature infants are at an increased risk for inguinal hernia, with the incidence ranging from 7 to 30%. Moreover, the associated risk of incarceration is more than 60% in this population. Most pediatric ventral and inguinal hernias are detected in the first year of life. Occasionally, hernias may remain asymptomatic and unnoticed by the parents until later in life. Finding an adult patient with an indirect inguinal hernia that has been present since birth is not unusual.

### Etiology of Inguinal Hernias in Children

The etiology of inguinal hernia in children can be termed an abnormality of embryologic development of the fetus. However, some children may present with an acquired form of inguinal hernia, also called a direct inguinal hernia. In this type of hernia, weakness of the inguinal floor is present, which allows for protrusion of viscera from the abdominal cavity. The hernia sac is composed of the peritoneal fold that contains the hernia.

- The following are associated with an increased risk of inguinal hernia:
  - Prematurity and low birth weight (Incidence approaches 50%)
  - Urologic conditions
    - Cryptorchidism
    - Hypospadias
    - Epispadias
    - Exstrophy of the bladder
    - Ambiguous genitalia
  - Patent processus vaginalis, which may be present because of increased abdominal pressure due to ventriculoperitoneal shunts, peritoneal dialysis, or ascites
  - Abdominal wall defects
    - Gastroschisis
    - Omphalocele
  - Family history
    - Meconium peritonitis
    - Cystic fibrosis
    - Connective tissue disease
    - Mucopolysaccharidosis
    - Congenital dislocation of the hip
    - Ehlers-Danlos syndrome
    - Marfan syndrome
    - Cloacal exstrophy
    - Fetal hydrops
    - Liver disease with ascites
    - Ventriculoperitoneal shunting for hydrocephalus

### Fast Facts

- Figures regarding inguinal hernia incarceration indicate the following risk patterns:
  - Incarceration occurs in 17% of right-sided hernias and 7% of left-sided hernias.
  - More than 50% of cases of incarceration occur within the first 6 months of life; the risk gradually decreases after age 1 year.
  - Premature infants have twice the risk of incarceration than the general pediatric population.
  - More than two-thirds of all incarcerations occur in children younger than 1 year.
- Girls are more likely to develop incarceration of an inguinal hernia; the incidence in girls is 17.2%, whereas the incidence in boys is 12%.

# DIFFERENTIAL DIAGNOSES OF INGUINAL HERNIA IN CHILDREN

## Hydrocele and Hernia in Children Varicocele in Adolescents

### Other

- Inguinal adenitis
- Femoral adenitis
- Psoas abscess
- Saphenous varix
- Hydrocele
- Retractile testis
- Varicocele
- Testicular tumor
- Undescended testis

### Classification—Inguinal

Inguinal hernia in children can be divided into two types:
1. Complete scrotal (Total funicular hernia of Herzfeld)
2. Incomplete bubonocele (Partial funicular hernia of Herzfeld)

About 5% of inguinal hernias in male infants are of the complete variety.

### Clinical Examination

Inguinal hernias are most easily observed while the child is bearing down in a standing position. The bulge may worsen throughout the day and disappear when the child is lying down. If the history suggests that a hernia is present, but the practitioner is unable to observe the groin bulge, a positive diagnosis may be made by eliciting a "silk glove" sign (Figs 13.2A to C). While the child is in a supine position, the inguinal area should be palpated. When the cord structures are rolled against the pubic bone, the practitioner may feel layers of processus vaginalis slipping over one another, as if made of silk. Alternatively, the child's caregiver could bring in a photograph of the bulge to confirm the diagnosis.

### Management

- Less than one-year-old should be operated on as urgent elective cases
- Older one-year-old surgery is less urgent
- Can often be performed as a day case procedure

**Clinical Presentations**

1. Hallmark of an indirect inguinal hernia is a groin bulge at the top of the scrotum or within the scrotum.
2. Bulge most visible during periods of increased intra-abdominal pressure.
3. Hernia may reduce spontaneously or may be manually reduced.
4. Physical examination may only reveal a thickened spermatic cord (silk-glove) sign.
5. Communicating hydroceles frequently present with a history of a scrotal mass that changes in size; the scrotal size increases during crying, defecation and decreases after periods of inactivity, e.g. sleeping. This is due to the exchange of fluid from the peritoneal cavity to the scrotum through a narrow communication (persistent patency of the processus).
6. In males, the most common content is bowel, in females, the ovary.
7. Hernias are often first discovered by parents who notice a bulge in groin area during diaper changes.
8. Most hernias are painless, but at times the initial presentation may be an incarcerated loop of bowel.
9. Hydroceles may be differentiated from incarcerated hernias by the absence of pain and symptoms of bowel obstruction.
10. Increased fat in the pubic area may make the diagnosis difficult. A hernia not felt on careful examination is unlikely to incarcerate.
11. Must differentiate from retractable testes that may appear as an inguinal bulge.
12. Most hydroceles disappear during the first year of life.

- Inguinal herniotomy is performed
- Transverse incision made in lowest inguinal skin crease
- 20% children develop a contralateral hernia
- Controversial as to whether contralateral exploration should be performed.

### Irreducible Hernias

- Initial management should be with reduction by taxis
- Required gentle pressure usually without sedation
- Forcible reduction under general anesthesia is contraindicated
- If remains irreducible should be operated on within 24 hours
- If intestinal obstruction present preoperative resuscitation is essential.

### Surgical Care

For inguinal hernia, elective herniorrhaphy is indicated to prevent incarceration and subsequent strangulation. Hernia repair is an outpatient procedure in the otherwise healthy full-term infant or child. Postpone the operation in the event of upper respiratory tract infection, otitis media, or significant rash in the groin.

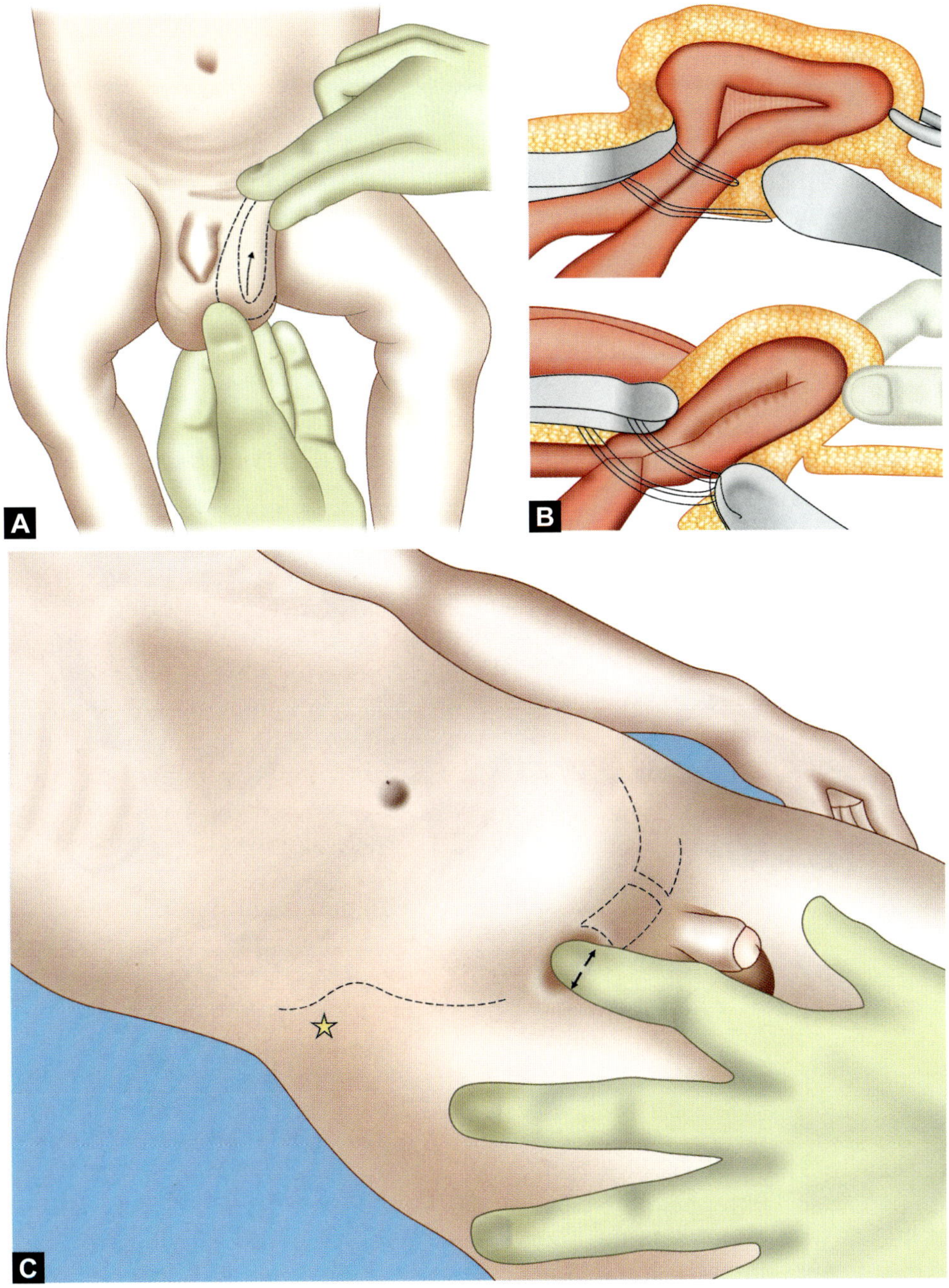

**Figs 13.2A to C:** Silk glove sign

- The abdominal wall in the groin area is made up of different structures going from deep to superficial layers (Figs 13.1 and 13.2):
  1. Peritoneum—the lining of the abdominal cavity (becomes the hernia sac)
  2. Subperitoneal fat—fat beneath the peritoneum
  3. Transversalis fascia—sheet of fibrous tissue that envelops the peritoneum
  4. Transversus abdominis muscle
  5. Internal oblique muscle
  6. External oblique muscle
  7. Subcutaneous fat
  8. Skin.

Although adult surgical procedures for correction of inguinal hernias are numerous and varied, only three procedures are necessary for the surgical repair of

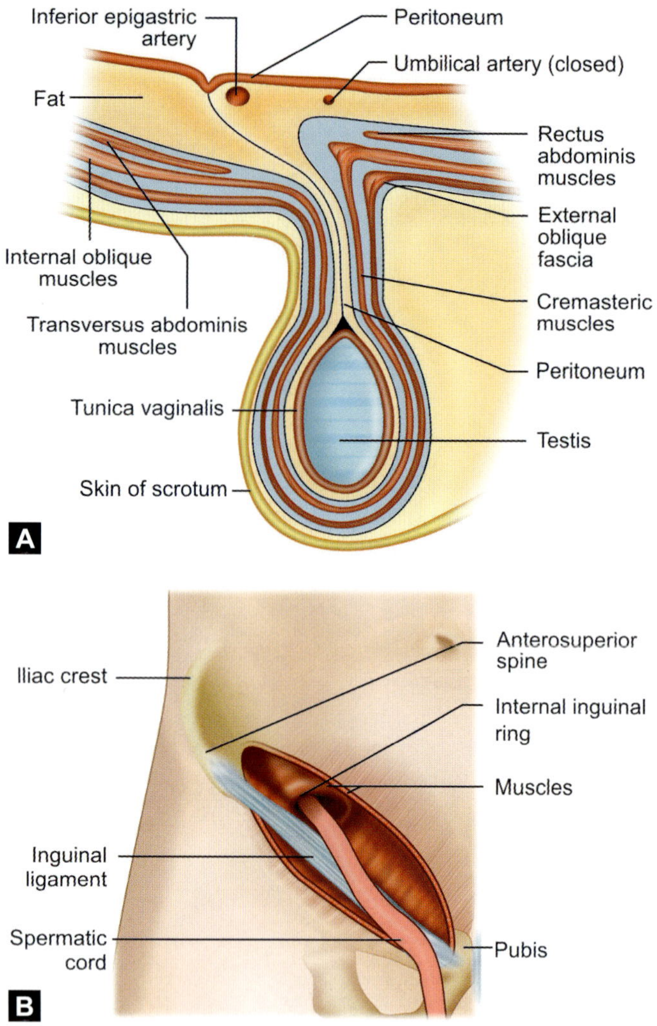


**Figs 13.3A and B:** Layers and anatomy of pediatric inguinal canal

indirect inguinal hernias in children: (1) high ligation and excision of the patent sac with anatomic closure, (2) high ligation of the sac with plication of the floor of the inguinal canal (the transversalis fascia), and (3) high ligation of the sac combined with reconstruction of the floor of the canal (Figs 13.3A and B).

*The first procedure*, high ligation and excision of the patent sac with anatomic closure, is the most common operative technique. It is appropriate when the hernia is not very large and has not been present for long.

*The second procedure*, high ligation of the sac with plication of the floor of the inguinal canal (the transversalis fascia), is necessary when the hernia has repeatedly passed through the internal ring and has enlarged the ring, thus partially destroying the inguinal floor.

*The third procedure*, high ligation of the sac combined with reconstruction of the floor of the canal, is occasionally necessary in small children with large hernias or when the hernia is long-standing. The protruding hernia causes gradual enlargement of the ring, progressing to complete breakdown of the transversalis fascia that forms the floor of the inguinal canal. The McVay or Bassini technique of herniorrhaphy is preferred.

## Repair of the Pediatric Inguinal Hernia

In babies and young children, the inguinal canal has not yet developed its oblique adult anatomy. The superficial ring is directly anterior to the deep ring and the sac is indirect. There is no acquired deformity of the canal. In these cases the fascia transversalis is normal and a simple herniotomy is all that is necessary. Straightforward inguinal herniotomy should give a 100% success.

- *Position:* The patient should be placed on his back at the operating table with his or her legs slightly abducted. A light cotton blanket (or warming device) lies over the chest and upper abdomen and a similar on the lower limbs. This prevents heat loss on operating table. The hernia contents must be completely reduced into the peritoneal cavity before the procedure.
- *Draping:* Drapes are applied so that the groin area and scrotum are exposed throughout the operation.
- *Incision:* A horizontal transverse incision is made in the transverse skin crease just above and medial to the external inguinal ring.The incision should be 1.0 to 1.5 cm long. The superficial ring and the emerging spermatic cord can be readily palpated under anesthesia. The site for incision and the direction of the subsequent dissection are thus confirmed. Next, identify and incise the Scarpa fascia. In young children, the Scarpa fascia may be confused with the aponeurosis of the external oblique. However, the Scarpa fascia is smooth, does not have any fibrous bands, and does not glisten like the aponeurosis. In addition, a layer of fat is found beneath the Scarpa fascia but not under the external oblique.
- *Dissection (External ring):* The superficial ring and cord, which have already been identified by palpation, are approached by gently opening the

subcutaneous fat with a blunt hemostat. At this stage the superficial epigastric vessels are encountered and picked up in light hemostats, divided with scissors and ligated.

- *Dissection (Cord):* Once the cord has been identified its covering must be opened to give access to the hernia sac. The sac lies on the anterosuperior aspect of the cord as it emerges from the external inguinal ring. One should be careful not to injure the minute ilioinguinal nerve during this dissection. It is covered first by diaphanous external spermatic fascia, then by cremasteric fascia, which is readily identified by its neat intertwining pink fascicles of muscles, and more deeply by the very delicate internal spermatic fascia. These structures—the three layers of spermatic fascia are separated from the enclosed contents of the cord by careful blunt dissection with a fine hemostat. "Atrick of the trade" is most useful here—a closed hemostat is pushed through the fascial layers into the cord and then opened slowly in the long axis so that a rent is made. If hernia sac is present, it is immediately apparent in the rent. The rent is held open with the hemostat and the sac grasped with a second hemostat placed between the open blades of the first. The sac can be identified lying on the anterosuperior aspect of the contents of the cord. It is pale blue and much thicker than the fascial coverings of the cord. The most difficult maneuver in the operation must be now carried out. The components of the cord are in the posterolateral position. Therefore, one should not stray far from this location to minimize the risk of injury to the cord structures. The sac is either complete (total funicular hernia), i.e. it extends to the scrotum and encompasses the testicle, or incomplete (partial funicular hernia), that is it extends along only part of the length of the cord.

If the sac is complete, its posterior wall must be separated from the other cord contents—the vas deferens, the testicular artery and the pampiniform plexus of veins. This must be done very gently. Above all, the vas or pampiniform vessels must never be grasped in forceps. Its successful accomplishment is a benchmark by which surgical competence can be measured. First, internal spermatic fascia fixing the pampiniform plexus to the sac is divided by scalpel.

Then fine hemostat is gently insinuated between each structure and the thin peritoneal sac wall in turn to push them off the sac. When each structure has been pushed off, the proximal sac is held in hemostat and sac divided across. The distal sac, testicle, cord can now be manipulated back into place in the scrotum. Gentle traction on the testicle in the scrotum at this time will confirm that it has been returned to its normal site.

- *Division of sac:* The sac can then be clamped and divided. The proximal sac is mobilized to the internal ring, which is often signified by the presence of retroperitoneal fat.
- Once the sac is confirmed to be empty, it is twisted on itself and doubly suture-ligated with sutures (e.g. 4-0 or silk or vicryl sutures can be used).
- *Closure:* If the ring is not enlarged, the distal sac is opened to drain any residual fluid and the sac is partially excised. Then, closure is accomplished in layers with absorbable sutures.
- If the internal ring is enlarged, the cord must be elevated from its bed with a soft rubber drain. A silk suture between the transversalis fascia and the inguinal ligament can be used to tighten the ring. Alternatively, a modified Bassini type of repair can be used to reinforce the inguinal floor.
- *Reinforcement:* If destruction of the canal floor is present, a reconstructive procedure, such as that of Bassini or McVay, is necessary.
- The McVay type of repair incorporates a relaxing incision in the rectus sheath that allows the conjoined tendon to be pulled down to the Cooper ligament and the femoral sheath.
- The incised aponeurosis of the external abdominal oblique muscle is closed with interrupted 4-0 or 5-0 silk sutures or a continuous 4-0 polyglycolic acid suture.
- Typically one or two interrupted absorbable sutures are used to close the Scarpa fascia. The skin can be closed with absorbable sutures.

*Inguinal hernia surgery in girls:* In little girls, sometimes an ovary can slip into a similar weakness in the same general area, and may slip all the way down into the labium majorum. The ovary also can get twisted and strangulated, so it gets fixed promptly as well.

Surgeons have long believed that if a male infant or child develops an inguinal hernia on one side of the body, the other side should be explored and repaired if an early defect is found. A large study in Japan reported in the Journal of Pediatric Surgery in July 1998 refutes this idea. The low (11.7%) eventual incidence of subsequent hernia on the other side contrasted with the fairly significant risk of damage to reproductive structures on the side of exploration is high enough to lead the researchers to recommend: leave the apparently normal side alone.

- In girls, a sliding hernia may contain the ovary or a portion of the fallopian tube. These structures should be carefully dissected from the internal wall of the sac before suture ligation. An alternate procedure involves incising the sac along the ovary and tube on either side and folding the flap into the peritoneum. A pursestring suture can then be used to close the sac. In the female, the sac can be sutured closed after division of the round ligament because no important structures pass through the inguinal ring.

## Exploration of the Contralateral Side

- The question of when the contralateral side needs to be explored is much debated. Advantages for exploration of the opposite side during repair of a known inguinal hernia include the following:
  - Existence of a patent processus vaginalis on the contralateral side (also called asymptomatic hernia) in a significant number of patients
  - Avoidance of second surgery and anesthetic if contralateral patent processus vaginalis becomes symptomatic
  - Eliminated cost of second surgery, if needed.

### *Disadvantages*

- Occasional injury to the vas or testicular vessels during surgical exploration
- Increased operating time for contralateral procedure
- May be unnecessary in as many as 70% of all patients undergoing hernia surgery.

### *Management of Incarcerated Hernia*

- When an incarceration is encountered, manual reduction should be attempted if the patient has no signs of systemic toxicity, including leukocytosis, severe tachycardia, abdominal distention, bilious vomiting, and discoloration of the entrapped viscera. If the patient appears toxic, emergent surgical exploration is necessary.
- Some authors have proposed the use of relaxation maneuvers to relieve the pressure on the neck of the hernia sac and to allow for the incarceration to resolve spontaneously. This involves placement of the sedated patient in the Trendelenburg position of 30 to 40° to apply mild traction on the entrapped viscera, facilitating reduction. If the hernia has not spontaneously reduced during the 1 to 2 hours of sedation, gentle but forceful manual reduction by an experienced physician must be attempted.
- As a rule, forceful manual reduction is recommended in all cases of incarcerated hernia, unless the clinician suspects the possibility of inguinal hernia strangulation. Such attempts are successful in more than 90% of cases and pose minimal risk to the entrapped structure. Successful reduction of an incarcerated inguinal hernia results in immediate patient comfort, relief of obstruction, and prevention of strangulation. Immediate surgery is performed if the reduction is unsuccessful; otherwise, elective operation is scheduled within 24 to 72 hours after reduction because recurrent incarceration is quite common.

### *Manual Reduction of Incarcerated Hernia*

- Once incarceration of an inguinal hernia has been confidently diagnosed, the parents must be informed that reduction of the hernia will be attempted. The patient is placed in the supine position and his or her pelvis is grasped gently but firmly by an assistant to prevent any lateral movement of the buttocks. Depending on the side of the hernia, the ipsilateral leg is then externally rotated and completely flexed into the frog position. This position causes the external ring to ascend so that it more nearly, but not completely, overrides the internal inguinal ring.
- Once both of these conditions have been established, the first 2 fingers of the guiding hand are placed over the hernial bulge and overriding the upper margin of the external inguinal ring in such a fashion as to prevent the hernia subluxating upwards and over the margin of the ring. Next, the apex of the hernia is grasped between the first 2 fingers and thumb of the reducing hand, and prolonged, steady, firm pressure is applied.
- This last point is crucial; the reducing hand must not be withdrawn after only a few seconds. One indication of the correct application of this technique is the onset of stiffness in the first 2 fingers and an ache in the thenar eminence. After a given interval that may take minutes, a sudden reduction of the hernia occurs with an almost audible thud, accompanied by complete relief in the patient. Using this method of

reduction, open operation of incarcerated inguinal hernia is a rare event. By successfully reducing an incarcerated inguinal hernia, the open operation can be accomplished electively and with decreased morbidity.

- *Management of hernia strangulation:* Once an incarcerated hernia becomes strangulated, reduction without operative intervention is not possible. Because of significant swelling from the compromised bowel, the presence of intestinal ischemia secondary to incarceration precludes the possibility of reducing the hernia back into the peritoneal cavity. In such cases, immediate operative intervention is indicated, and the viability of the intestine must be carefully assessed at the time of surgery. If necrosis has developed, resect the affected segment of bowel. Incidence of hernia recurrence after emergent surgery for incarceration or strangulation is typically much higher than that reported for elective hernia repair.
- *Management of umbilical hernia:* Because many umbilical hernias spontaneously close in the first few years of life, elective surgical repair is rarely indicated before school age. Moreover, the occurrence of umbilical hernia incarceration is quite rare. Umbilical hernia repair is quite simple and is typically performed in an outpatient surgical suite. Simple primary closure of the fascial defect under the umbilicus is easily performed using absorbable sutures. A mesh is rarely necessary, only in cases of an extremely large umbilical hernia.

## Laparoscopic Needle-assisted Repair of Inguinal Hernia

- A new and innovative technique for repair of inguinal hernia in young children using a total laparoscopic approach has been described. The technique is described as laparoscopic needle-assisted repair.
- Standard laparoscopy is performed via a small 5 mm umbilical port with a 5 mm, 30º-angled laparoscope. Once the indirect inguinal hernia is identified, the laparoscopic repair is performed.
- The first step is to clearly define the inguinal hernia and the lateral and medial border of the open internal inguinal ring. This is accomplished by probing the groin region with a small 22-gauge needle.
- Under careful laparoscopic-guided visualization, a 22-gauge Tuhoe spinal needle with a 2-0 Prolene suture thread inside the barrel of the needle is inserted and passed underneath the peritoneum and the inguinal ligament, lateral to the internal inguinal ring, away from the spermatic vessels and vas. All needle movements are performed by the operating surgeon from outside the body cavity under direct laparoscopic control so that the position of the tip of the needle can be precisely placed at the desired location inside the peritoneal cavity. The Prolene thread is than pushed through the barrel of the needle into the abdominal cavity, creating an internal "loop." The needle is pulled out, leaving the Prolene loop of the thread inside the abdomen.
- From the outside, the patient's body, one of the threaded ends is introduced again into the barrel of the spinal needle, and the needle is passed through the same skin puncture point, through the medial aspect of the internal inguinal ring, under the peritoneum. Again, the vas and vessels are mobilized to stay away from the needle, in order to prevent any injury. Once the tip of the needle is in the desired position next to the loop of Prolene, the thread is pushed in so that it passes through the loop. At this point, the thread-loop is pulled out of the abdomen, with the thread end caught by the loop. In this way, the suture thread of Prolene is placed around the internal inguinal ring under the peritoneum, creating a complete purse-string suture with the ends of the suture coming out of the same skin needle hole in the groin region. The knot is tied to close the internal inguinal ring and hernia opening. With this technique the knot is buried in the subcutaneous tissue.
- If an open internal inguinal ring is identified in the contralateral side, it is closed using the same technique through a small needle hole in the opposite groin.

## Further Inpatient Care

Most patients who undergo elective repair of an inguinal or umbilical hernia are discharged from the hospital shortly after surgery. Overnight observation is indicated only in small premature babies who are at risk for postoperative apnea. Such patients are usually admitted for 24-hour observation and monitoring in the hospital.

## Complications

- Few complications result from operative repair of an inguinal hernia. Possible consequences of hernia repair include decreased testicular size (£ 20% of patients), testicular atrophy (1-2%), vas injury (<1%), and development of sperm-agglutinating antibodies. The risk of gonadal injury in females is low. Fortunately, in the hands of pediatric surgeons, such complications are quite rare.

- The incidence of wound infection is 1 to 2%.
- Hernia recurrence rates are less than 1% when experienced pediatric surgeons perform the operation. Factors associated with recurrence of inguinal hernia include an unrecognized tear in the sac, failure to repair an enlarged inguinal ring, damage to the canal and inguinal floor, infection, history of incarceration, and conditions producing increased intra-abdominal pressure, such as chronic respiratory problems.
- The vas deferens and ilioinguinal nerve occasionally may be injured and should be repaired with 7-0 or 8-0 Maxon sutures. This may be technically difficult because of the extremely small vas lumen not traversed by semen. One infertility expert advises marking the ends of the vas with permanent suture and performing vasovasotomy after puberty with a 2-layer closure. It is also important to remember that the finding of vas or epididymis on the surgical pathology report does not necessarily imply injury because embryonal müllerian remnants have been recognized in 1 to 6% of surgical specimens. Specific histologic features of the remnant include a smaller diameter and failure to show a prominent muscular wall with Masson trichrome staining.

## Prognosis

Overall prognosis is excellent; most patients do extremely well after operative repair of their inguinal hernia. Mortality is extremely rare but, unfortunately, continues to be reported as a consequence of delayed recognition of an incarcerated and strangulated inguinal hernia.

# Chapter 14

# Femoral Hernia

## Surgery

Femoral hernias occur just below the inguinal ligament, when abdominal contents pass through a naturally occurring weakness called the femoral canal (Fig. 14.1).

## Anatomy

The femoral canal is located below the inguinal ligament on the lateral aspect of the pubic tubercle. It is bounded by the inguinal ligament anteriorly, pectineal ligament posteriorly, lacunar ligament medially, and the femoral vein laterally. It normally contains a few lymphatics, loose areolar tissue and occasionally a lymph node called Cloquet's node. The function of this canal appears to be to allow the femoral vein to expand when necessary to accommodate increased venous return from the leg during periods of activity. Femoral hernias are more common in females than in males (Fig. 14.2).

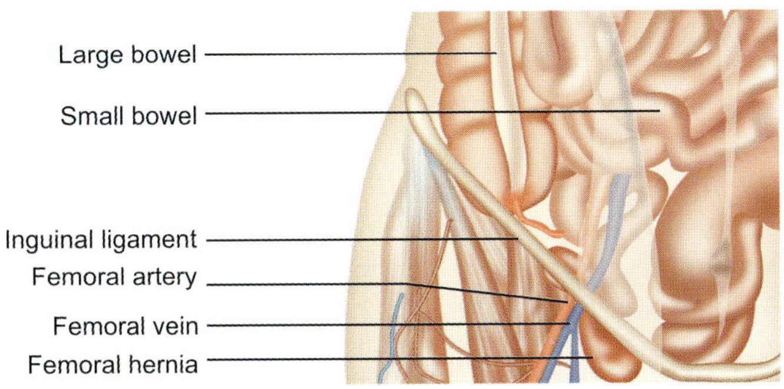


**Fig. 14.1:** Femoral hernia

The borders of the femoral triangle are the inguinal ligament (superior), the sartorious muscle (lateral) and the adductor longus muscle (medial). It contains, from lateral to medial, the femoral nerve and branches, the femoral artery and branches, and the femoral vein and tributaries. The following specializations of abdominal fascia in this region are also important:

- *Femoral sheath*: A diverticulum of the transversalis fascia. It wraps the femoral vessels for the first 2 or 3 cm of their trip through the femoral triangle. The femoral sheath does not wrap around the femoral nerve. It has three compartments. The lateral compartment contains the femoral artery, the middle compartment has the femoral vein, and the medial compartment is designated as the femoral canal.
- *Femoral canal*: The medial compartment of the femoral sheath. It usually contains fat, a few lymph vessels, and maybe a deep inguinal lymph node (node of Cloquet).
- *Femoral ring*: The opening at the superior end of the femoral canal.

The adductor canal allows passage of the femoral vessels and the saphenous nerve through the middle one-third of the thigh. The quadriceps femoris muscles are separated from the adductor muscles by a deep groove. Put a roof on that baby, let's say the sartorious muscle, and you have the adductor canal. The canal ends at the adductor hiatus, which is a split in the adductor magnus muscle.

The femoral artery supplies a major portion of the thigh (analogously, the femoral vein drains a good deal of the thigh). The femoral artery gives off the superficial epigastric artery, the superficial circumflex

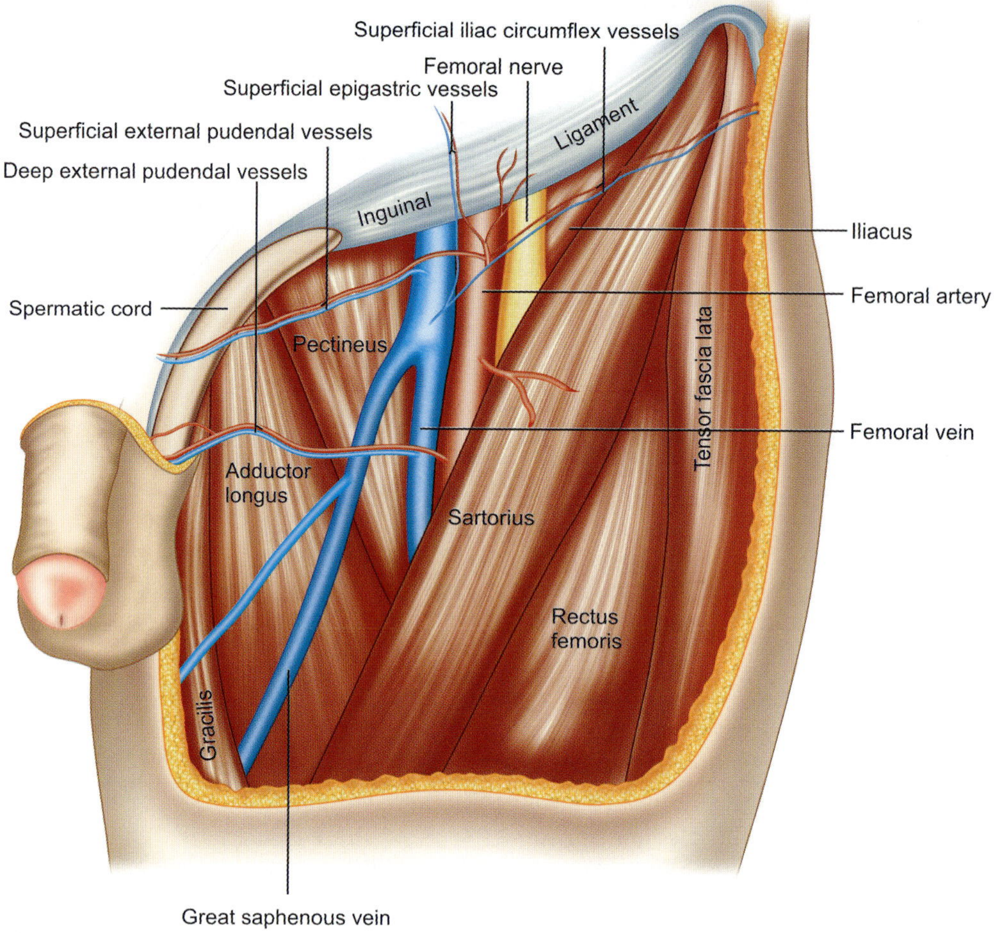


**Fig. 14.2:** Anatomy of femoral canal

iliac artery, the superficial external pudendal artery (all three just distal to the inguinal ligament), the deep external pudendal artery, the deep femoral artery, and the descending genicular artery. The largest and most important of these is the deep femoral artery.

The deep femoral artery supplies the hip joint, proximal thigh, and posterior thigh, including the neck of the femur. It gives off two important branches. The medial femoral circumflex artery supplies the iliopsoas muscle, pectineus muscle, and the hip joint via ascending and descending branches. The lateral femoral circumflex artery supplies the lateral hip, thigh, and knee via ascending, transverse, and descending branches. The descending branch anastomoses with both the descending genicular branch of the femoral artery as well as the lateral superior genicular branch of the popliteal artery, to provide collateral circulation to the knee (Latin, poples = ham of the knee, genu = knee).

The obturator artery supplies the medial thigh and hip, including the head of the femur (to a limited degree). It accomplishes this via anterior and posterior branches.

## Femoral Hernia

Femoral hernia is always acquired and descends through the femoral canal beneath Poupart's ligament to make its appearance at the saphenous opening on the thigh. Beneath the inner end of Poupart's ligament is the iliopectineal line of the horizontal ramus of the pubic bone. The two form an angle with the spine of the pubis as its apex. Gimbernat's ligament is the prolongation of Poupart's ligament from the spine of the pubis for about 2 cm (3/4 inch) out on the iliopectineal line. From the iliopectineal line the pectineus muscle proceeds downward and outward beneath Poupart's ligament to below and behind the lesser trochanter of the femur. Farther out beneath Poupart's ligament run the femoral vein and artery, the latter being to the outer side of the vein. Between the femoral vein and Gimbernat's ligament is left a space 1 to 2 cm (2/5 to 4/5 inch) wide. This space is called the femoral canal. It is through this canal or opening that femoral hernia descends. The femoral sheath is the continuation downward of the transversalis fascia which is prolonged from the interior of the pelvis over the femoral artery and vein and between the vein and Gimbernat's ligament so as to form three compartments. The outer contains the femoral artery, the middle the femoral vein, and the inner is the femoral canal. The femoral canal is from 1 to 2 cm (2/5 to 4 inch) long and runs from the abdominal side of Poupart's ligament to the upper edge of the saphenous opening and lies between the femoral vein and Gimbernat's ligament. Its lower extremity is closed by the meeting of its sides. Above, or superficial to it, is Poupart's ligament, and beneath it is the horizontal ramus of the pubis and pectineal fascia covering the pectineus muscle. It is filled with loose connective tissue, fat, and lymphatics, and sometimes contains a lymphatic node, forming all together what has been called the septum crurale. It will thus be seen that the septum crurale is continuous with the subperitoneal fatty tissue (Fig. 14.3).

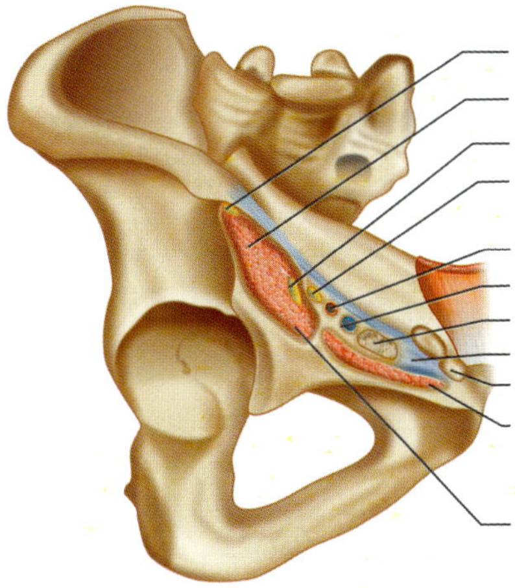


**Fig. 14.3:** Crural arch and the structures which pass beneath it

## Coverings of a Femoral Hernia

When a femoral hernia descends, the intestine pushes in front of it the peritoneum, septum crurale (subperitoneal tissue), and the femoral sheath (transversalis fascia) and makes its appearance at the saphenous opening. The cribriform fascia closing the saphenous opening gives it a covering, and also the subcutaneous tissue and skin above.

## Saphenous Opening

This has its centre 4 cm (1¼ inch) below and to the outer side of the spine of the pubis. Its margin blends above with Poupart's ligament to proceed to the spine of the pubis. Its outer and upper edge is marked, forming the falciform process or ligament (of Burns). The upper inner portion of the falciform process is attached to the iliopectineal line and spine of the pubis and, blending with Poupart's ligament above, is called Gimbernat's ligament (ligamentum lacunare).

The part of the fascia lata forming the falciform process thins out over the femoral artery and becomes the cribriform fascia (fascia cribrosa) as it passes from the inner side of the femoral artery on to the femoral vein to blend with the pubic fascia to the inner side. The superficial epigastric, superficial circumflex iliac, and superficial external pubic arteries and veins all pierce this cribriform fascia, as do also the superficial lymphatics and the long or internal saphenous vein.

- The saphenous opening (fossa ovalis).
- View of the inguinal and femoral regions from within; the peritoneum has been removed (Fig. 14.4).

## Causes of Femoral Hernia

- Metabolic, storage disorders
  - Obesity, massive
  - Obesity
- Deficiency disorders
  - Malnutrition/Starvation
- Anatomic, foreign body, structural disorders
  - Hernia, femoral
- Functional, physiologic variant disorders
  - Coughing, vigorous/effects
  - Heavy lifting
  - Weight lifting activity
  - Weight loss

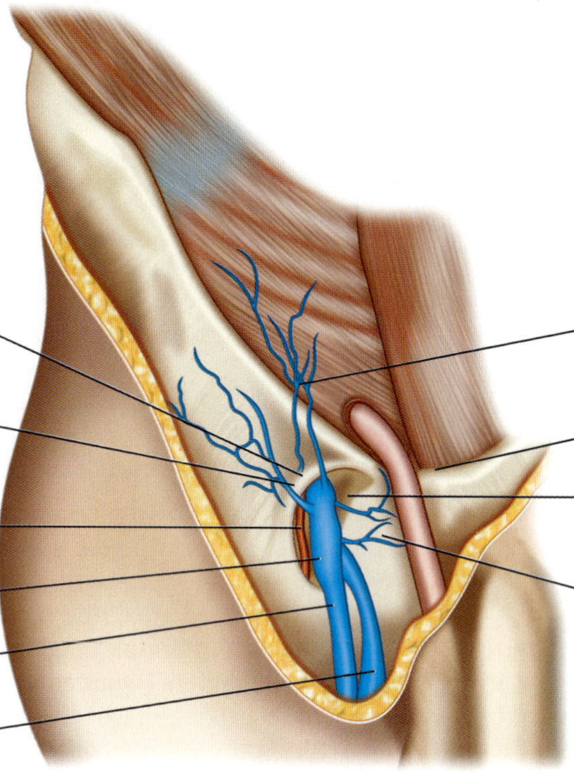


**Fig. 14.4:** Veins of femoral canal

## Demographics

Femoral hernias are a relatively uncommon type, accounting for only 3% of all hernias. While femoral hernias can occur in both males and females, almost all of them develop in women because of the wider bone structure of the female pelvis. Femoral hernias usually grow larger over time; any activity that involves straining, such as heavy lifting or a chronic cough, may cause the hernia to enlarge. Poor abdominal muscle tone,obesity, and pregnancy also increase a woman's risk of developing a femoral hernia. Most femoral hernias develop on only one side of the patient's abdomen, but about 15% of femoral hernias are bilateral. These bilateral hernias are more likely to become strangulated. An additional 20% of femoral hernias become incarcerated (Figs 14.5A and B).

Femoral hernias are more common in adults than in children. Those that do occur in children are more likely to be associated with a connective tissue disorder or with conditions that increase intra-abdominal pressure. Seventy percent of pediatric cases of femoral hernias occur in infants under the age of one.

### Classification

One subtype, De Garengeot's hernia, has been described. This is a vermiform appendix trapped within the hernial sac.

#### *Signs and Symptoms*

They typically present as a groin lump. They may or may not be associated with pain. Often, they present with a varying degree of complication ranging from irreducibility through intestinal obstruction to frank gangrene of contained bowel. The incidence of strangulation in femoral hernias is high. A femoral hernia has often been found to be the cause of unexplained small bowel obstruction.

The obvious finding may be a lump in the groin. Cough impulse is often absent and should not be relied on solely when making a diagnosis of femoral hernia. The lump is more globular than the pear shaped lump of the inguinal hernia. The bulk of a femoral hernia lies below an imaginary line drawn between the anterior superior iliac spine and the pubic tubercle (which essentially

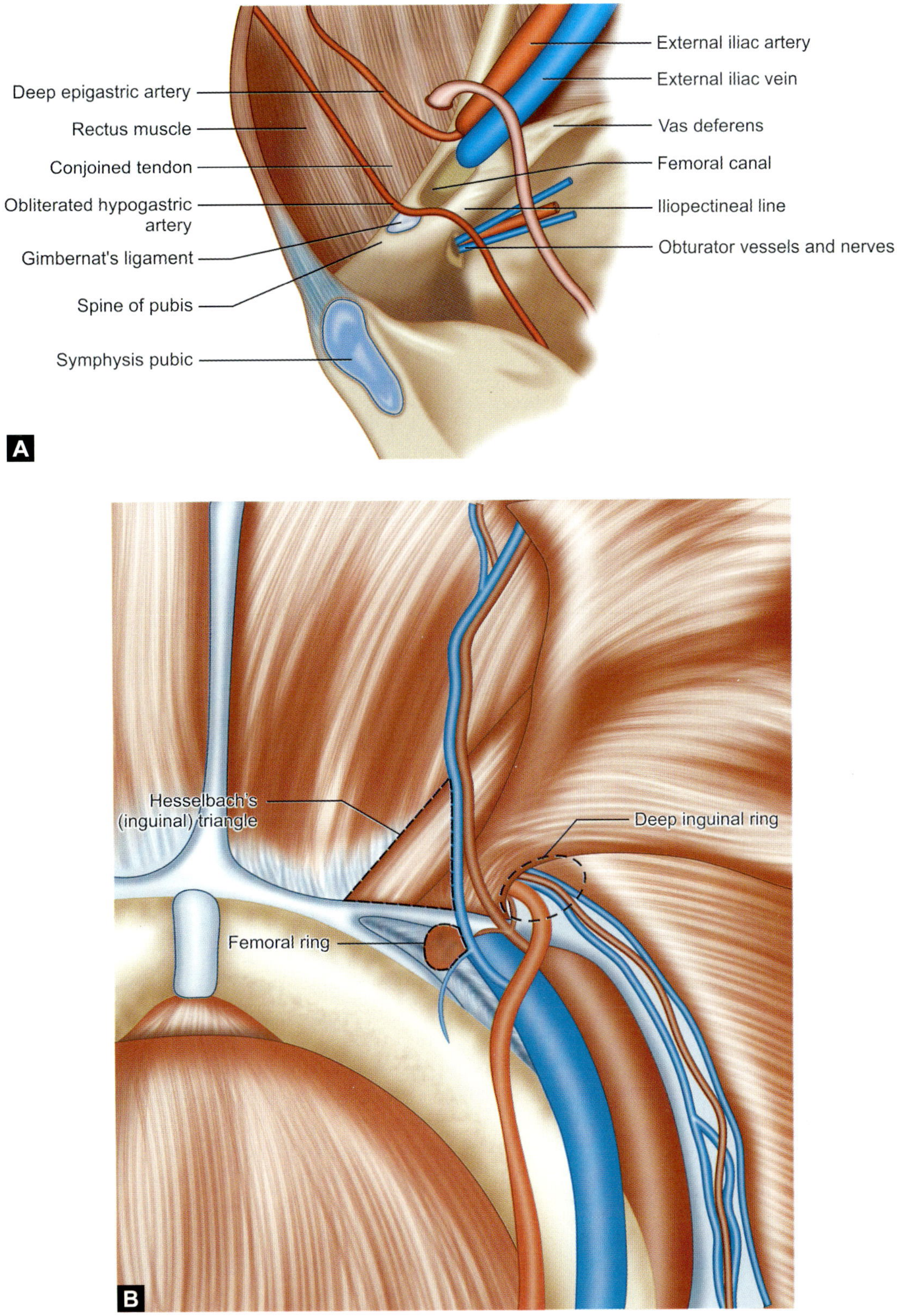


**Figs 14.5A and B:** Arteries in femoral canal

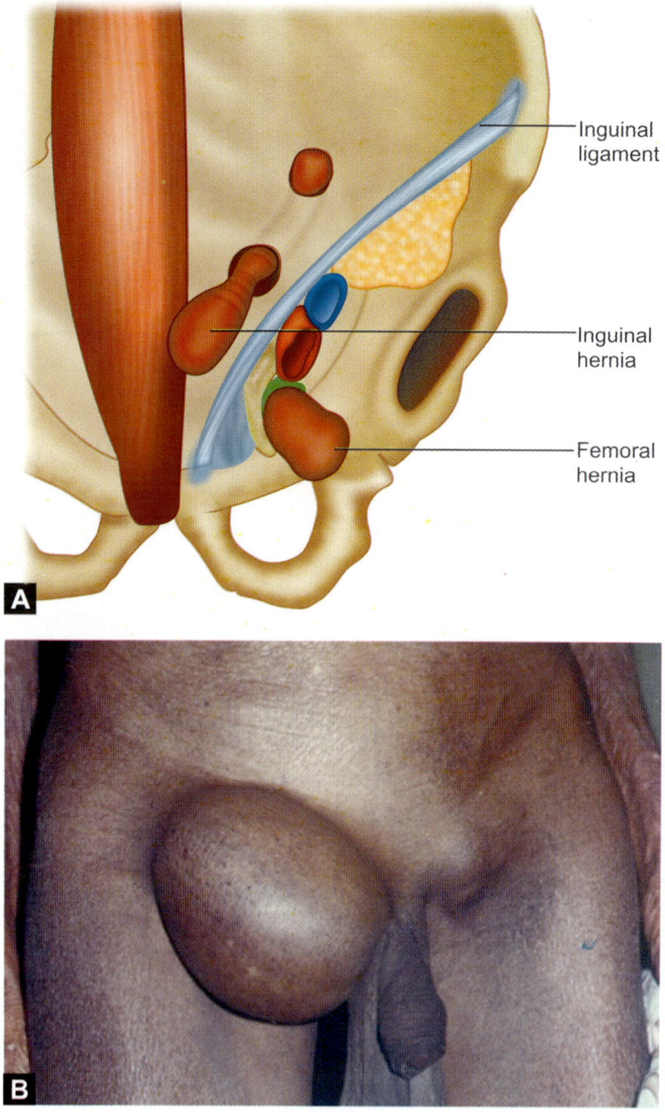


Figs 14.6A and B: Femoral hernia

represents the inguinal ligament) whereas an inguinal hernia starts above this line. Nonetheless, it is often impossible to distinguish the two preoperatively.

### *Diagnosis*

The diagnosis is largely a clinical one, generally done by physical examination of the groin. However, in obese patients, imaging in the form of ultrasonography, CT or MRI may aid in the diagnosis. An abdominal X-ray showing small bowel obstruction in a female patient with a painful groin lump needs no further investigation. Several other conditions have a similar presentation and must be considered when forming the diagnosis: inguinal hernia, an enlarged inguinal lymph node, aneurysm of the femoral artery, saphena varix, and an abscess of the psoas.

**Clinical Tips**

1. All patients with a hernia should be examined standing up then lying down.
2. Both sides must be examined.
3. All possible hernia sites should be examined
4. The patient is asked to cough with their head turned away from the examiner and any cough impulse is noted.
5. Then the hernia or swelling is palpated to confirm whether it is a hernia. Reduction is attempted by gentle pressure.
6. In overweight patients, the hernia may be difficult to see or even palpate. Both the external ring and the femoral canal can be examined with the tip of the fingers and the patient coughing. Sometimes, an squelch can be felt.

A differential diagnosis should be considered.

## Femoral Hernias (Figs 14.6A and B)

- Inguinal hernia
- Lymph nodes
- Lipomata
- Abscess.

Femoral and inguinal hernias can occasionally occur together therefore must examine both sites, the inguinal canal and the femoral canal.

**Clinical Tips**

*Note*: The large femoral hernia expands and actually appears to be anterior to the femoral vein as well. This is important when making a surgical incision.

Differential diagnosis of a strangulated femoral hernia is an abscess in the groin.

## Management of Femoral Hernias

Absolutely surgery is always advised for femoral hernias as there is hardly any truss that can support femoral hernias and chances of strangulation in femoral hernias are very high. The strangulation of femoral hernias carry a high degree of morbidity.

Femoral hernias, like most other hernias, usually need operative intervention. This should ideally be done as an elective (nonemergency) procedure. However, because of the high incidence of complications, femoral hernias often need emergency surgery.

## Surgery

Surgery may be performed under general or regional anesthesia. Three approaches have been described.

1. Lockwood's infrainguinal approach
2. Lotheissen's transinguinal approach
3. McEvedy's high approach.

## Lockwood's Infrainguinal Approach

Charles Barrett Lockwood (September 23, 1856-November 8, 1914) was a British surgeon and anatomist who practiced surgery at St Bartholomew's Hospital in London. Lockwood was a member of the Royal College of Surgeons.

Lockwood is remembered for his surgical work with femoral and inguinal hernias. He developed an infra-inguinal approach for femoral hernia operations that is known today as the low approach or Lockwood's operation. In 1893, he published an important book titled *Radical Cure of Femoral and Inguinal Hernia*.

### *Preoperative Management*

In the uncomplicated case no special preoperative management is required. The bladder is frequently a sliding component of the medial wall of the femoral hernia, and preoperative catheterization is sensible precaution.

In strangulated or obstructed hernia, nasogastric aspiration and fluid balance correction is essential.

### *Anesthesia (Figs 14.7 to 14.12)*

General anesthesia is preferred, however, local anesthesia can be employed.

- *Position*: Patient is placed supine on operating table and head tilt is 15° down.
- *Draping*: In normal circumstances the draping is done only to the groin but in case of strangulation the whole abdomen with groin is exposed for possible requirement of laparotomy.
- *Incision*: A 6 cm long and parallel to inguinal ligament incision is taken possibly directly over the femoral hernia. Incision is deepened dissecting the fascia and subcutaneous fat till the coverings of the sac are seen.
- *Sac mobilization*: The sac is coming from the femoral canal contains coverings of (from inside out) fascia transversalis, extraperitoneal fat, attenuated cribriform fascia, femoral fascial layer. The fundus of the sac is lying at the inguinal ligament. With a gauze swab a blunt dissection is started to eliminate the fascial layers.
- *Identification of femoral opening*: For identifying the boundaries of the femoral canal, neck of the sac is cleared of fat and fascial layers. Lateral boundary of the canal is identified and care is taken not to injure the femoral vein and artery which is covered by thick and opaque sheath of fascia.The lateral boundary is cleared with metzenbaum scissors for sac dissection. Neck of the sac is exposed, which finishes the dissection and identification of sac.
- *Contents of sac*: 'Trick of the trade' is to open the lateral side of the fundus of the sac whilst medial side is avoided as it may contain bladder. Hemostasis is mandatory here as the lateral fat contains the veins which may bleed confusing the anatomy. After opening the fat (extraperitoneal) the peritoneal layer will be seen which is lifted with a hemostat and opened as said earlier. After opening the sac the contents, if free are reduced to abdomen; else adhesiolysis is done and reduction of contents is done. If in a strangulated hernia, blackish, dead omentum is encountered then the blood supply is ligated and excision of the same is done.
- *Sac closure and excision*: Empty sac with free neck is ready to be closurd and ligated, excised. The neck of the sac is pulled and traction is applied. Then the absorbable suture like Vicryl 0/00 is used to transfix the sac and remaining sac is excised with good stump. The remaining stump of the sac will automatically recede through the femoral canal and away from sight.
- *Femoral canal repair*: Figure-of-eight suture is employed to repair the canal with polypropylene suture (2/0 or 3/0). With the use of retractor femoral vein is retracted laterally. First suture is taken at the pectineal ligament at its deeper aspect towards the medial margin of femoral vein. Second suture should be taken at inguinal ligament and iliopubic tract of fascia transversalis at a distance from its pubic attachment. Next the pectineal ligament is picked up, again from the deep to superficial halfway between the first pectineal suture and the lacunar ligament and finally the inguinal ligament is picked up, again halfway between the first suture and the attachment of the ligament to the pubis. Now the free end of the suture is passed deep to the two loops and two ends are tied securely. When the suture is pulled tight, the

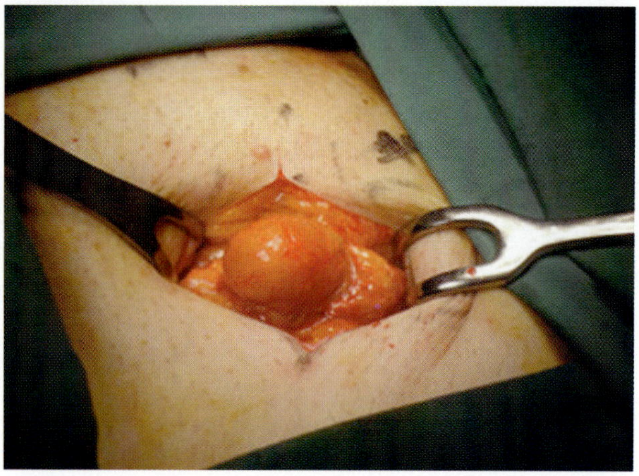

Fig. 14.7: The hernia is exposed

## Clinical Tips

Note: The large femoral hernia expands and actually appears to be anterior to the femoral vein as well. This is important when making a surgical incision.

Differential diagnosis of a strangulated femoral hernia is an abscess in the groin.

## Surgical Tips

The femoral hernia looks just like a lump of fat. To expose the hernia the deep fascia of the thigh is divided. There may be venous tributaries of the long sapnenous vein or branches of the femoral artery such as the superficial epigastric. Lymph nodes may also be encountered.

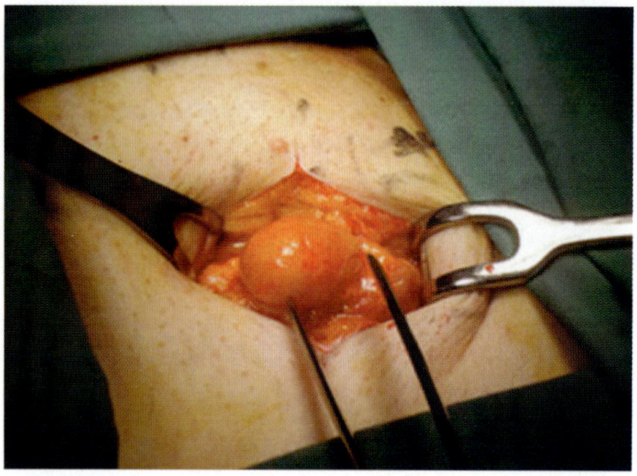

Fig. 14.8: Exposed—I

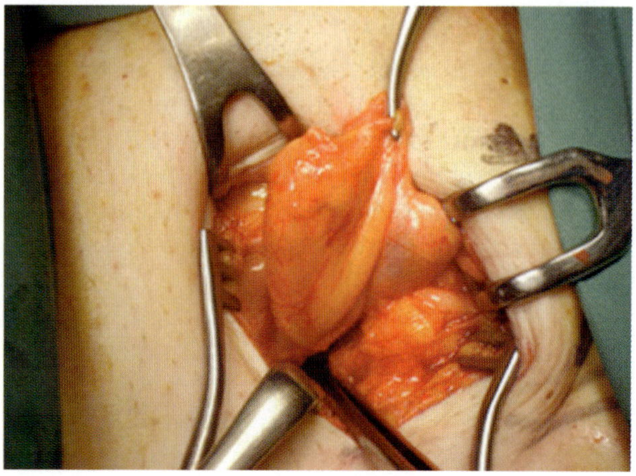

Fig. 14.9: Narrow neck demonstrated. Sac has been dissected free

## Surgical Tips

Femoral hernias are very commonly irreducible and may easily strangulate.

To reduce the hernia the surrounding fat is excised so that the sac can be gently manipulated back in.

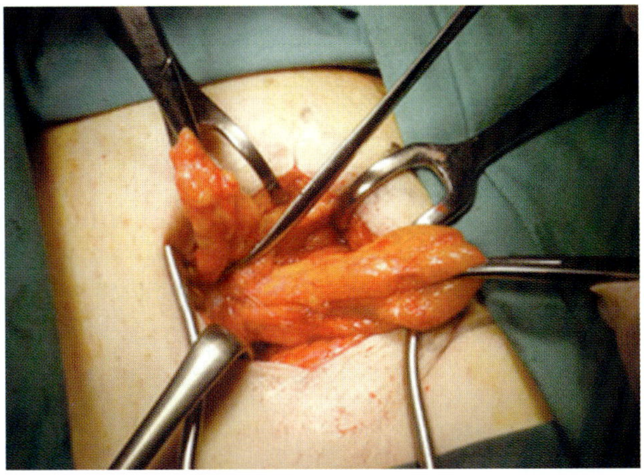

**Fig. 14.10:** Sac being demonstrated. Fat being dissected free. Sac is transfixed and excised or even maybe just reduced. Fat is excised

**Surgical Tips**

Femoral hernias are very commonly irreducible and may easily strangulate.

To reduce the hernia the fat is removed and the sac is narrowed down.

The contents must be reduced. The sac is then opened and by this stage the hernia can be readily reduced. The sac is then transfixed and excised.

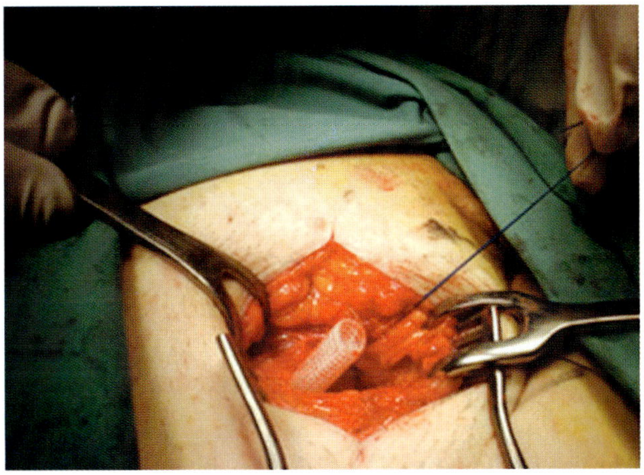

**Fig. 14.11:** Mesh plug placed into femoral canal

**Surgical Tips**

Previously, femoral hernias were repaired by suturing. However, this causes tension with a higher rate of recurrence. There was also the risk of narrowing or injuring the femoral vein. Now a popular technique described by Lichtenstein is to insert a rolled up mesh like a cigarette. Commonly polypropylene. This avoids tension and is readily fixed into position with a low recurrence rate.

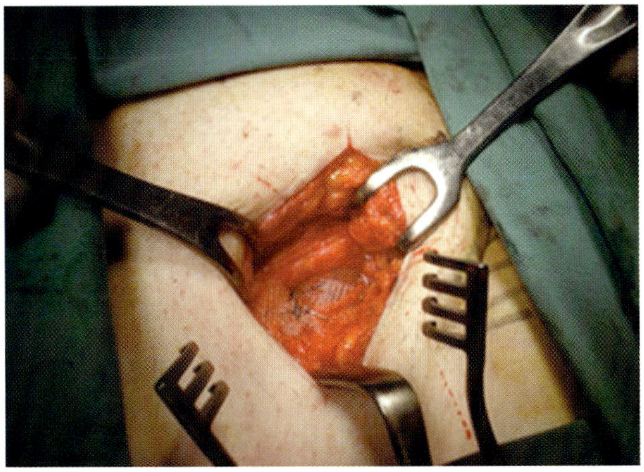

**Fig. 14.12:** Mesh plug fixed into position

medial 0.75 cm or so of the inguinal ligament will be approximated to the pectineal line and the femoral canal closed.

Patient in theater recumbent and the surface markings shown. Transverse upper line is the previous incision. Triangle is the external ring. The swelling is outlined and the vertical lines are the femoral nerve, artery and vein. Note that the swelling overlies the vein.

## Conclusion

- Thus, femoral hernias are not common compared to inguinal hernias. They occur relatively more frequently in females. Because of the narrow rigid walls of the femoral ring they are commonly irreducible and may readily strangulate. Thus, they should be repaired in most cases to avoid the risk of strangulation and emergency surgery. They are sometimes confused with inguinal hernias and other lumps which may occur in the femoral triangle.

### Lotheissen's Transinguinal Approach

Georg Lotheissen (September 14, 1868-October 28, 1941) was an Austrian surgeon who was born in Geneva, Switzerland.

In 1892, he earned his medical doctorate in Vienna, and following graduation was an assistant to Emil Zuckerkandl (1849-1910), and a surgical apprentice under Theodor Billroth (1829-1894) and Carl Gussenbauer (1842-1903). From 1895 to 1901 he was first assistant to Viktor von Hacker (1852-1933) at the surgical clinic at Innsbruck, where in 1899 he was habilitated for surgery. In 1902, he returned to Vienna, where in 1915 he became an associate professor (extraordinarius).

Lotheissen made important contributions in his work involving esophageal surgery and herniorrhaphy. In 1897, he was the first surgeon to suture the conjoint tendon to Cooper's (pectineal) ligament, which he performed on a patient with a recurrent inguinal hernia. Decades later, American surgeon Chester McVay (1911-1987) popularized this operation, and this procedure is now referred to as a "Lotheissen-McVay herniotomy".

His name is also associated with "Lotheissen's operation", which is also known as "Lotheissen's trans-inguinal approach". This surgery involves operating for femoral hernia through the posterior wall of the inguinal canal.

### Procedure

*Aim*: Closure of the medial portion of femoral canal.

*Incision and dissection*: Inguinal incision same as for inguinal hernia surgery by Shouldice method.

*Procedure*: Repair is done by opening the fascia transversalis in the posterior wall of inguinal canal. Then extraperitoneal fat on the neck of femoral hernia is identified and removed by blunt dissection.

*Sac*: Identification and delivery of the sac of femoral hernia is done above the inguinal ligament or it also can be opened below the inguinal ligament. Then the contents of the sac are reduced. This is followed by transfixation and ligation of the sac.

*Repair*: The medial part of the inguinal ligament is sutured to the pectineal ligament in figure-of-eight fashion by nonabsorbable sutures like Prolene Polypropylene).

*Inguinal repair*: Repair of inguinal canal is done by tension free method or Shouldice type repair.

*In females*: In female patients the Coopeer's ligament repair is advised.

This is a technically difficult surgery. It is a time consuming surgery.

### McEvedy's High Approach (Extraperitoneal Operation)

This operation illustrates the genius of an expert surgical anatomist. Exploiting the fascial plane dissection at its most elegant. Henry's extraperitoneal approach to the anterior pelvis gives an excellent exposure of both femoral canals simultaneously, but it is not an operation for the tyro. In the hands of an expert it is a fine operation enabling bilateral femoral hernia to be dealt with simultaneously through one incision.

*Repair*: The patient is placed on the operating table and bladder emptied by catheterization. A vertical midline suprapubic incision is made, the aponeurotic layer is opened and peritoneum is exposed. The recti are retracted to either side and the space between the peritoneum and the abdominal wall muscles is opened by gentle blunt dissection in order to approach the femoral canal on the either side. Femoral sacs are dealt with by reduction of their contents, transfixation of their necks and resection of redundant sacs. If strangulation is present the subjacent peritoneum is opened, the contents of the sac inspected, and so forth. The femoral canal is repaired using a nonabsorbable suture as described in inguinal operation. The anterior abdominal wall is closed layer by layer.

## Laparoscopic Repair for Femoral Hernia

For femoral hernia laparoscopic techniques described in inguinal hernioplasty are employed. There is no difference in the technique.

TEP: Totally extraperitoneal repair

TAPP: Transabdominal preperitoneal repair

## Morbidity and Mortality Rates

The mortality rate following an uncomplicated femoral hernia repair is essentially zero. The mortality rate for repair of a strangulated hernia that has necessitated a bowel resection is higher, however, ranging from 5 to 19%. Morbidity following an uncomplicated herniorrhaphy is low; one Danish study reported that the most common complication, reported by 8% of patients, was pain during procedures performed under local anesthesia. A British study of laparoscopic hernia repairs found that only 22 out of 3017 patients reported recurrence of the hernia. The incidence of postoperative swelling and bruising was 8%.

# Chapter 15

# Umbilical Hernia

## Umbilical Hernias (Figs 15.1A and B)

"Omphalos was the center stone in the Temple of Apollo at Delphi. The term was modified to name the center point of a newborn infant, from which the term umbilical cord emanated. In Latin, *umbo* denoted the ornamental stud at the center of a shield, from which the term for the umbilicus area was derived. The Anglo-Saxon, *nafe,* meaning hub of a wheel, was converted to navel."

An umbilical hernia is a protrusion around the navel (umbilicus) that may contain part of the intestine and/or the fatty membrane found inside the abdomen (omentum). Hernias often protrude through areas of muscle weakness such as around the navel. This is the area where blood vessels from the mother supply the developing fetus with nutrients through the umbilical cord. After birth, the umbilical cord is severed, leaving the belly button as its lifetime reminder. Umbilical hernias in babies (congenital) usually resolve spontaneously by ages 1 to 2.

An adult umbilical hernia (acquired) occurs when the connective tissue (fascia) of the abdominal wall becomes weak around the area of the navel. The weakening occurs over a period of years until eventually the abdominal contents, encased in a sac, protrude through the abdominal wall, and a bulge forms around the umbilicus. A newly formed umbilical hernia is usually small and contains only the fatty omentum. However, as more of the abdominal contents (transverse colon, small intestine, greater omentum) push into the sac, the umbilical hernia can grow in size.

A reducible hernia can easily be returned to the abdominal cavity. When the hernia can no longer be reduced, it is called "incarcerated"; these hernias have a high risk for losing the blood supply that keeps the tissue alive (strangulation). For that reason, repair of an umbilical hernia is recommended as soon as possible after it is discovered.

### Risk

Umbilical hernias are the most common in infants. In an adult, any condition that causes build-up of pressure against the abdominal wall may contribute to umbilical hernia formation. This includes extreme obesity, heavy lifting, accumulation of abdominal fluids (ascites), coughing, straining with urination or defecation, chronic obstructive pulmonary disease (COPD), or even multiple pregnancies.

### Incidence and Prevalence

Of the half million hernia operations performed in the US every year, about 14% are umbilical hernia repairs (Golladay). Congenital umbilical hernias generally close spontaneously by age 1 or 2 (Nicks).

Slightly more females than males are treated for umbilical hernias, with a ratio of 1.7 to 1 (Golladay). As with all abdominal hernias, the prevalence of umbilical hernia increases with age, and umbilical hernias are more common in individuals of African ancestry (Golladay).

## Diagnosis

### History

Individuals with umbilical hernia report a central mid-abdominal bulge that may expand when the individual

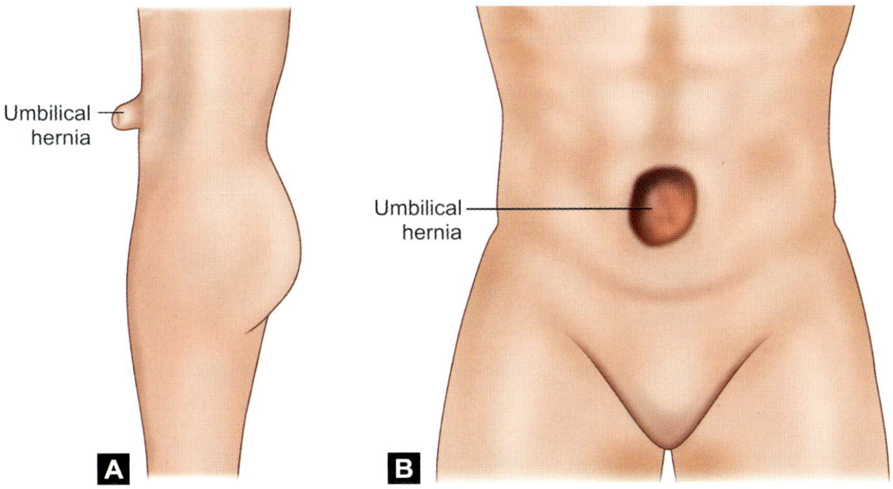


**Figs 15.1A and B:** Umbilical hernias

coughs or strains the abdomen. Pain in the area of the hernia is not uncommon with coughing or straining. A careful review of symptoms should seek other medical conditions that may be associated with increased intra-abdominal pressure.

### Physical Examination

The presence of an umbilical hernia is identified by a bulge or a palpable defect at the level of the umbilicus. There may be discoloration of the skin overlying the hernia.

### Tests

The diagnosis is made based on the history and physical examination, and tests are usually not needed. However, the physician may use CT imaging, ultrasound, or X-ray aided by contrast material to visualize the herniated contents.

## Treatment (Figs 15.2A to E)

A small umbilical hernia that is easily pushed back into the abdomen (reduced) in an adult of normal weight may be watched closely, particularly if the individual is a poor surgical risk or elderly. Repair of umbilical hernias is recommended in all other adults. Large umbilical hernias are often treated with the Mayo procedure, which uses an implanted polyurethane mesh to provide support and hold the herniated sac inside the abdomen.

### Truss

Trusses were sometimes used in the past when surgery was a more dangerous proposition but have fallen out of favor since they can injure delicate skin and bowel and mask signs of strangulation. Corsets and binders are sometimes used on a temporary basis before surgery or for individuals who are not surgical candidates.

Umbilical hernia repair in the adult is indicated for incarceration, a small neck in relation to the size of the hernia, ascites, chromatic skin change, or rupture. The approach to management of an umbilical hernia in a child relates to the natural history of umbilical hernias and their importance in adulthood. Most umbilical hernias close spontaneously in children during the preschool-aged period. Therefore, repair of an umbilical hernia is not indicated in children younger than 5 years unless the child has a large proboscoid hernia with thin, hyperpigmented skin or is undergoing an operation for other reasons or if the hernia causes familial or social problems. The size of the fascial defect rather than the size of the external protrusion predicts potential for spontaneous closure. Walker demonstrated that fascial rings measuring less than 1 cm in diameter usually close, while rings larger than 2 cm seldom close spontaneously. Therefore, many pediatric surgeons will repair umbilical

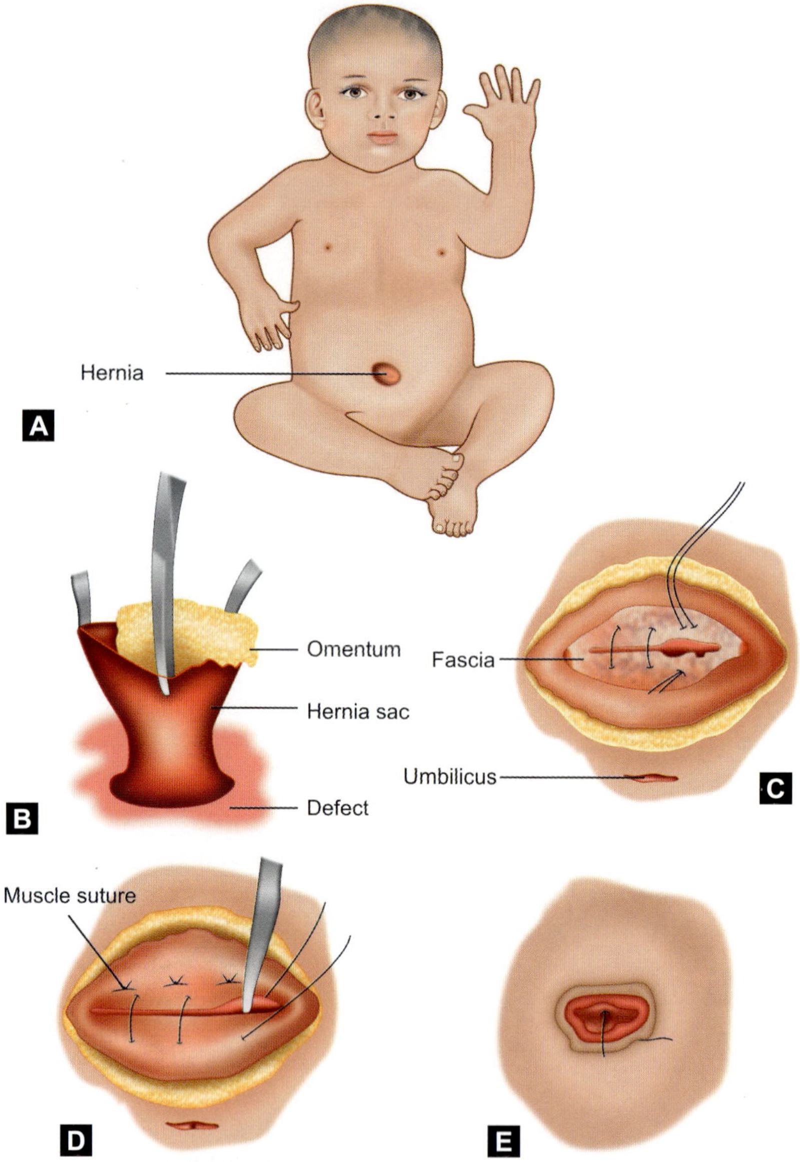


**Figs 15.2A to E:** Umbilical hernia repair

hernias with large fascial defects (>2.5 cm) earlier than the smaller counterparts.

The umbilicus is a natural hernial opening in the abdominal wall. It can develop a hernia at any age. In children, umbilical hernias are the third most common disorder after hydroceles and inguinal hernias. The hernia is present in about one to every five birth, the incidence in black infants being up to eight times higher than in white infants. Predisposing factors are a low birth weight and prematurity. A familial predisposition appears in 9 to 12%, but no genetic pattern of inheritance has been identified. In children most umbilical hernias are asymptomatic beside the obvious cosmetic defect. Infantile umbilical hernias rarely enlarge over time and will disappear in 90% of children by the age of 2 years. The spontaneous resolution appears to be directly influenced by the size of the umbilical ring. Defects with an umbilical ring larger than 1.5 cm are unlikely to resolve spontaneously. Complications such as strangulation of omentum or intestine and evisceration are seldom and occur approximately in 4% of cases. Indication for surgical repair are occurrence of complaints and complications or a persistence of the hernia beyond the age of 2 years. If the fascial defect is less than 1.5 cm in diameter or is asymptomatic a herniorrhaphy may be delayed until the child is 5 years old.

Umbilical hernias in adults are indirect herniations through the umbilical canal, and there have a high tendency to incarcerate and strangulate and do not resolve spontaneously. Most of these patients are females.

Because the risk of incarceration rises to 30%, operation is advised. Management includes operative therapy with repositioning of the hernial content and continuous suture, using local anesthesia in elective repair in adults or general anesthesia in children or in an emergency situation.

An exception is acquired umbilical hernias, that may occur in patients with acute abdominal distension. Reasons for an acute elevation of the intra-abdominal pressure include ascites from cirrhosis, congestive heart failure or nephrosis. Patients undergoing peritoneal dialysis also have a high incidence of these hernias. As the majority of these patients have serious underlying problems, a surgical repair is not indicated unless complications, such as incarceration or spontaneous rupture, occur.

## Epidemiology and Pathology

Umbilical hernia has not received as much attention as other abdominal wall defects. Prevalence in the adult population is 2% and is much more common in cirrhotic patients and obese middle-aged multiparous females. Adult umbilical hernias have an acquired origin as a consequence of increases in pressure (pregnancy, ascites, etc.), the pull of the abdominal muscles, and the deterioration of connective tissue. Attention needs to be paid to the development of umbilical hernias after laparoscopic trocar insertion. All trocar sites larger than 10 mm should be properly closed after operation.

### Outlook

The high morbidity and mortality associated with incarcerated umbilical hernias demand an elective repair in all circumstances. There is a lack of control trials evaluating the results of surgical repairs based on the tight overlapping closure of the umbilical ring described by Mayo, while recurrence after umbilical herniorrhaphy is thought to be a common event. The possibility of the application of biomaterials to the surgical correction of umbilical hernias that have been successfully used in the inguinal canal opens a new field for further clinical investigation. Control studies with long follow-up are now required in order to establish evidence-based umbilical surgery.

## Mayo's Procedure for Umbilical Hernia

William Mayo used first time an overlapping procedure for umbilical hernia repair in 1895. Mayo advocated his technique of overlapping the adjucent tissues in vertical plane.

### Indications of Umbilical Hernia Surgery

1. Discomfort and pain at the umbilicus
2. Protrusion at umbilicus
3. Association with inguinal hernia
4. Strangulation
5. Obstruction
6. Incarceration
7. Damaged and ulcerated overlying skin.

### Absolute Contraindications for Surgery

- Obesity
- Ascites
- Chronic cardiovascular of thoracic disease.

### The Surgery

#### *Open Technique of Repair*

a. *Position of patient*: Supine position on operating table and draping is done to adequately expose the umbilicus and surrounding area in case if incision has to extended.
b. *Incision*: Incision is planned according to size of hernia. A circumlinear incision is employed for hernias around the size of 2 to 3 cm. For larger size hernias than this; the incision needs to be modified as the extension of the circumlinear incision on the lateral boundary of umbilicus. The incision will cover all area around umbilicus and section of umbilicus can be done by prior consent from the patient with this type of incision.The lateral boundaries of the incision should be decided by the surgeon according to size of hernia.
c. *Progression of incision*: Removal of redundant fat and skin is done to deepen the incision. The

muscular aponeurosis is exposed by dissection. With the help of electrocautery the incision is deepened not to harm the blood supply of the skin at right angle to fibers of aponeurosis.

d. *Neck of sac*: "Trick of the trade here is to identify the neck of the sac first and incise it". Upon dissection to the level of muscular aponeurosis the sac is freed of the fat and tissue to determine its margins. The aponeurosis is also cleared off the tissue and margins are clear cut visualized. Then the sac is opened at neck and the contents are visualized. Adhesions are frequently present in the sac with the visceral organs like omentum and intestines. Adhesions should be dissected and freed by careful ligation. The important thing to remember here is the partially ischemic omentum should not be left in peritoneal cavity; but excised. Bowel if present in the sac should be carefully preserved intact otherwise post-operative fistula will follow. Return of organs in sac to perineal cavity should be done after satisfying hemostasis. While dissecting the sac it should be taken affirmatively that the adhesions are always present more at the neck than fundus and one should insert the finger into the sac at the neck incision and start separating the adhesions and not at fundus.

e. *Sac closure*: Closure of the sac is commenced after the above mentioned procedure. Sac should be closed with absorbable sutures and returned to abdomen after hemostasis.

f. *Enlarging the aponeurosis*: The aponeurotic defect is enlarged 1 to 3 cm on either side in a transverse line to facilitate the repair and for the insertion of prosthetic mesh. This does not apply to PHS (prolene hernia system).

g. *Defect repair:* (1) Pure tissue repair—Mayo's technique is employed to repair the defect by pure tissue repair method. This involves holding of the structures like margins of the opening, aponeurosis, posterior rectus sheath and peritoneum in hemostats. The deep sutures are placed with round body needle of the non-absorbable sutures like polypropylene. The suture enters the upper flap from without, between 2 and 3 cm from its margin. The needle is then grasped on the deep surface of the upper flap, passed across the defect and then from the outside to the lower flap. Then the needle is pulled back through the lower flap, across the defect and through the deep surface of the upper flap. The suture thus placed is held in a clip. Many more such sutures are inserted and held untied until all are in place. Once all have been placed then tied. After the sutures have all been placed the flaps are brought together, the upper being railroaded down the sutures until it lies overlapping the lower flap. The sutures are now tied, fixing the tissues firmly together. A triple layer, double throw knot is used. When all the knots are complete the ends are cut. The edge of the upper flap is sutured to the anterior surface of the lower flap using the polypropylene sutures after placement of the suction drain in between the two flaps. The umbilicus is reposited and sutured to muscular aponeurosis with absorbable sutures. Underlying fascia and fat layer are sutured in separate layers with absorbable sutures. Skin is closed with sutures or staples.

(2) Prosthetic repair of the defect—Flat polypropylene or other biomaterial mesh is used to give support to the umbilicus after the repair of the defect to prevent recurrence. As Mayo's repair has high failure rates this is now widely used. The mesh is placed in onlay and inlay fashion. This involves the placement of the mesh above the repair of the defect which is called an onlay mesh repair. The onlay mesh of appropriate size is placed over the repaired defect and sutured to the aponeurosis with continuous nonabsorbable sutures along the circumference of the mesh. The mesh can be cut to made fit in the defective area at least covering 3 to 4 cm around the defect. Rest of the procedure is followed to close the incision. The inlay mesh is used on the principle of PASCAL. The inlay mesh serves more for the support of the abdominal contents. This mesh is put into the defect behind the posterior aponeurotic sheath by clearing the space between the peritoneum and the posterior rectus sheath. The mesh is placed there and held in place with four main principle sutures with nonabsorbable material from inside out fashion. The knots are securely and firmly tightened and it should be tension free. Then the defect is closed in transverse fashion with running continuous suture of polypropylene. Rest of

the procedure follows. This inlay mesh is very useful for preventing the recurrence in most of the patients.

h. *Repair with prolene hernia system (PHS)*—This PHS is revolutionizing the umbilical hernia surgery in today's world. There are now scientific evidences regarding the use of PHS in this surgery without recurrences. This system prevents recurrence in most of the cases and gaining popularity very fast.

### *Incision*

For small to medium sizes hernias incision can be placed circumlinear inside the umbilicus. Like the incision for laparoscopic port insertion. Incision is deepened till surgeon faces the aponeurosis.

### *Sac*

The sac is dealt with as described in previous topic. Closure of the sac is done and returned to the abdomen.

### *Repair with Prolene Hernia System (Figs 15.3A and B)*

At the time of dissection the margins of the defect are cleared off any tissue by surgeon. Then the finger or a rolled gauze piece is inserted into the preperitoneal space to create the adequate space for placement of the prolene hernia system (PHS) device. The size of the device is chosen according to the defect size. The blunt and blind dissection by finger or gauze piece is commenced with a sweeping like action. The preperitoneal space is created on either side of the defect facilitating at least 4 to 6 cm of free space. Hemostasis is highly important here. The preperitoneal space must be dissected more than that is needed for the plug so that the underlay will lay open and flat. It is best to ensure that that portion of the product is flat because any wrinkle of any flat mesh can incite the development of adhesions in that area. Once this is placed the overlay will lie over the linea alba and the anterior rectus sheath. The overlay part of the PHS can be cut short to cover only defect and the edges of the overlay are sutured to the margins of the defect; with interrupted nonabsorbable sutures. Rest of the closure process of the incision can be left to surgeons choice.

## Laparoscopic Repair

There is no consensus on the best technique for the repair of umbilical hernia in adults. The role of laparoscopic hernioplasty of umbilical hernia remains controversial. Laparoscopic onlay patch hernioplasty is a safe and efficacious technique for the repair of umbilical hernia. Compared to Mayo repair, the laparoscopic approach confers the advantages of reduced postoperative pain, shorter hospital stay, and a diminished morbidity rate.

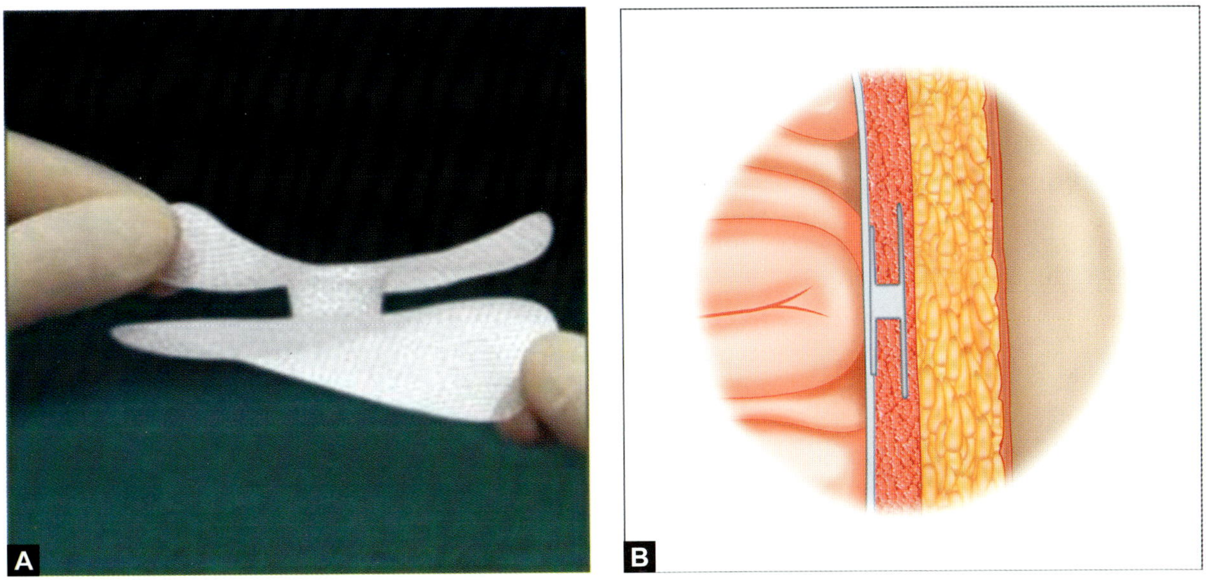


**Figs 15.3A and B:** Prolene hernia system

# Chapter 16

# Epigastric Hernia

An epigastric hernia happens, when weakness in the abdominal muscle allows the tissues of the abdomen to protrude through the muscle. An epigastric hernia is usually present at birth, and may heal without treatment as the infant grows and the abdominal muscles strengthen. An epigastric hernia is similar to a umbilical hernia, except the umbilical hernia forms around the belly button and the epigastric hernia is usually between the belly button and the chest.

An epigastric hernia is typically small enough that only the peritoneum, or the lining of the abdominal cavity, pushes through the muscle wall. In severe cases, portions of an organ may move through the rent in the muscle.

## Epigastric Hernia

*Epigastric hernia:* Occurring between the navel and the lower part of the rib cage in the midline of the abdomen, epigastric hernias are composed usually of fatty tissue and rarely contain intestine. Formed in an area of relative weakness of the abdominal wall, these hernias are often painless and unable to be pushed back into the abdomen when first discovered (Figs 16.1 and 16.2).

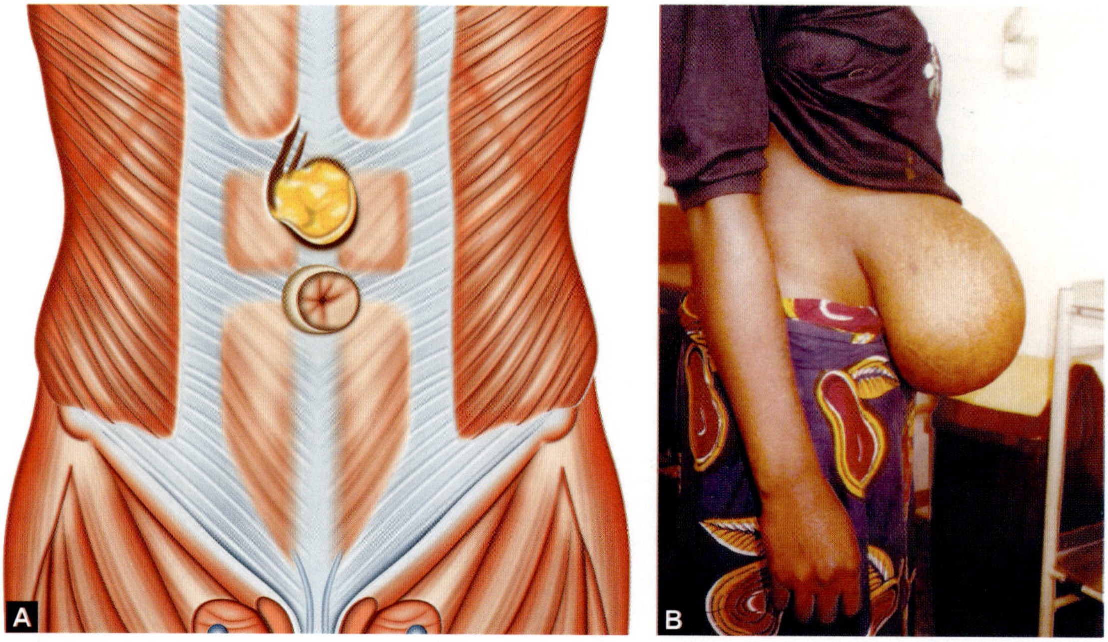


**Figs 16.1A and B:** Epigastric hernia—I

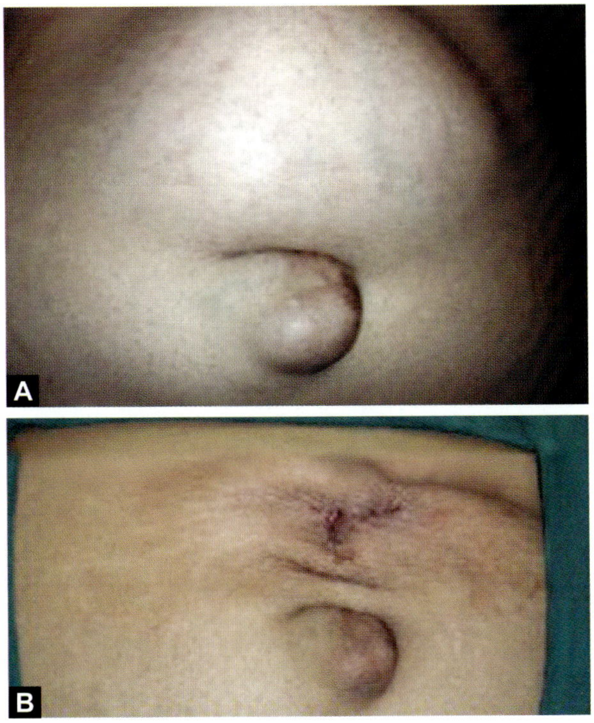


**Figs 16.2A and B:** Epigastric hernia—II

A linea alba hernia protrudes anywhere between the xiphoid process and the umbilicus, but usually in the midline between these two structures. About 3 to 5% of people develop epigastric hernias. They are common between the ages of 20 and 50, and occur more often in men than in women. About 20% of the hernias are multiple and 80% occur just off the midline.

The epigastric hernia commences as a protrusion of extra-peritoneal fat where the linea alba is pierced by a small blood vessel. The swelling enlarges and drags a pouch of peritoneum with it. Frequently, the sac is empty or contains a small portion of greater omentum because the mouth of the hernia is usually small.

## Investigations

Diagnosis of an epigastric hernia is confirmed by any maneuver which increases intra-abdominal pressure and makes the mass bulge anteriorly. The mass is often difficult to palpate, so that ultrasound or a CT scan may be necessary.

### Clinical Features

The patient with an epigastric hernia may be asymptomatic. The abdominal mass is discovered as a part of a routine examination.
The features in a symptomatic patient may include:

- Pain - which varies from mild epigastric pain to a deep burning pain radiating to the back or the lower abdomen
- An abdominal mass - which may be palpable and tender
- Abdominal bloating
- Vomiting
- Nausea
- Aggravated by eating
- Relieved by reclining so that the mass falls away from the anterior abdominal wall

Smaller hernia are prone to incarceration and strangulation. They frequently contain only extraperitoneal fat. Large ones seldom strangulate and additionally contain omentum.

## Pathological Anatomy

### *The Muscles and Fasciae of the Abdomen*

The muscles of the abdomen may be divided into two groups: (1) the anterolateral muscles; (2) the posterior muscles (Fig. 16.3).

1. *The anterolateral muscles of the abdomen:* The muscles of this group are:
   - Obliquus externus

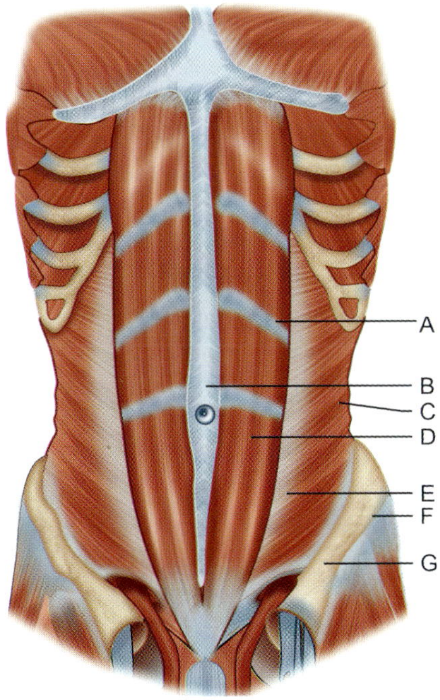


**Fig. 16.3:** A. Intersection tendineae; B. Linea alba; C. Muscles transversus abdominis; D. Muscle rectus abdominis; E. Vagina muscle recti abdominis (lamina anterior); F. Spina iliaca anterior superior; G. Ligamentum inguinale

- Transversus
- Obliquus internus
- Rectus
- Pyramidalis.

*The Superficial Fascia:* The superficial fascia of the abdomen consists, over the greater part of the abdominal wall, of a single layer containing a variable amount of fat; but near the groin it is easily divisible into two layers, between which are found the superficial vessels and nerves and the superficial inguinal lymph glands.

The superficial layer (*fascia of Camper*) is thick, areolar in texture, and contains in its meshes a varying quantity of adipose tissue. Below, it passes over the inguinal ligament, and is continuous with the superficial fascia of the thigh. In the male, Camper's fascia is continued over the penis and outer surface of the spermatic cord to the scrotum, where it helps to form the dartos. As it passes to the scrotum, it changes its characteristics, becoming thin, destitute of adipose tissue, and of a pale reddish color, and in the scrotum, it acquires some involuntary muscular fibers. From the scrotum, it may be traced backward into continuity with the superficial fascia of the perineum. In the female, Camper's fascia is continued from the abdomen into the labia majora.

The deep layer (*fascia of scarpa*) is thinner and more membranous in character than the superficial, and contains a considerable quantity of yellow elastic fibers. It is loosely connected by areolar tissue to the aponeurosis of the obliquus externus abdominis, but in the middle line it is more intimately adherent to the linea alba and to the symphysis pubis, and is prolonged on to the dorsum of the penis, forming the fundiform ligament; above, it is continuous with the superficial fascia over the rest of the trunk; below and laterally, it blends with the fascia lata of the thigh a little below the inguinal ligament; medially and below, it is continued over the penis and spermatic cord to the scrotum, where it helps to form the dartos. From the scrotum, it may be traced backward into continuity with the deep layer of the superficial fascia of the perineum (*fascia of Colles*). In the female, it is continued into the labia majora and thence to the fascia of Colles.

The obliquus externus abdominis (*external or descending oblique muscle*) situated on the lateral and anterior parts of the abdomen, is the largest and the most superficial of the three flat muscles in this region (Fig. 16.4). It is broad, thin, and irregularly quadrilateral, its muscular portion occupying the side, its aponeurosis the anterior wall of the abdomen. It arises, by eight fleshy digitations, from the external surfaces and inferior borders of the lower eight ribs; these digitations are arranged in an oblique line which runs downward and backward, the upper ones being attached close to the cartilages of the corresponding ribs, the lowest to the apex of the cartilage of the last rib, the intermediate ones to the ribs at some distance from their cartilages. The five superior serrations increase in size from above downward, and are received between corresponding processes of the Serratus anterior; the three lower ones diminish in size from above downward and receive between them corresponding processes from the Latissimus dorsi. From these attachments, the fleshy fibers proceed in various directions. Those from the lowest ribs pass nearly vertically downward, and are inserted into the anterior half of the outer lip of the iliac crest; the middle and upper fibers, directed downward and forward, end in an aponeurosis, opposite to a line drawn from the prominence of the ninth costal cartilage to the anterior superior iliac spine.

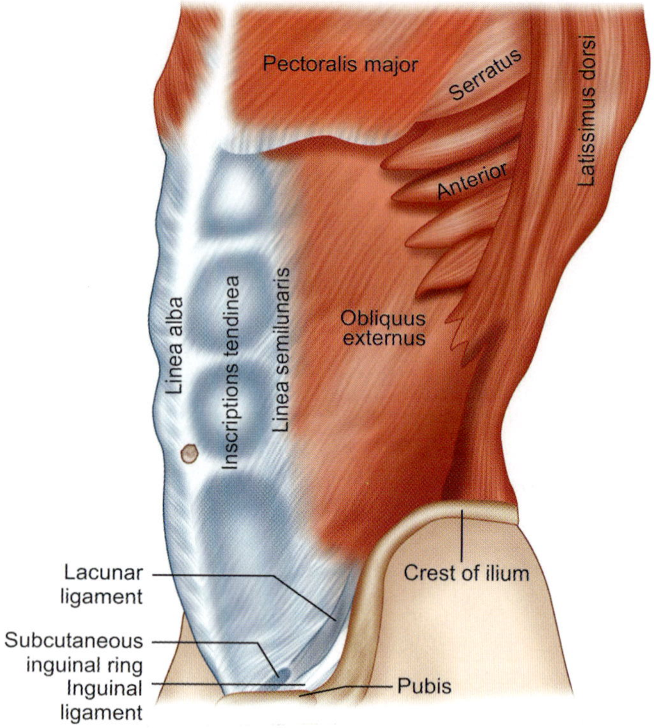


**Fig. 16.4:** The obliquus externus abdominis

The aponeurosis of the obliquus externus abdominis is a thin but strong membranous structure, the fibers of which are directed downward and medialward. It is joined with that of the opposite muscle along the middle line, and covers the whole of the front of the abdomen; above, it is covered by and gives origin to the lower fibers of the pectoralis major; below, its fibers are closely aggregated together, and extend obliquely across from the anterior superior iliac spine to the public tubercle and the pectineal line. In the middle line, it interlaces with the aponeurosis of the opposite muscle, forming the linea alba, which extends from the xiphoid process to the symphysis pubis.

That portion of the aponeurosis which extends between the anterior superior iliac spine and the pubic tubercle is a thick band, folded inward, and continuous below with the fascia lata; it is called the inguinal ligament. The portion which is reflected from the inguinal ligament at the pubic tubercle is attached to the pectineal line and is called the lacunar ligament. From the point of attachment of the latter to the pectineal line, a few fibers pass upward and medialward, behind the medial crus of the subcutaneous inguinal ring, to the linea alba; they diverge as they ascend, and form a thin triangular fibrous band which is called the reflected inguinal ligament.

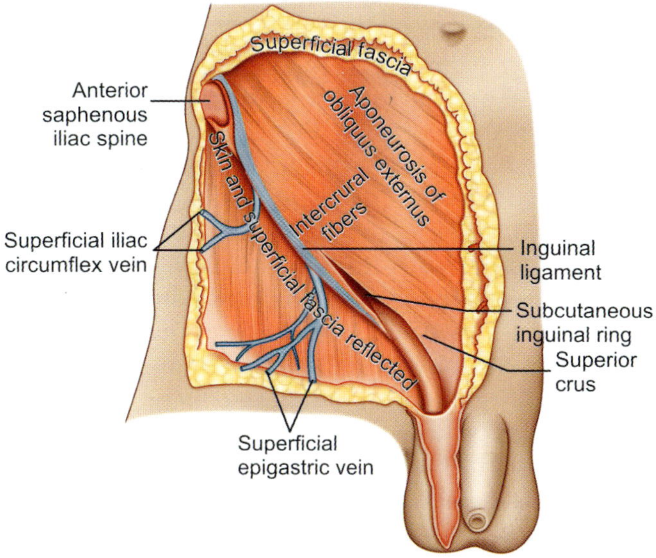


**Fig. 16.5:** The subcutaneous inguinal ring

In the aponeurosis of the obliquus externus, immediately above the crest of the pubis, is a triangular opening, the subcutaneous inguinal ring, formed by a separation of the fibers of the aponeurosis in this situation.

The following structures require further description, viz., the subcutaneous inguinal ring, the intercrural fibers and fascia, and the inguinal, lacunar, and reflected inguinal ligaments.

*The subcutaneous inguinal ring (annulus inguinalis subcutaneus; external abdominal ring) (Fig. 16.5)*: The subcutaneous inguinal ring is an interval in the aponeurosis of the obliquus externus, just above and lateral to the crest of the pubis. The aperture is oblique in direction, somewhat triangular in form, and corresponds with the course of the fibers of the aponeurosis. It usually measures from base to apex about 2.5 cm, and transversely about 1.25 cm. It is bounded below by the crest of the pubis; on either side by the margins of the opening in the aponeurosis, which are called the crura of the ring; and above, by a series of curved intercrural fibers. The inferior crus (*external pillar*) is stronger and is formed by that portion of the inguinal ligament which is inserted into the pubic tubercle; it is curved so as to form a kind of groove, upon which, in the male, the spermatic cord rests. The superior crus (*internal pillar*) is a broad, thin, flat band, attached to the front of the symphysis pubis and interlacing with its fellow of the opposite side.

The subcutaneous inguinal ring gives passage to the spermatic cord and ilioinguinal nerve in the male, and to the round ligament of the uterus and the ilioinguinal nerve in the female; it is much larger in men than in women, on account of the large size of the spermatic cord.

*The intercrural fibers (fibrae intercrurales; intercolumnar fibers)*: The intercrural fibers are a series of curved tendinous fibers, which arch across the lower part of the aponeurosis of the obliquus externus, describing curves with the convexities downward. They have received their name from stretching across between the two crura of the subcutaneous inguinal ring, and they are much thicker and stronger at the inferior crus, where they are connected to the inguinal ligament, than superiorly, where they are inserted into the linea alba. The intercrural fibers increase the strength of the lower part of the aponeurosis, and prevent the divergence of the crura from one another; they are more strongly developed in the male than in the female.

As they pass across the subcutaneous inguinal ring, they are connected together by delicate fibrous tissue, forming a fascia, called the intercrural fascia. This intercrural fascia is continued down as a tubular prolongation around the spermatic cord and testis, and encloses them in a sheath; hence it is also called the external spermatic fascia. The subcutaneous inguinal ring is seen as a distinct aperture only after the intercrural fascia has been removed.

*The inguinal ligament* (*ligamentum inguinale* (*Pouparti*)*; Poupart's ligament*): The inguinal ligament is the lower border of the aponeurosis of the obliquus externus, and extends from the anterior superior iliac spine to the pubic tubercle. From this latter point, it is reflected backward and lateralward to be attached to the pectineal line for about 1.25 cm, forming the lacunar ligament. Its general direction is convex downward toward the thigh, where it is continuous with the fascia lata. Its lateral half is rounded, and oblique in direction; its medial half gradually widens at its attachment to the pubis, is more horizontal in direction, and lies beneath the spermatic cord.

*The lacunar ligament* (*ligamentum lacunare* [*Gimbernati*]*; Gimbernat's ligament*)*:* The lacunar ligament is that part of the aponeurosis of the obliquus externus which is reflected backward and lateralward, and is attached to the pectineal line. It is about 1.25 cm long, larger in the male than in the female, almost horizontal in direction in the erect posture, and of a triangular form with the base directed lateralward. Its base is concave, thin, and sharp, and forms the medial boundary of the femoral ring. Its apex corresponds to the pubic tubercle. Its posterior margin is attached to the pectineal line, and is continuous with the pectineal fascia. Its anterior margin is attached to the inguinal ligament. Its surfaces are directed upward and downward (Fig. 16.6).

*The reflected inguinal ligament* (*ligamentum inguinale reflexum* [*Collesi*]*; triangular fascia*)*:* The reflected inguinal ligament is a layer of tendinous fibers of a triangular shape, formed by an expansion from the lacunar ligament and the inferior crus of the subcutaneous inguinal ring. It passes medialward behind the spermatic cord, and expands into a somewhat fan-shaped band, lying behind the superior crus of the subcutaneous inguinal ring, and in front of the inguinal aponeurotic falx, and interlaces with the ligament of the other side of the linea alba.

*Ligament of Cooper:* This is a strong fibrous band, which was first described by Sir Astley Cooper. It extends lateralward from the base of the lacunar ligament along the pectineal line, to which it is attached. It is strengthened by the pectineal fascia, and by a lateral expansion from the lower attachment of the linea alba (*adminiculum lineae albae*).

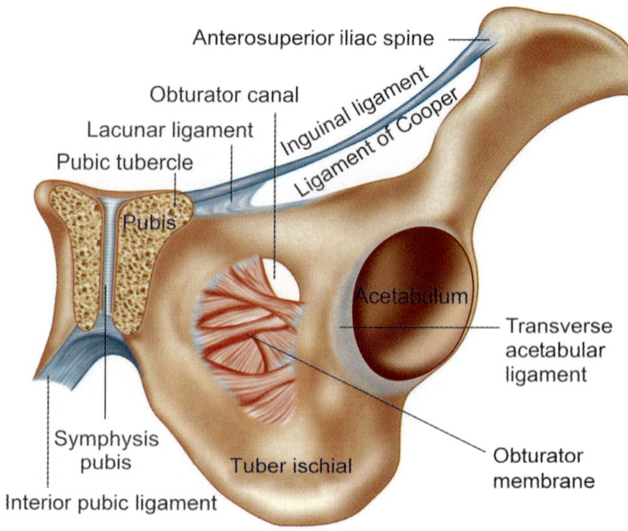


**Fig. 16.6:** The inguinal and lacunar ligaments

*Variations:* The obliquus externus may show decrease or doubling of its attachments to the ribs; addition slips from lumbar aponeurosis; doubling between lower ribs and ilium or inguinal ligament. Rarely tendinous inscriptions occur.

The obliquus internus abdominis (*internal or ascending oblique muscle*) (Fig. 16.7), thinner and smaller than the Obliquus externus, beneath which it lies, is of an irregularly quadrilateral form, and situated at the lateral and anterior parts of the abdomen. It arises, by fleshy fibers, from the lateral half of the grooved upper surface of the inguinal ligament, from the anterior two-thirds of the middle lip of the iliac crest, and from the posterior lamella of the lumbodorsal fascia. From this origin, the fibers diverge; those from the inguinal ligament, a few in number and paler in color than the rest, arch downward and medialward across the spermatic cord in the male and the round ligament of the uterus in the female, and, becoming tendinous, are inserted, conjointly with those of the transversus, into the crest of the pubis and medial part of the pectineal line behind the lacunar ligament, forming what is known as the inguinal aponeurotic falx. Those from the anterior third of the iliac origin are horizontal in their direction, and, becoming tendinous along the lower fourth of the linea semilunaris, pass in front of the rectus abdominis to be inserted into the

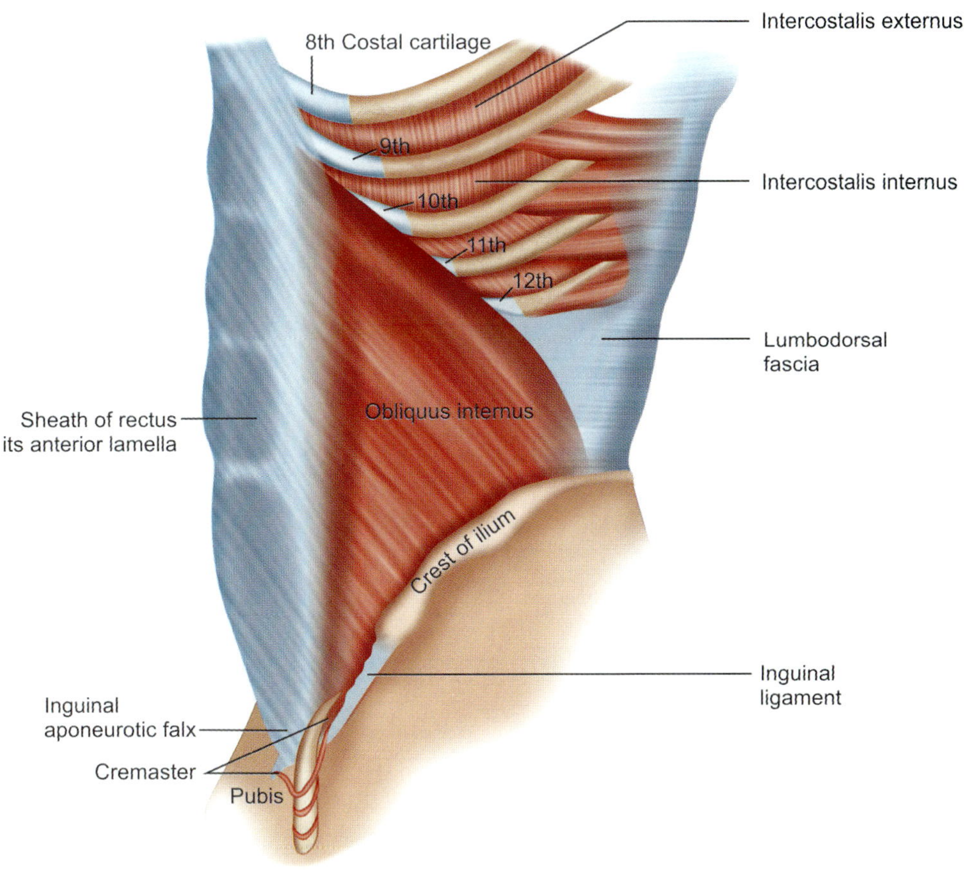


**Fig. 16.7:** The obliquus internus abdominis

linea alba. Those arising from the middle third of the iliac origin run obliquely upward and medialward, and end in an aponeurosis; this divides at the lateral border of the rectus into two lamellae, which are continued forward, one in front of and the other behind this muscle, to the linea alba: the posterior lamella has an attachment to the cartilages of the seventh, eighth, and ninth ribs. The most posterior fibers pass almost vertically upward to be inserted into the inferior borders of the cartilages of the three lower ribs, being continuous with the intercostales interni.

*Variations:* Occasionally, tendinous inscriptions occur from the tips of the tenth or eleventh cartilages or even from the ninth; an additional slip to the ninth cartilage is sometimes found; separation between iliac and inguinal parts may occur.

The cremaster is a thin muscular layer, composed of a number of fasciculi which arise from the middle of the inguinal ligament where its fibers are continuous with those of the obliquus internus and also occasionally with the transversus. It passes along the lateral side of the spermatic cord, descends with it through the subcutaneous inguinal ring upon the front and sides of the cord, and forms a series of loops which differ in thickness and length in different subjects. At the upper part of the cord the loops are short, but they become in succession longer and longer, the longest reaching down as low as the testis, where a few are inserted into the tunica vaginalis. These loops are united together by areolar tissue, and form a thin covering over the cord and testis, the cremasteric fascia. The fibers ascend along the medial side of the cord, and are inserted by a small pointed tendon into the tubercle and crest of the pubis and into the front of the sheath of the rectus abdominis (Fig. 16.8).

The transversus abdominis (*transversalis muscle*), so called from the direction of its fibers, is the most internal of the flat muscles of the abdomen, being placed immediately beneath the Obliquus internus. It arises,

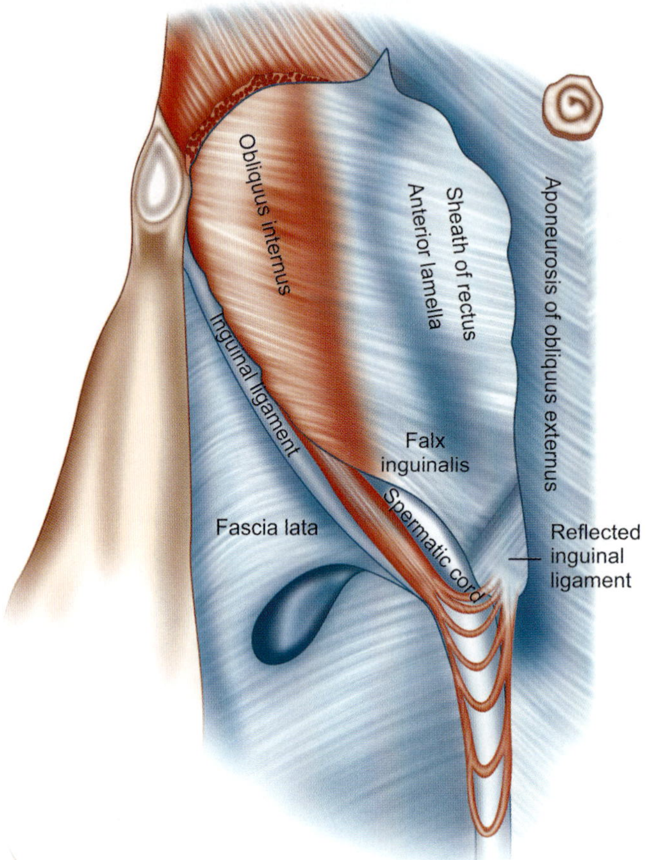


**Fig. 16.8:** The cremaster

by fleshy fibers, from the lateral third of the inguinal ligament, from the anterior three-fourths of the inner lip of the iliac crest, from the inner surfaces of the cartilages of the lower six ribs, interdigitating with the diaphragm, and from the lumbodorsal fascia. The muscle ends in front in a broad aponeurosis, the lower fibers of which curve downward and medialward, and are *inserted,* together with those of the obliquus internus, into the crest of the pubis and pectineal line, forming the inguinal aponeurotic falx. Throughout the rest of its extent the aponeurosis passes horizontally to the middle line, and is inserted into the linea alba; its upper three-fourths lie behind the rectus and blend with the posterior lamella of the aponeurosis of the obliquus internus; its lower fourth is in front of the rectus.

*Variations:* It may be more or less fused with the obliquus internus or absent. The spermatic cord may pierce its lower border. Slender muscle slips from the iliopectineal line to transversalis fascia, the aponeurosis of the transversus abdominis or the outer end of the linea semicircularis and other slender slips are occasionally found.

The inguinal aponeurotic falx (*falx aponeurotica inguinalis; conjoined tendon of internal oblique and transversalis muscle*) of the obliquus internus and transversus is mainly formed by the lower part of the tendon of the transversus, and is inserted into the crest of the pubis and pectineal line immediately behind the subcutaneous inguinal ring, serving to protect what would otherwise be a weak point in the abdominal wall. Lateral to the falx is a ligamentous band connected with the lower margin of the Transversus and extending down in front of the inferior epigastric artery to the superior ramus of the pubis; it is termed the interfoveolar ligament (Fig. 16.10) of Hesselbach and sometimes contains a few muscular fibers.

The rectus abdominis is a long flat muscle, which extends along the whole length of the front of the abdomen, and is separated from its fellow of the opposite side by the linea alba (Fig. 16.9). It is much broader, but thinner, above than below, and arises by two tendons; the lateral or larger is attached to the crest of the pubis, the medial interlaces with its fellow of the opposite side, and is connected with the ligaments covering the front of the symphysis pubis. The muscle is inserted by three portions of unequal size into the cartilages of the fifth, sixth, and seventh ribs. The upper portion, attached principally to the cartilage of the fifth rib, usually has some fibers of insertion into the anterior extremity of the rib itself. Some fibers are occasionally connected with the costoxiphoid ligaments, and the side of the xiphoid process.

The rectus is crossed by fibrous bands, three in number, which are named the tendinous inscriptions; one is usually situated opposite the umbilicus, one at the extremity of the xiphoid process, and the third about midway between the xiphoid process and the umbilicus. These inscriptions pass transversely or obliquely across the muscle in a zigzag course; they rarely extend completely through its substance and may pass only halfway across it; they are intimately adherent in front to the sheath of the muscle. Sometimes one or two additional inscriptions, generally incomplete, are present below the umbilicus.[27]

The rectus is enclosed in a sheath formed by the aponeuroses of the obliqus and transversus, which are arranged in the following manner. At the lateral margin of the rectus, the aponeurosis of the obliquus internus divides into two lamellae, one of which passes in front

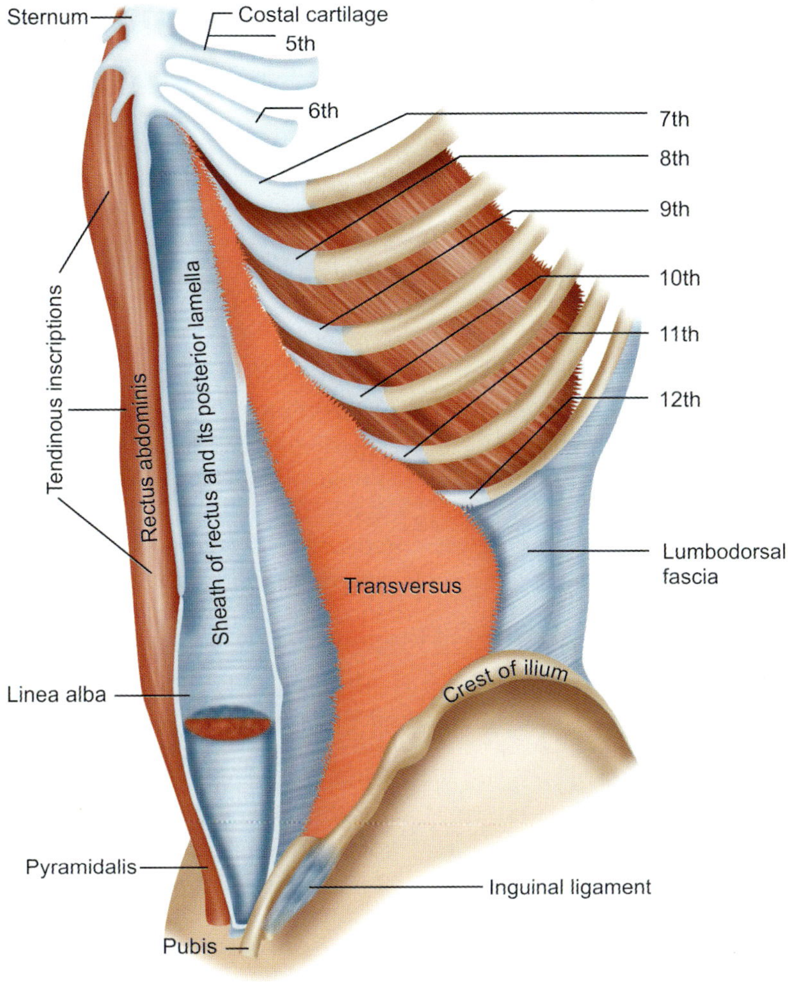


**Fig. 16.9:** The transversus abdominis, rectus abdominis, and pyramidalis

of the rectus, blending with the aponeurosis of the obliquus externus, the other, behind it, blending with the aponeurosis of the transversus, and these, joining again at the medial border of the rectus, are inserted into the linea alba. This arrangement of the aponeurosis exists from the costal margin to midway between the umbilicus and symphysis pubis, where the posterior wall of the sheath ends in a thin curved margin, the linea semicircularis (Fig. 16.12), the concavity of which is directed downward: below this level the aponeuroses of all three muscles pass in front of the rectus. The rectus, in the situation where its sheath is deficient below, is separated from the peritoneum by the transversalis fascia. Since the tendons of the obliquus internus and transversus only reach as high as the costal margin, it follows that above this level the sheath of the rectus is deficient behind, the muscle resting directly on the cartilages of the ribs, and being covered merely by the tendon of the obliquus externus.

The pyramidalis is a small triangular muscle, placed at the lower part of the abdomen, in front of the rectus, and contained in the sheath of that muscle. It *arises* by tendinous fibers from the front of the pubis and the anterior pubic ligament; the fleshy portion of the muscle passes upward, diminishing in size as it ascends, and ends by a pointed extremity which is *inserte*d into the linea alba, midway between the umbilicus and pubis. This muscle may be wanting on one or both sides; the lower end of the rectus then becomes proportionately

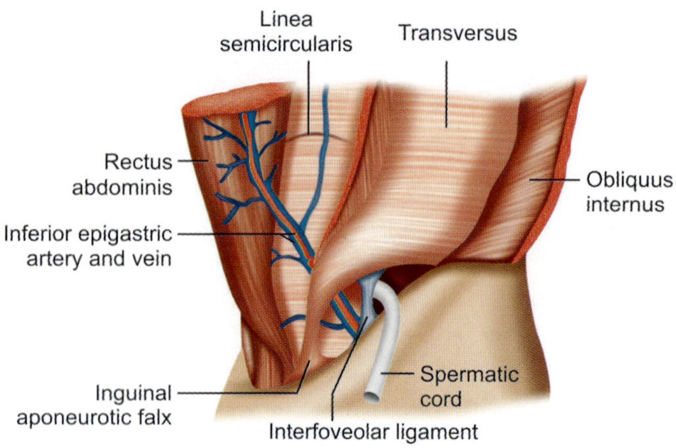


**Fig. 16.10:** The interfoveolar ligament, seen from front side (Modified from Braune)

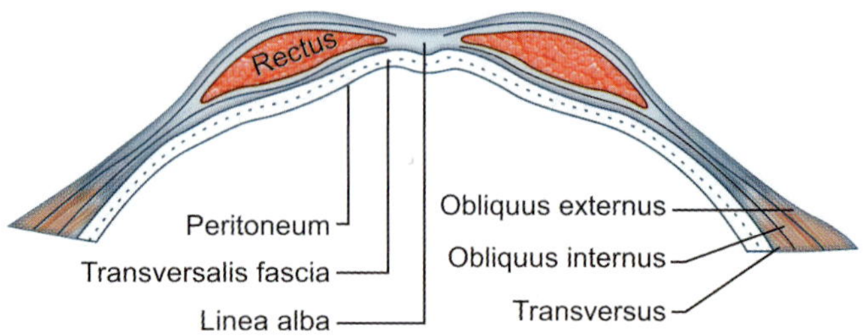


**Fig. 16.11:** Diagram of sheath of rectus

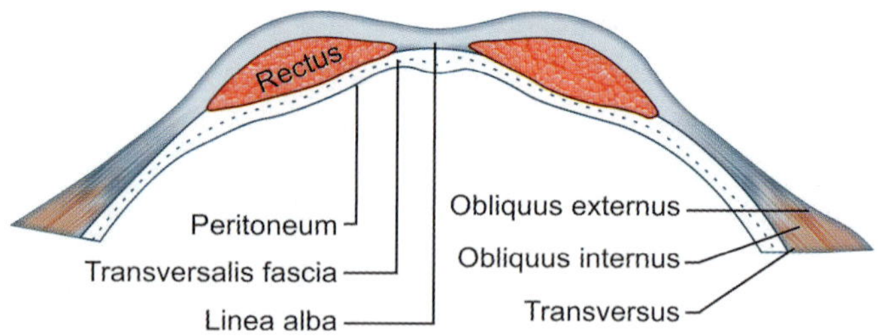


**Fig. 16.12:** Diagram of a transverse section through the anterior abdominal wall, below the linea semicircularis

increased in size. Occasionally it is double on one side, and the muscles of the two sides are sometimes of unequal size. It may extend higher than the level stated.

Besides the rectus and pyramidalis, the sheath of the rectus contains the superior and inferior epigastric arteries, and the lower intercostal nerves (Fig. 16.11).

*Variations:* The rectus may insert as high as the fourth or third rib or may fail to reach the fifth. Fibers may spring from the lower part of the linea alba.

*Nerves:* The abdominal muscles are supplied by the lower intercostal nerves. The obliquus internus and transversus also receive filaments from the anterior branch of the iliohypogastric and sometimes from the ilioinguinal. The cremaster is supplied by the external spermatic branch of the genitofemoral and the pyramidalis usually by the twelfth thoracic.

*The linea alba:* The linea alba is a tendinous raphé in the middle line of the abdomen, stretching between the xiphoid process and the symphysis pubis. It is placed between the medial borders of the recti, and is formed by the blending of the aponeuroses of the obliqus and transversus. It is narrow below, corresponding to the linear interval existing between the recti; but broader above, where these muscles diverge from one another. At its lower end the linea alba has a double attachment—its superficial fibers passing in front of the medial heads of the recti to the symphysis pubis, while its deeper fibers form a triangular lamella, attached behind the recti to the posterior lip of the crest of the pubis, and named the adminiculum lineae albae. It presents apertures for the passage of vessels and nerves; the umbilicus, which in the fetus exists as an aperture and transmits the umbilical vessels, is closed in the adult.

*The lineae semilunares:* The lineae semilunares are two curved tendinous lines placed one on either side of the linea alba. Each corresponds with the lateral border of the rectus, extends from the cartilage of the ninth rib to the pubic tubercle, and is formed by the aponeurosis of the obliquus internus at its line of division to enclose the rectus, reinforced in front by that of the obliquus externus, and behind by that of the transversus.

*Actions:* When the pelvis and thorax are fixed, the abdominal muscles compress the abdominal viscera by constricting the cavity of the abdomen, in which action they are materially assisted by the descent of the diaphragm. By these means assistance is given in expelling the feces from the rectum, the urine from the bladder, the fetus from the uterus, and the contents of the stomach in vomiting.

If the pelvis and vertebral column be fixed, these muscles compress the lower part of the thorax, materially assisting expiration. If the pelvis alone be fixed, the thorax is bent directly forward, when the muscles of both sides act; when the muscles of only one side contract, the trunk is bent toward that side and rotated toward the opposite side.

If the thorax be fixed, the muscles, acting together, draw the pelvis upward, as in climbing; or, acting singly, they draw the pelvis upward, and bend the vertebral column to one side or the other. The recti, acting from below, depress the thorax, and consequently flex the vertebral column; when acting from above, they flex the pelvis upon the vertebral column. The pyramidales are tensors of the linea alba.

*The transversalis fascia:* The transversalis fascia is a thin aponeurotic membrane which lies between the inner surface of the transversus and the extraperitoneal fat. It forms part of the general layer of fascia lining the abdominal parietes, and is directly continuous with the iliac and pelvic fasciae. In the inguinal region, the transversalis fascia is thick and dense in structure and is joined by fibers from the aponeurosis of the transversus, but it becomes thin as it ascends to the diaphragm, and blends with the fascia covering the under surface of this muscle. Behind, it is lost in the fat which covers the posterior surfaces of the kidneys. *Below,* it has the following attachments: posteriorly, to the whole length of the iliac crest, between the attachments of the transversus and iliacus; between the anterosuperior iliac spine and the femoral vessels it is connected to the posterior margin of the inguinal ligament, and is there continuous with the iliac fascia. Medial to the femoral vessels it is thin and attached to the pubis and pectineal line, behind the inguinal aponeurotic falx, with which it is united; it descends in front of the femoral vessels to form the anterior wall of the femoral sheath. Beneath the inguinal ligament it is strengthened by a band of fibrous tissue, which is only loosely connected to the ligament, and is specialized as the deep crural arch. The spermatic cord in the male and the round ligament of the uterus in the female pass through the transversalis fascia at a spot called the abdominal inguinal ring. This opening is not visible externally, since the transversalis fascia is prolonged on these structures as the infundibuliform fascia.

*The abdominal inguinal ring* (*annulus inguinalis abdominis; internal or deep abdominal ring*) (Fig. 16.13)*:* The abdominal inguinal ring is situated in the transversalis fascia, midway between the anterosuperior iliac spine and the symphysis pubis, and about 1.25 cm above the inguinal ligament. It is of an oval form, the long axis of the oval being vertical; it varies in size in different subjects, and is much larger in the male than in the female. It is bounded, above and laterally, by the arched lower margin of the transversus; below and medially, by the inferior epigastric vessels. It transmits the spermatic cord in the male and the round ligament of the uterus in the female. From its circumference a thin funnel-shaped membrane, the infundibuliform fascia, is continued

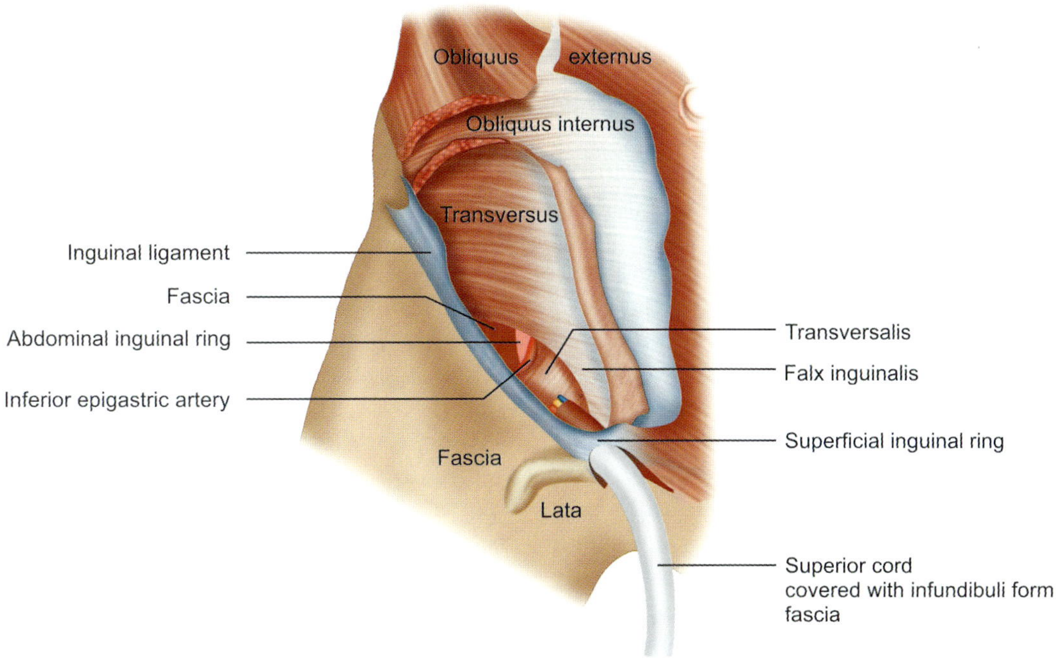


**Fig. 16.13:** The abdominal inguinal ring

around the cord and testis, enclosing them in a distinct covering.

*The inguinal canal (canalis inguinalis; spermatic canal):* The inguinal canal contains the spermatic cord and the ilioinguinal nerve in the male, and the round ligament of the uterus and the ilioinguinal nerve in the female. It is an oblique canal about 4 cm long, slanting downward and medialward, and placed parallel with and a little above the inguinal ligament; it extends from the abdominal inguinal ring to the subcutaneous inguinal ring. It is bounded, in front, by the integument and superficial fascia, by the aponeurosis of the obliquus externus throughout its whole length, and by the obliquus internus in its lateral third; behind, by the reflected inguinal ligament, the inguinal aponeurotic falx, the transversalis fascia, the extraperitoneal connective tissue and the peritoneum; above, by the arched fibers of obliquus internus and transversus abdominis; below, by the union of the transversalis fascia with the inguinal ligament, and at its medial end by the lacunar ligament.

*Extraperitoneal connective tissue:* Between the inner surface of the general layer of the fascia which lines the interior of the abdominal and pelvic cavities, and the peritoneum, there is a considerable amount of connective tissue, termed the extraperitoneal or subperitoneal connective tissue.

The parietal portion lines the cavity in varying quantities in different situations. It is especially abundant on the posterior wall of the abdomen, and particularly around the kidneys, where it contains much fat. On the anterior wall of the abdomen, except in the public region, and on the lateral wall above the iliac crest, it is scanty, and here the transversalis fascia is more closely connected with the peritoneum. There is a considerable amount of extraperitoneal connective tissue in the pelvis.

The visceral portion follows the course of the branches of the abdominal aorta between the layers of the mesenterics and other folds of peritoneum which connect the various viscera to the abdominal wall. The two portions are directly continuous with each other.

*The deep crural arch:* Curving over the external iliac vessels, at the spot where they become femoral, on the abdominal side of the inguinal ligaments and loosely connected with it, is a thickened band of fibers called the deep crural arch. It is apparently a thickening of the transversalis fascia joined laterally to the center of the lower margin of the inguinal ligament, and arching across the front of the femoral sheath to be inserted by a broad attachment into the pubic tubercle and pectineal line, behind the inguinal aponeurotic falx. In some subjects this structure is not very prominently marked, and not infrequently it is altogether wanting.

2. *The posterior muscles of the abdomen*
    - Psoas major
    - Iliacus
    - Psoas minor
    - Quadratus lumborum.

The psoas major, the psoas minor, and the iliacus, with the fasciae covering them, will be described with the muscles of the lower extremity.

*The fascia covering the quadratus lumborum:* This is a thin layer attached, medially, to the bases of the transverse processes of the lumbar vertebrae; below, to the iliolumbar ligament; above, to the apex and lower border of the last rib. The upper margin of this fascia, which extends from the transverse process of the first lumbar vertebra to the apex and lower border of the last rib, constitutes the lateral lumbocostal arch. Laterally, it blends with the lumbodorsal fascia, the anterior layer of which intervenes between the quadratus lumborum and the sacrospinalis.

The quadratus lumborum is irregularly quadrilateral in shape, and broader below than above. It arises by aponeurotic fibers from the iliolumbar ligament and the adjacent portion of the iliac crest for about 5 cm, and is inserted into the lower border of the last rib for about half its length, and by four small tendons into the apices of the transverse processes of the upper four lumbar vertebrae. Occasionally a second portion of this muscle is found in front of the preceding. It arises from the upper borders of the transverse processes of the lower three or four lumbar vertebrae, and is inserted into the lower margin of the last rib. In front of the quadratus lumborum are the colon, the kidney, the psoas major and minor, and the diaphragm; between the fascia and the muscle are the twelfth thoracic, ilioinguinal, and iliohypogastric nerves.

*Variations:* The number of attachments to the vertebrae and the extent of its attachment to the last rib vary.

*Nerve supply:* The twelfth thoracic and first and second lumbar nerves supply this muscle.

*Actions:* The quadratus lumborum draws down the last rib, and acts as a muscle of inspiration by helping to fix the origin of the diaphragm. If the thorax and vertebral column are fixed, it may act upon the pelvis, raising it toward its own side when only one muscle is put in action; and when both muscles act together, either from below or above, they flex the trunk.

In the ventral rectus sheath essentially oblique fibril bundles intermingle with each other, while the dorsal rectus sheath consists chiefly of transverse fibril bundles. In the linea alba three different zones of fiber orientation follow each other from ventral to dorsal. The lamina fibrae obliquae consists of intermingling oblique fibers. The lamina fibrae transversae contains mainly transverse fibril bundles, while an inconstant, small lamina fibrae irregularium is composed of oblique fibers. Different regions can be distinguished in the craniocaudal course of the linea alba: supraumbilical part, umbilical part, transition zone, and infra-arcuate part.

The various muscle bundle and aponeurotic fiber directions give the anterior abdominal wall a reinforced criss-cross plywood structure particularly in the upper abdomen. The anterior abdominal wall can be divided into two structural-functional zones, an upper parachute area aiding respiratory movement and a lower belly support area. The anatomy of the midline aponeurosis is related to epigastric hernia formation. Epigastric hernia formation is found exclusively in patients with single anterior and single posterior lines of decussation. Uncoordinated tearing strains on the aponeurotic fibers of linea alba, for instance in vigorous sports, coughing or vomiting, will stretch the decussations and allow the development of fatty protrusions between their bundles.

The differential diagnosis of an epigastric hernia includes:

- Peptic ulcer
- Gallbladder disease
- Hiatus hernia
- Pancreatitis
- Upper small bowel obstruction
- Subcutaneous lipoma
- Neurofibroma.

## Epigastric Hernia Surgery

Surgery should always be advised and preformed for epigastric herniations of all sizes. Now, it should be observed that whatever the size of the defect presents, one should always go for tension-free repair with prosthesis implant. The days of fascial darning are over.

1. *Anesthesia*: General anesthesia is employed.
2. *Suture material*: Nonabsorbable polypropylene for suture repair and implant fixation.
3. *Procedure*:
    - Draping should be done so as to expose xiphisternum till umbilicus (Wide area)
    - *Incision:* Two types of incisions can be employed for the surgery viz vertical and transverse. If the surgeon knows the defect of epigastric hernia that it is either solitary or multiple, then vertical incision should be taken. If the surgeon knows that the defect is solitary and small then a transverse incision should be taken as it helps for the cosmetic purpose. The latter heals well and securely.
    - *Dissection:* The abdominal fat surrounding the fatty hernia is dissected and the hernia is freed from all directions up to neck. Sometimes the defect in linea alba needs to be enlarged by incision on it. This should be done in opposite directions in lateral directions. All additional defects should be looked for and extension of incision on linea alba should be made. This is best done in vertical incisions.
    - *Sac:* The neck of the sac is opened and the contents of the sac are returned to the abdomen. Nowadays the whole sac along with the contents are reduced to the abdomen. It is seldom practiced to transfix the sac and excise it. However, it should be completely observed that the contents and the sac are completely reduced to abdomen. There should be no constriction on the contents at all.

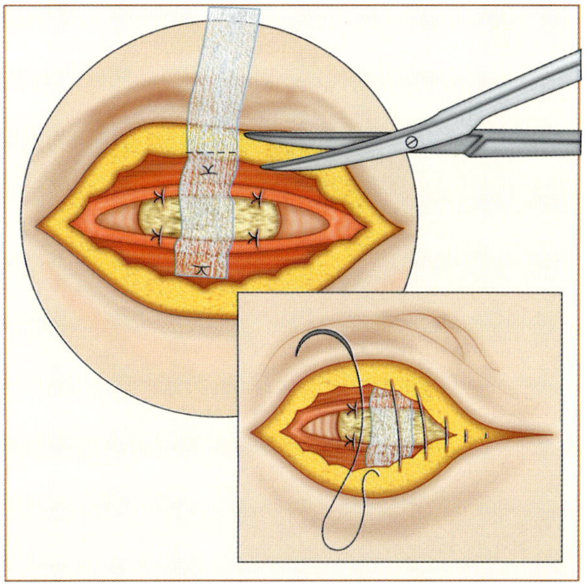

**Fig. 16.14:** Prosthesis implant—a suitable and available prosthesis should be implanted as inlay (in between the preperitoneal space)

- *Other defects:* A strict lookout for other corresponding defects should be made and they are reduced effectively as well.
- *Prosthesis implant:* A suitable and available prosthesis should be implanted as inlay (in between the preperitoneal space). It should be fixed to the aponeurosis by four anchoring sutures from inside out. The prosthesis should be covering the defect area and it should be at least 4 cm cover after defect line. The preperitoneal space should be well prepared for this. There should be no kinking of the mesh material. The light weight mesh which is partly absorbable with large pores is preferred (Fig. 16.14).
- *Closure of defect:* The defect is now closed with simple continuous or interrupted non-absorbable polypropylene sutures in adults and for children the PDS suture is preferred.
- *Drain:* The suction drain is placed so as to absorb the serous collection. This keeps the incision free of discharges.
- *Subcutaneous tissue:* The subcutaneous tissue is closed with absorbable sutures of surgeon's preference. This is not mandatory. The subcutaneous tissue can be left without suturing.
- *Skin:* Skin is closed with nonabsorbable sutures or staples,subcuticular sutures.

The surgery is more or less similar to umbilical hernia surgery.

## Complications of Epigastric Hernia Operation

Major complications of epigastric hernia surgery include recurrence of hernia, wound infection, bleeding, bruising, swelling, numbness, injury to intestine or other intra-abdominal organs.

# Chapter 17

# Incisional/Ventral Hernias

## Incisional/Ventral Hernia Surgery

An incisional hernia occurs in an area of weakness caused by an incompletely-healed surgical wound. Since median incisions in the abdomen are frequent for abdominal exploratory surgery, ventral incisional hernias are termed ventral hernias. These can be among the most frustrating and difficult hernias to treat (Fig. 17.1).

Clinically, incisional hernias present as a bulge or protrusion at or near the area of a surgical incision. Virtually any prior abdominal operation can develop an incisional hernia at the scar area (provided adequate healing does not occur), from large abdominal procedures (intestinal surgery, vascular surgery), to small incisions (appendix removal, or abdominal exploratory surgery).

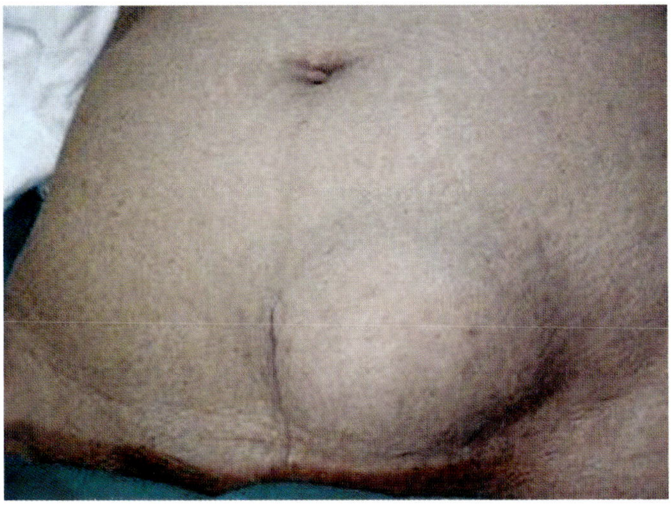

**Fig. 17.1:** Incisional/ventral hernia

While these hernias can occur at any incision, they tend to occur more commonly along a straight line from the xiphoid process of the sternum straight down to the pubic bone, and are more complex in these regions. Hernias in this area have a high rate of recurrence if repaired via a simple suture technique under tension. For this reason, it is especially advised that these be repaired via a tension free repair method using mesh.

- *Incisional hernia*: Abdominal surgery causes a flaw in the abdominal wall. This flaw can create an area of weakness in which a hernia may develop. This occurs after 2 to 10% of all abdominal surgeries, although some people are more at risk. Even after surgical repair, incisional hernias may return.
- These hernias may occur after large surgeries such as intestinal or vascular (heart, arteries, and veins) surgery, or after smaller surgeries such as an appendectomy or a laparoscopy, which typically requires a small incision at the navel. Incisional hernias themselves can be very small or large and complex, involving growth along the scar tissue of a large incision. They may develop months after the surgery or years after, usually because of inadequate healing or excessive pressure on an abdominal wall scar.

## Demographics

Because incisional hernias can occur at the site of any type of abdominal surgery previously performed on a wide range of individuals, there is no outstanding profile of an individual most likely to have an incisional hernia. Men, women, and children of all ages and ethnic backgrounds may develop an incisional hernia after abdominal surgery. Incisional hernia occurs more commonly among adults than among children.

### Symptoms and Signs

1. Many patients do not have any symptoms
2. Difficulty in bending
3. Cosmetic deformity
4. Persistent abdominal pain
5. Discomfort in abdomen
6. Occasional episodes of subacute intestinal obstruction
7. Incarceration
8. Strangulation
9. Unusually it may rupture
10. Dermatitis due to friction of bulge on clothes
11. The first symptom a person may have with an incisional hernia is pain, with or without a bulge in the abdomen at or near the site of the original surgery. Incisional hernias can increase in size and gradually produce more noticeable symptoms.

### Etiological Factors of Incisional Hernia

The factors that increase the risk of incisional hernia are conditions that increase strain on the abdominal wall, such as obesity, advanced age, malnutrition, poor metabolism (digestion and assimilation of essential nutrients), pregnancy, dialysis, excess fluid retention, and either infection or hematoma after a prior surgery.

Tension created when sutures are used to close a surgical wound may also be responsible for developing an incisional hernia. Tension is known to influence poor healing conditions because of related swelling and wound separation. Tension and abdominal pressure are greater in people who are overweight, creating greater risk of developing incisional hernias following any abdominal surgery, including surgery for a prior inguinal (groin) hernia. People who have been treated with steroids or chemotherapy are also at greater risk for developing incisional hernias because of the affect these drugs have on the healing process.

1. Sepsis is the main cause which occurs in post operative status giving rise to incisional hernia within first year of surgery.
2. Drainage tubes placement.
3. Repeated surgeries within 6 months.
4. Inflammatory bowel disease.
5. Early wound dehiscence.
6. Laparoscopic Surgery-Port sites.
7. Following specific surgeries on abdomen and pelvis cause incisional hernia in excess number of Patients:
   - Hysterectomy
   - Cholecystectomy and Biliary tract surgery
   - Appendectomy
   - Colorectal surgery
   - Gastric operations
   - Cesarean Surgery
8. Midline incisions taken are at high-risk developing hernia.
9. Lower midline incision have high-risk of developing hernia.

## Diagnosis

Reviewing the patient's symptoms and medical history are the first steps in diagnosing an incisional hernia. All prior surgeries will be discussed. The doctor will ask how much pain the patient is experiencing, when it was first noticed, and how it has progressed. The doctor will palpate the area, looking for any abnormal bulging or mass, and may ask the patient to cough or strain in order to see and feel the hernia more easily. To confirm the presence of the hernia, an ultrasound examination or other scan such as computed tomography (CT) may be performed. Scans will allow to visualize the hernia and to make sure that the bulge is not another type of abdominal mass such as a tumor or enlarged lymph gland. The doctor will be able to determine the size of the defect and whether or not surgery is an appropriate way to treat it.

Patients with hernias present to the emergency department (ED) secondary to a complication associated with the hernia. Hernias also may be detected in the ED on routine physical examination. However, in relation to the chief complaint, the following clinical issues must be considered:

- Asymptomatic hernia
  - Presents as a swelling or fullness at the hernia site
  - Aching sensation (radiates into the area of the hernia)
  - No true pain or tenderness upon examination
  - Enlarges with increasing intra-abdominal pressure and/or standing
- Incarcerated hernia
  - Painful enlargement of a previous hernia or defect

- Cannot be manipulated (either spontaneously or manually) through the fascial defect
- Nausea, vomiting, and symptoms of bowel obstruction (possible)

• Strangulated hernia
  - Symptoms of an incarcerated hernia present combined with a toxic appearance
  - Systemic toxicity secondary to ischemic bowel is possible
  - Strangulation is probable if pain and tenderness of an incarcerated hernia persist after reduction
  - Suspect an alternative diagnosis in patients who have a substantial amount of pain without evidence of incarceration or strangulation

## Physical

In general, the physical examination should be performed with the patient in both the supine and standing positions, with and without the Valsalva maneuver. The examiner should attempt to identify the hernia sac as well as the fascial defect through which it is protruding. This allows proper direction of pressure for reduction of hernia contents. The examiner should also identify evidence of obstruction and strangulation.

## Examination

The sac and fibrous margins of the sac are examined with patient supine, relaxed, and then standing erect.
The strength of the abdominal wall musculature should be assessed. The divarication, if any should be noted.

## Classification

### *Lateral Hernias (Fig. 17.2)*

The borders of the lateral area are defined as

1. *Cranial*: the costal margin
2. *Caudal*: the inguinal region
3. *Medially*: the lateral margin of the rectal sheath
4. *Laterally*: the lumbar region.

Thus, four L-zones on each side are defined as:

1. *L1*: subcostal (between the costal margin and a horizontal line 3 cm above the umbilicus)
2. *L2*: flank (lateral to the rectal sheath in the area 3 cm above and below the umbilicus)
3. *L3*: iliac (between a horizontal line 3 cm below the umbilicus and the inguinal region)
4. L4: lumbar (laterodorsal of the anterior axillary line)

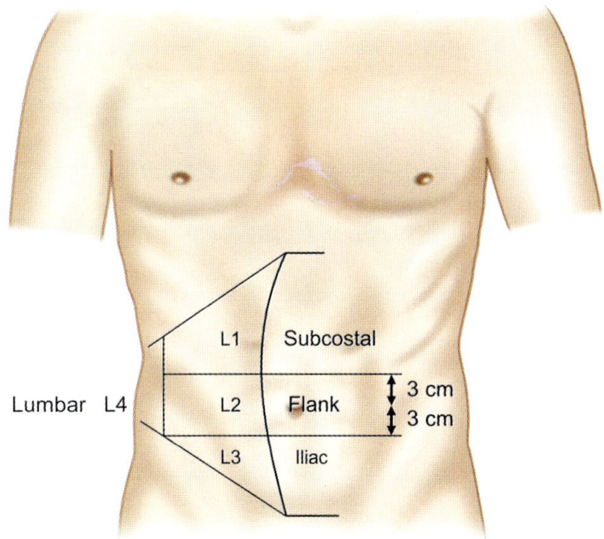


**Fig. 17.2:** Classification—lateral hernias

In contrast to primary abdominal wall hernias, incisional hernias come in many different sizes and shapes. So the size of an incisional hernia is not easily captured in only one variable or measurement. For classification in the two dimensional grid format, it is essential to bring the variable "size of the hernia defect" in one quantitative or semiquantitative measure. Chevrel solved this problem by choosing the width of the hernia defect as the one parameter to classify, stating that the width is the most important measurement of size to determine the difficulty of successfully repairing the hernia. The width of the hernia defect was defined as the greatest horizontal distance in cm between the lateral margins of the hernia defect on both sides (Figs 17.3 and 17.4).

### *Preparation for Surgery*

Many months before the surgery, the patient's doctor may advise weight loss to help reduce the risks of surgery and to improve the surgical results. Control of diabetes and smoking cessation are also recommended for a better surgical result.

## Indications for Incisional Hernia Repair

Patients having discomfort, pain, recurrent colic, occasional episodes of subacute episodes of subacute intestinal obstruction, irreducible hernias, narrow neck defects.

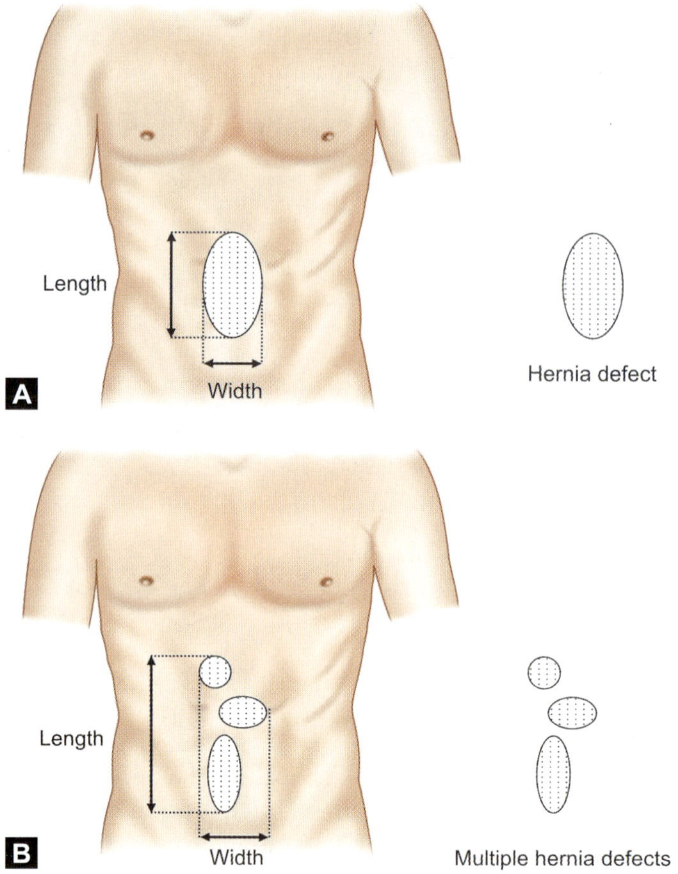


**Figs 17.3A and B:** (A) Single hernia defect; (B) Multiple hernia defects

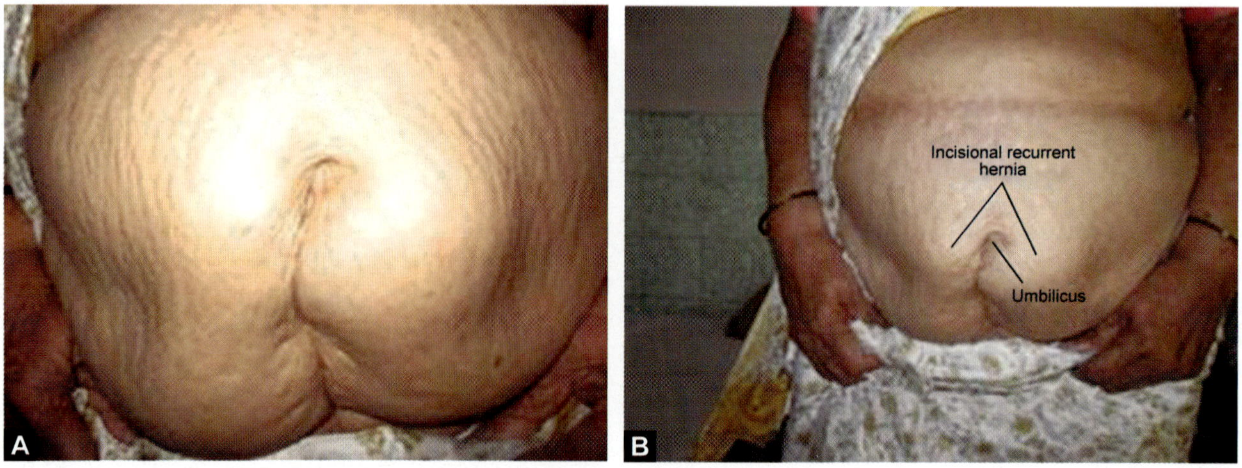


**Figs 17.4A and B:** Incisional hernia with multiple defects

## Treatment

Incisional hernias are repaired most of the times due to above said indications. However, in patients with extreme obesity the repair should be undertaken after weight control according to height and age.

*Procedure:* Two types of procedure are practiced :

1. Open prosthetic incisional hernia repair.
2. Laparoscopic Incisional hernia repair.

*Types of Repair:* Primary, primary with relaxing incisions, primary with onlay mesh reinforcement, onlay mesh only, inlay mesh placement, retrorectus mesh placement, and intraperitoneal mesh placement.

- Primary repair
  - Usually for facial defects less than 5 cm in diameter
  - Recurrence rates of approximately 50% have been reported
  - There is tension present in this repair. May use relaxing incisions to reduce tension (e.g. Keel procedure, separation-of-parts technique)
- Mesh products
  - Absorbable meshes only used in cases where mesh infection is a significant risk and cannot perform primary closure
  - Polyester mesh associated with higher rates of entero-cutaneous fistula formation and mesh infection
  - Polypropylene has greatest tissue ingrowth of all meshes available
  - PTFE has fewest bowel complications due to its nonadhesiveness to bowel

## Open Prosthetic Incisional Hernia Repair

### Position: Supine on Operating Table

Incision and dissection: An elliptical incision made on the scar. This incision should enclose the scar. This incision should be spread adequately to access the defect effectively. Minimum excision of the skin is done (Figs 17.5A and B).

*Dissection*: The redundant skin and scar are separated from the underlying hernia sac, which is often just subcutaneous especially near the fundus of the hernia. Redundant skin and scar tissue is removed. Now, the hernia is dissected from the surrounding subcutaneous fat. The scar tissue is incised in an elliptical fashion around the hernia neck, where it merges with the stretched aponeurosis. The peritoneal hernia sac is thus defined all around at its attachment to the muscle/aponeurotic layer (Figs 17.6A and B).

The dissection is carried to the neck of the sac. If the contents of the sac are reducible then those contents are reduced in the abdomen. The sac is transfixed and excised. Remaining part is sutured and closed. If the contents are not reducible, then the aponeurosis is excised 1 to 2 cm

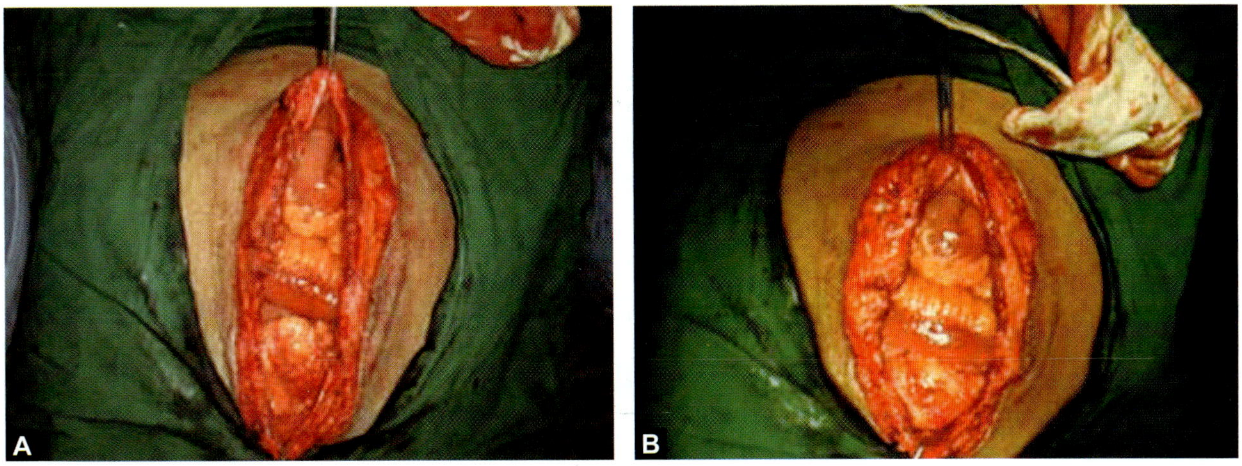

**Figs 17.5A and B:** All defects opened up to form a single vertical defect

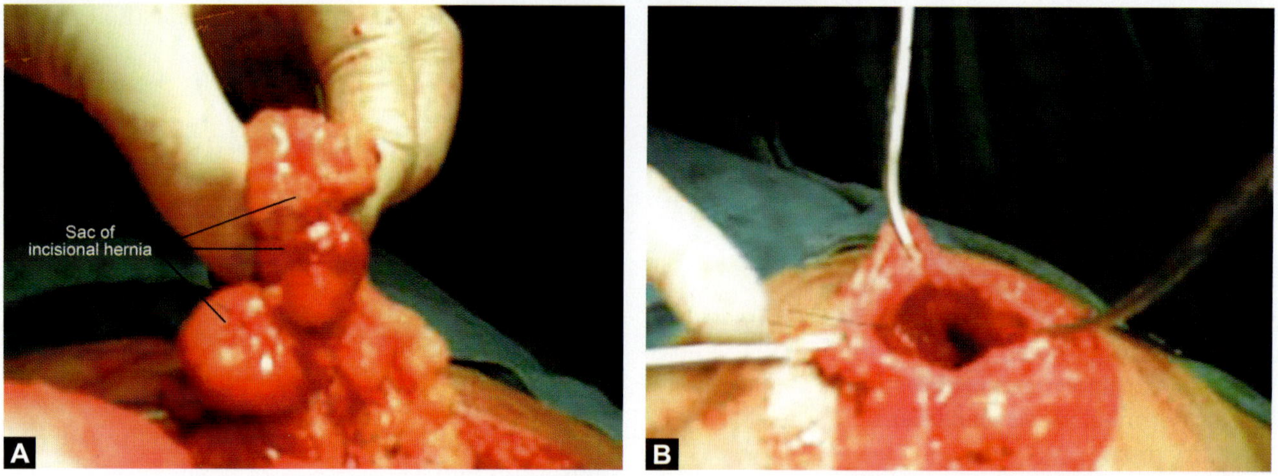


**Figs 17.6A and B:** (A) Sac of incisional hernia; (B) Opened sac of incisional hernia

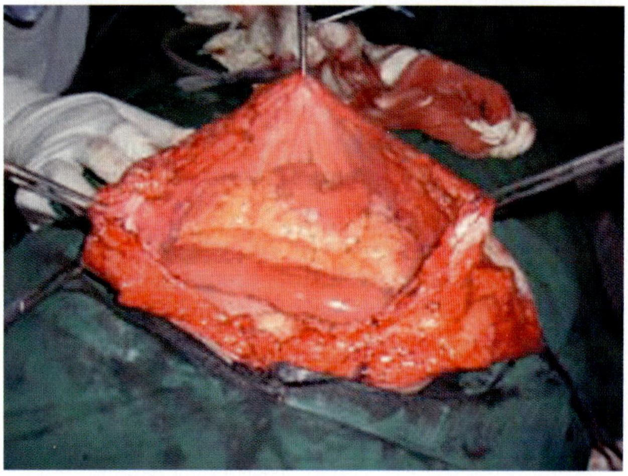

**Fig. 17.7:** Peritoneal suturing done

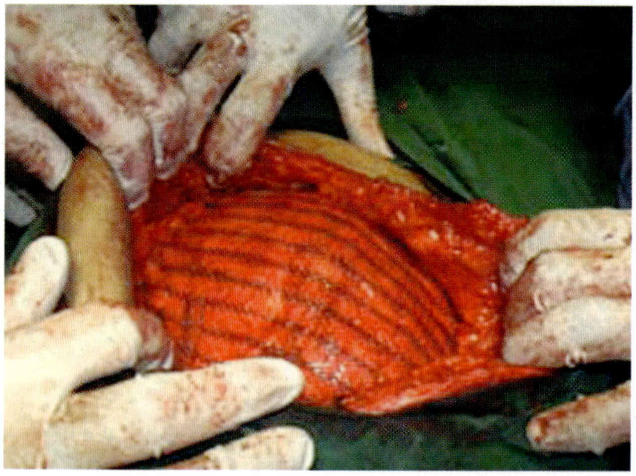

**Fig. 17.8:** Vyproll mesh implanted properitoneally

on either side in transverse fashion and the defect is made bigger, so as to reduce its contents. After reduction of the contents, if the sac is bigger then it is excised; however if the sac is small then it is returned to the abdomen.

*Closure of peritoneum*: If the peritoneum is free from visceral organs and can be approximated then closure of peritoneum is done with the absorbable suture. If the peritoneum is not amenable to approximation then omentum is placed over the intestines.

In the latter case a bilayered mesh with absorbable inner layer is to be used for this type of repair to prevent adhesions and fistula (Fig. 17.7).

## Repair of Defect

The aponeurotic defect is examined. If the defect can not be closed by approximation without tension then small multiple or solo incisions should be taken on the lateral parts of aponeurosis on both sides of the defect. This procedure with allow sliding of the edges of the aponeurosis so as to approximate the defect. Non-absorbable interrupted or continuous sutures are taken to close the defect in case of onlay prosthetic mesh placement. In case of inlay mesh placement, the mesh is placed prior to the closure (Figs 17.8 and 17.9).

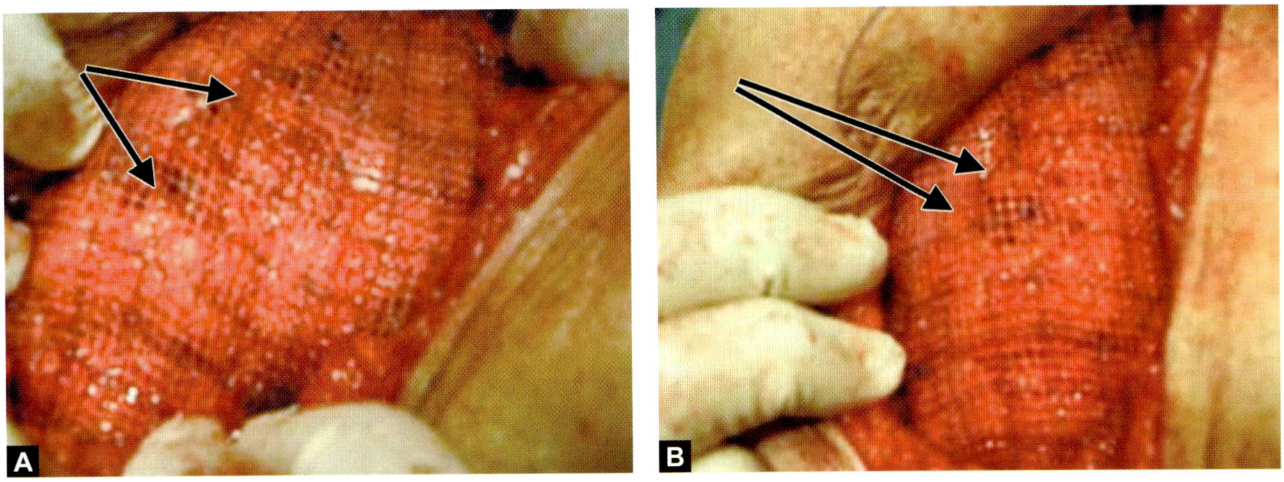

**Figs 17.9A and B:** Vyproll mesh implanted properitoneally complete (arrows)

*Choice of mesh*: The choice of mesh is guided by the characteristics of the patient and hernia defect(s) and ultimately the surgeon's preference. The mesh should be sized to provide an overlap of at least 4 to 5 cm around the circumference of the defect. Large central defects should be repaired with wider overlap to allow fixation to normal abdominal wall to avoid eventration of the mesh. Small, Swiss cheese-type defects may require a lesser margin. The potential for prosthetic mesh contraction should always be considered when sizing the mesh. Depending on the type of mesh the degree of contraction may vary considerably.

*Onlay mesh repair*: After closure of the peritoneum, the edges of the aponeurotic defects are approximated and closed with nonabsorbable sutures. The onlay mesh is taken and assured that the edges of the mesh cover 5 cm over the defect area on all sides.

*Inlay mesh repair*: Intraperitoneal-hernia sac is excised and fascial margin is identified around the hernia defect. Either polypropylene or ePTFE is sutured circumferentially to fascial edge. Polypropylene would be used when omentum can be placed between intestine and mesh;ePTFE should be used when there is no omentum available (Figs 17.10 and 17.11).

## Preparation of Mesh

Onlay mesh is prepared for the defect which should cover the defect on all sides at least up to 4 to 5 cm. Then the mesh is divided in center with the defect line parallel. Then onlay mesh is put over the defect evenly and 4 lines of sutures or staplers are placed on the mesh. Two lines of staples or sutures on either side of the defect. Once all the sutures are placed in 4 lines then the mesh along with the defect is mobilized towards the center and then the defect in the mesh is sutured (Fig. 17.15).

*Drain*: A suction drain is inserted along the suture line of mesh and around the mesh. In case of the inlay preperitoneal mesh insertion the drain is put on the defect closure line. The drain is fixed with the non absorbable sutures

*Closure*: Subcutaneous fat along with the fascia is closed with absorbable sutures,interrupted fashion. skin can be closed with the nonabsorbable sutures or staplers (Figs 17.12 to 17.14).

*Dressing*: Dry dressing is applied and the wound is dressed with long elastic dressing so as to provide stability to incision.

*Drain removal*: This is decided according to the collection in drain. Usually drain is removed on 3 to 4th postoperative day provided there is no or minimal collection.

## Laparoscopic Incisional Hernia Repair

In general, the procedure for laparoscopic incisional hernia repair (LIHR) consists of four steps: appropriate port placement, adhesiolysis, intraperitoneal measurement of the hernia size, and anchoring of the mesh. The first trocar should be placed away from scars and sites of previous surgery to prevent intraoperative bowel injury as well as to enable easy access to adhesiolysis.

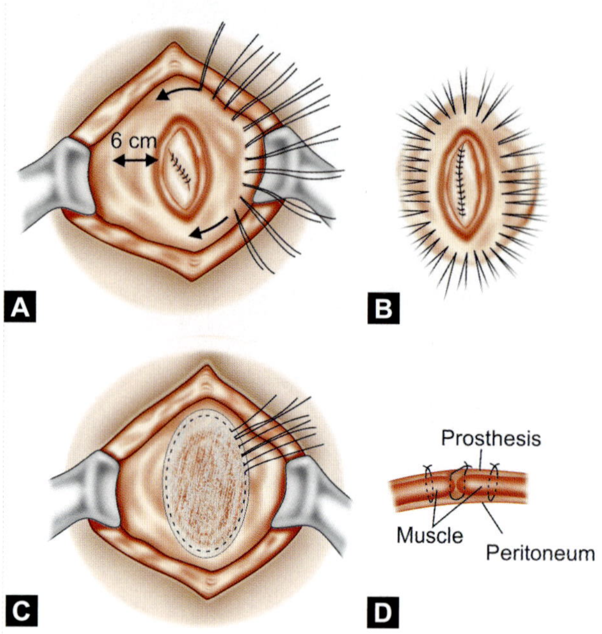


Figs 17.10A to D

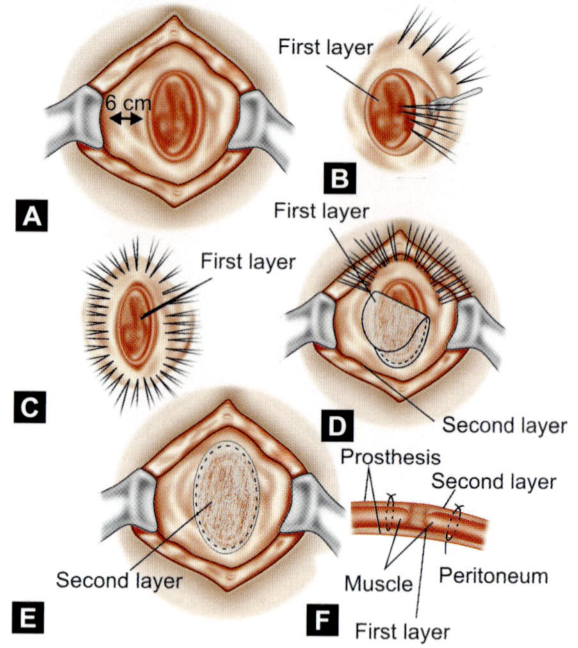


Figs 17.11A to F

**Figs 17.10 and 17.11:** Inlay mesh repair—intraperitoneal hernia sac is excised and fascial margin is identified around the hernia defect. Either polypropylene or ePTFE is sutured circumferentially to fascial edge

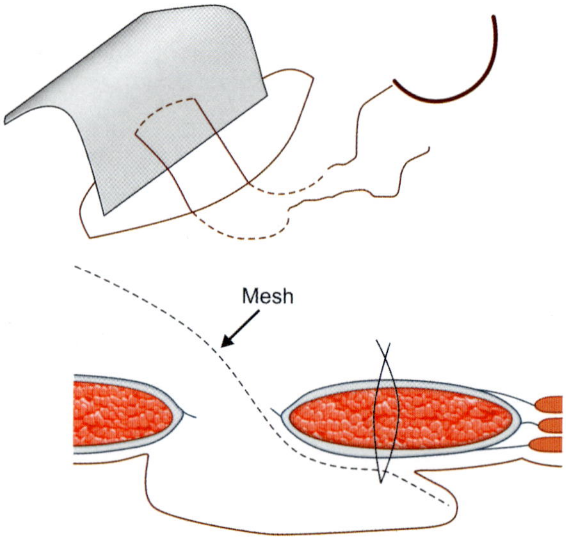


**Fig. 17.12:** 1 to 1.5 cm tangential bite of mesh is taken about 2.5 cm from its margin and the needle is then passed back along a path retrograde to the first pass of the needle and about 1 to 1.5 cm from it. When the suture is drawn and tied, mesh is tucked into the retrofascial position

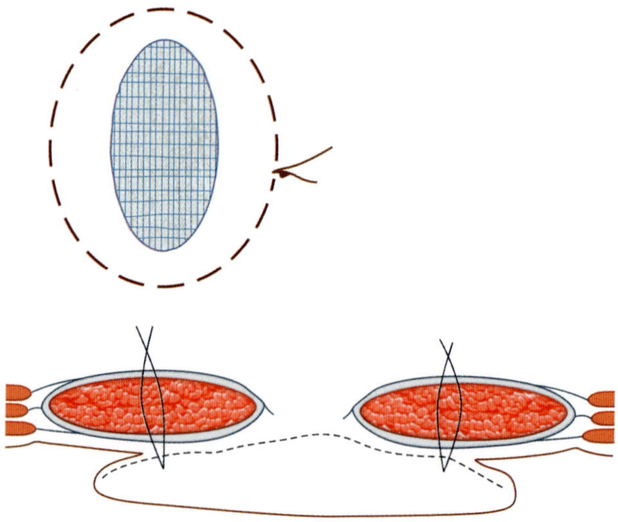

**Fig. 17.13:** Suturing in like fashion is continued until the entire piece of mesh has been tucked into position posterior to the defect and myofascial layer

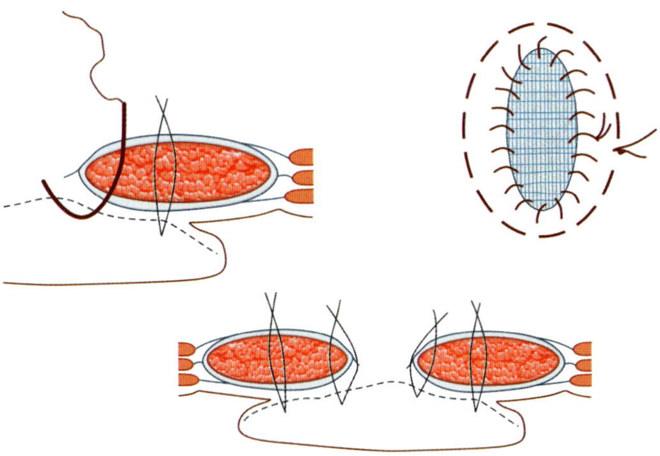

**Fig. 17.14:** The overhang is sutured to the mesh with continuous radial stitches, completing the repair

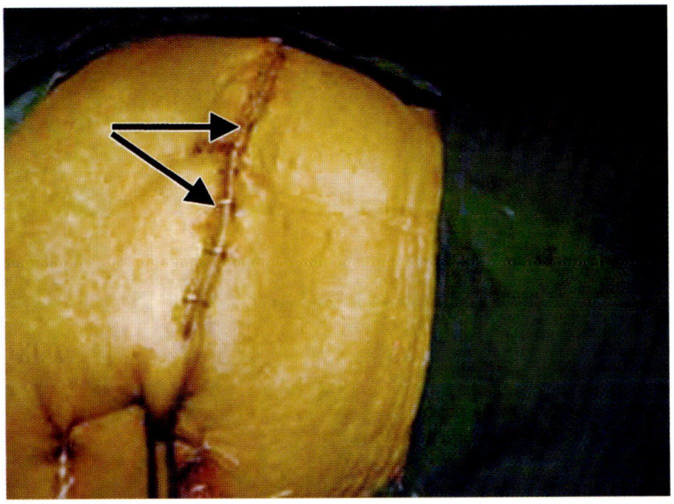

**Fig. 17.15:** Skin sutured with staplers in a horizontal incision (arrows)

## Laparoscopic Ventral Hernia Repair

### *Patient Selection and Preoperative Care*

The success of laparoscopic ventral hernia repair begins with careful patient selection. Exclusion criteria are not absolute and may diminish with the experience of the surgeon. A history of multiple previous repairs does not exclude a laparoscopic approach but the more inexperienced surgeon wisely may choose to defer these patients, particularly those with previous intraperitoneal polypropylene mesh. Patients with previous major wound or mesh infection may not be candidates for laparoscopic repair with synthetic mesh until it is clear that the infection is completely cleared. Even then, caution should be exercised as a latent bacterial infection may "reactivate" after hernia repair. Patients with loss of domain combined with obesity must be approached cautiously, given the limited working space and the risk for compartment syndrome. Patients with acute incarceration with bowel obstruction may be candidates for laparoscopic repair; however, those with significant abdominal distention, large defects, previous hernia repairs, or hemodynamic instability may be better served by open repair (Figs 17.16A to E).

The process of informed consent should include a careful preoperative discussion of the risks, benefits, possible complications, and postoperative expectations of seroma formation and pain. Particular attention should be given to the risk for bowel injury and the surgeon's algorithm for management. Safe methods range from conversion to laparotomy to repair the bowel to laparoscopic repair. A staged procedure may be performed with completion of the adhesiolysis and later placement of the mesh. Alternatively, an open tissue repair, such as components separation with biologic mesh reinforcement, may be an option.

### *Preparation and Instrumentation*

Preoperative antibiotic prophylaxis, such as a first generation cephalosporin, and subcutaneous heparin prophylaxis is recommended. The patient is placed in a supine position with the arms carefully padded, positioned, and tucked to the sides. The abdomen is prepped widely to allow lateral port placement. The surgeon may also select to place an occlusive skin barrier over the abdomen to avoid contact of the mesh with the skin and skin flora. The patient is placed under general anesthesia.

Essential laparoscopic instrumentation includes atraumatic graspers, laparoscopic scissors, irrigation/ suction device, and a suture passer. Three trocars are needed,including a 10- to 12-mm port and two 5-mm ports (Fig. 17.17). Additional 5-mm trocars may be placed as needed to facilitate adhesiolysis and mesh fixation from both sides of the abdomen. A 5-mm, 30-degree laparoscope is more versatile than the 10-mm laparoscope, allowing movement from trocar to trocar, which may facilitate adhesiolysis and mesh fixation from various angles.

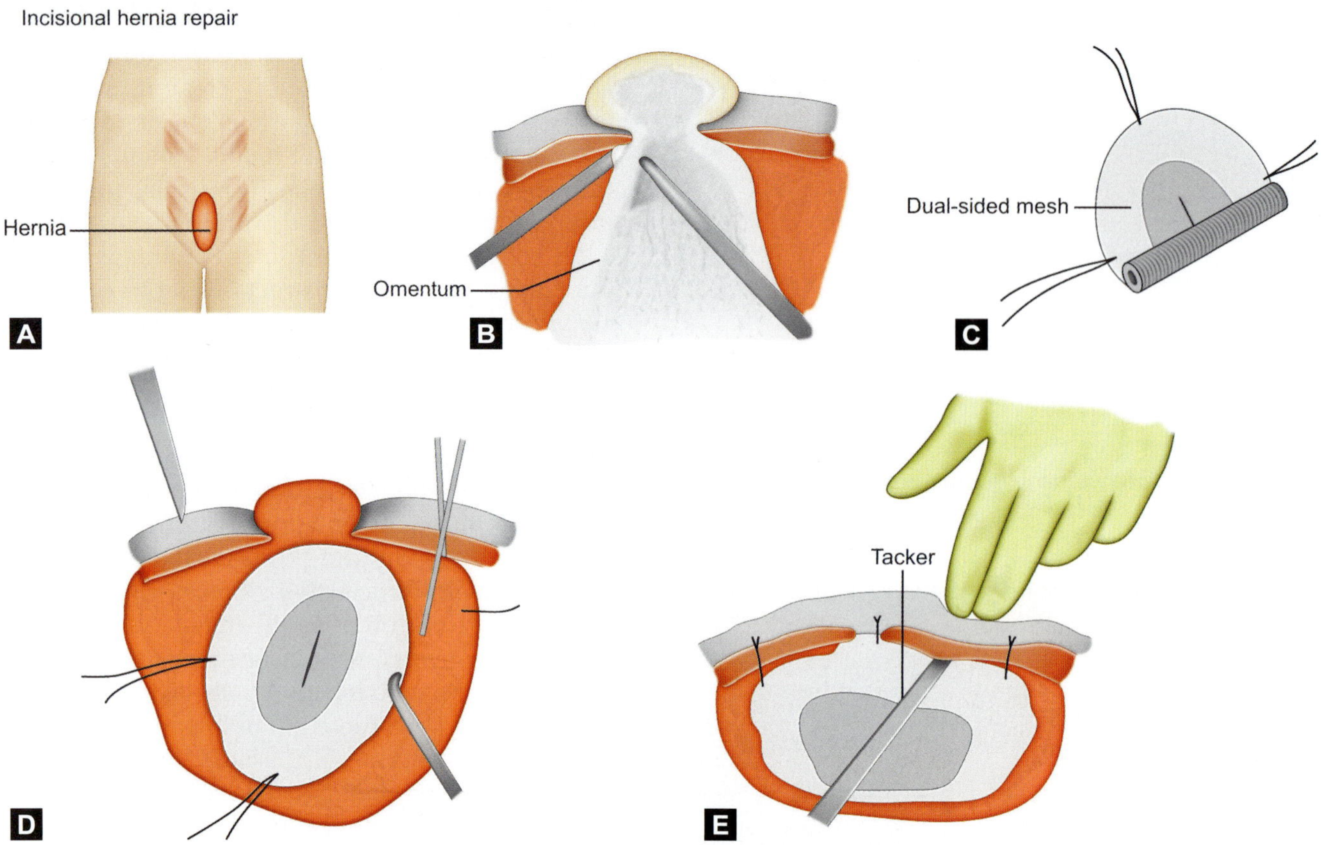


**Figs 17.16A to E:** An incisional hernia occurs at the site of a previous incision. (A) Intestinal contents break through the abdominal wall and bubble up under the skin; (B) In a laparoscopic repair, the surgeon uses laparoscopic forceps to pull the material, omentum, from the hernia site; (C and D) A mesh pad is inserted into the site to line the hernia site; (E) and is tacked into place

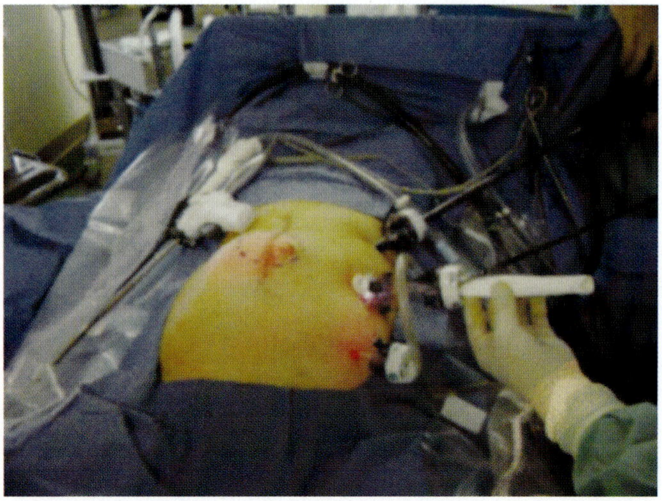

**Fig. 17.17:** Placement of trocars for laparoscopic incisional hernia repair. The rolled mesh is inserted through a 12-mm port

### *Operative Procedure*

Abdominal access may be achieved via the closed Veress needle technique in a virgin area just below the costal margin or via open Hasson technique. This is a matter of surgeon preference and experience. Both techniques are associated with a risk for visceral or vascular injury. If the Veress needle technique is used, it is helpful to use an optiview trocar with camera visualization as the first port. This should be placed in the lateral abdomen away from the defect. Lateral placement is important in terms of later allowance for wide mesh overlap of the defect. The Veress needle entry site is inspected for any intra-abdominal injury. If the open Hasson technique is used, S retractors, serially grasping, and division of the fascial layers in the lateral abdomen facilitate peritoneal entry. The remaining 5-mm ports are also placed laterally under direct camera visualization.

Adhesiolysis is the key portion of the repair. This should be conducted with great care, ever mindful of the potential for bowel injury. Grading of the adhesions in terms of tenacity guides the surgeon to perform blunt dissection for the filmy adhesions and sharp dissection for denser adhesions. Thermal energy sources should be used judiciously. Clips or sutures are used as needed where hemostasis is required close to the intestine.

Adhesiolysis can be challenging in patients who have undergone previous mesh repair. If the intestine is densely adherent to the abdominal wall or previous mesh, the plane of dissection should be superficial to this, leaving a medallion of mesh on the intestine rather than injuring the bowel during an attempt to separate the two. After taking down adherent intestine, it is imperative to closely inspect the bowel for any injury before proceeding. Additionally, the abdomen should be inspected for bleeding and bowel injury at the completion of the adhesiolysis and at the end of the procedure. The finding of no bowel injury should be appropriately documented.

Reduction of the incarcerated hernia often requires gentle hand-over-hand atraumatic retraction with sharp division of fibrous bands or the hernia sac. External palpation over the defect may facilitate reduction of hernia contents (Fig. 17.18). Care should be taken to reduce the hernia entirely of its contents so as not to leave necrotic material in the hernia sac if possible.

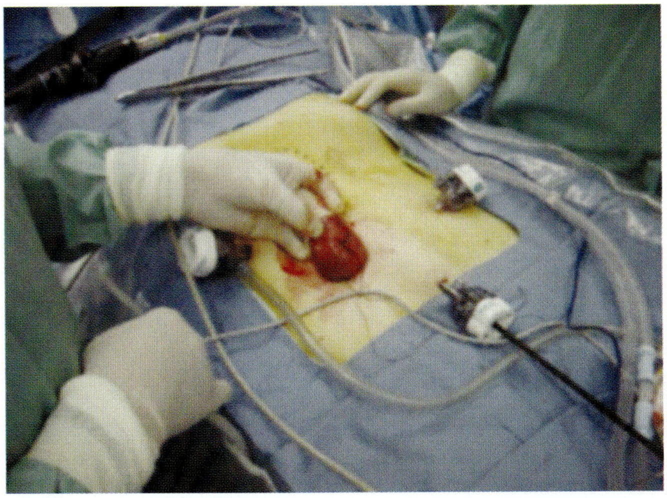

**Fig. 17.18:** The "incarceration technique" any serosal defect created during adhesiolysis is repaired extraperitoneally by delivering the lesion through a 12-mm port site maintaining a pneumoperitoneum

Once the entire abdominal wall is cleared of all adhesions, it is inspected for hemostasis and for fascial defects. These are measured for appropriate mesh sizing. Internal measurement is more accurate than external measurement of the defect, particularly in the obese patient where the thick abdominal wall will exaggerate the defect size, resulting in an inappropriately oversized and unwieldy mesh. Should the patient have multiple defects, the borders of the most extremely located defects should determine the size.

The choice of mesh is guided by intraperitoneal placement with exposure to bowel, the characteristics of the patient and hernia defect(s) and ultimately the surgeon's preference. The mesh should be sized to provide an overlap of at least 4 to 5 cm around the circumference of the defect. Large central defects should be repaired with wider overlap to allow fixation to normal abdominal wall to avoid eventration of the mesh. Small, Swiss cheese–type defects may require a lesser margin. The potential for prosthetic mesh contraction should always be considered when sizing the mesh. Depending on the type of mesh, the degree of contraction may vary considerably.

The mesh is appropriately oriented according to the size of the mesh and defect, also considering the side of the mesh that will be exposed to the viscera. The orientation of the mesh is further maintained by marking with ink a notation on 1 or 2 borders of the mesh. One stay suture of heavy, permanent monofilament suture is placed at each of the 4 sides of the mesh with the knots on the noncoated or macroporous side of the mesh. Only 2 or 3 knot throws should be placed to avoid a bulky knot that may separate the mesh from the abdominal wall. In certain cases, placement of 4 sutures at the edges of the mesh may not be possible. Epigastric hernias, for example, will require additional superior overlap of the defect with placement of the mesh between the liver and the diaphragm (Figs 17.19 and 17.20).

The mesh is rolled so that the visceral side of the mesh is outside. This can be rolled in a scroll fashion from both sides or from 1 edge of the mesh to the other. A smaller mesh may be inserted within a 12-mm trocar (Fig. 17.17). Otherwise, it can be pushed or pulled into the port incision with the trocar removed under camera visualization. The mesh is unrolled and appropriately oriented. The stay sutures are brought out in a serial fashion so the mesh is centered under the single or multiple defects.

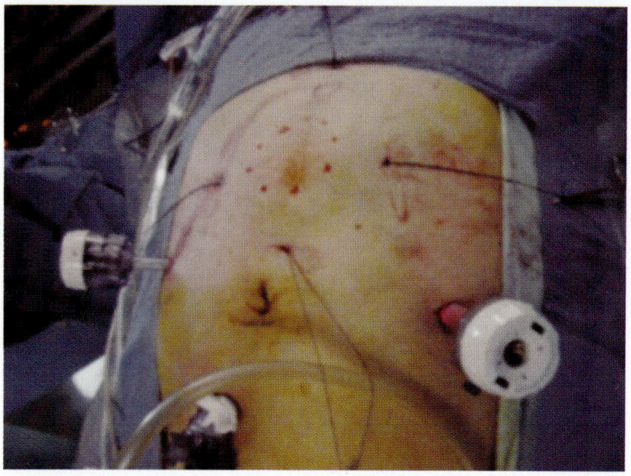

**Fig. 17.19:** Four stitches corresponding to the cardinal points of the hernia defect are taken outside by using an EndoClose™

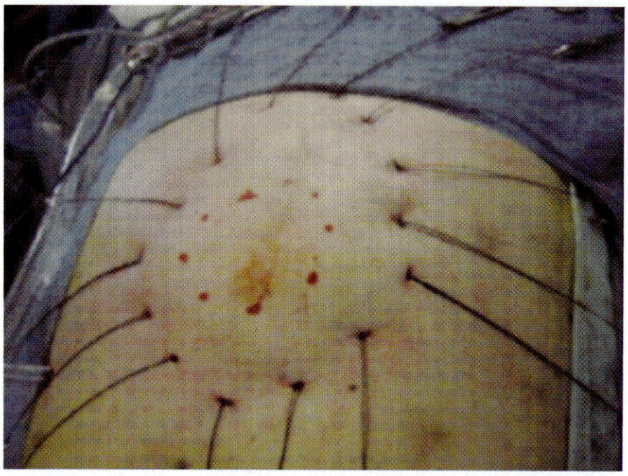

**Fig. 17.20:** Anchoring the mesh by the circumferential transfascial sutures using 2-0 nylon with a straight needle

The most critical suture is placed first, for example, where there is little room for adjustment. Each planned suture site is anesthetized with local anesthetic, bupivacaine, and a small stab incision is made. Each end of the suture is brought out with the suture passer taking care to leave a 1 cm fascial bridge between the 2 ends. The sutures are clamped and not tied until all stay sutures have been externalized and the mesh is in a good position. External markings on the patient's abdomen, noting the median point in the vertical and horizontal directions over the defect, may serve as a guide to appropriate suture placement.

Once the mesh is in an appropriate position with wide overlap and the stay sutures are located so that the mesh lies taut and smooth, the sutures are tied. The mesh is further fixated in between sutures with tacks to avoid intestinal herniation above the mesh during its incorporation. The tacks should be placed flush with the mesh to limit any adherence to the bowel and should be placed from 0.5 to 1.0 cm apart. Tacks that are not properly set should be removed from the abdomen. It is important to note that the tacks alone do not provide adequate purchase of the abdominal wall or secure fixation of the mesh. Additional heavy, monofilament, permanent sutures should be placed around the circumference of the mesh every 3 to 4 cm apart with the suture passer.

Pre-emptive analgesia with injection of local anesthetic may reduce postoperative pain. Care should also be taken to avoid undue tension when tying down the sutures to avoid local ischemia, postoperative pain, and recurrent herniation at the suture sites.

The hernia repair concludes with final inspection of the abdomen for any bleeding or bowel injury. The trocars are removed and the sites are inspected for bleeding. The fascia at the larger trocar site is closed with absorbable suture. The incisions are closed with subcuticular suture closure. The small stab incision suture sites may be treated with steristrips or skin sealant. An abdominal binder postoperatively may provide the patient some abdominal support to facilitate ambulation and pulmonary toilet (Fig. 17.21).

### *Rives-Stoppa Ventral Hernia Repair*

The Rives-Stoppa hernia repair revolutionized herniorrhaphy, creating a tension-free repair with a widely overlapping prosthetic mesh. This repair is the basis for

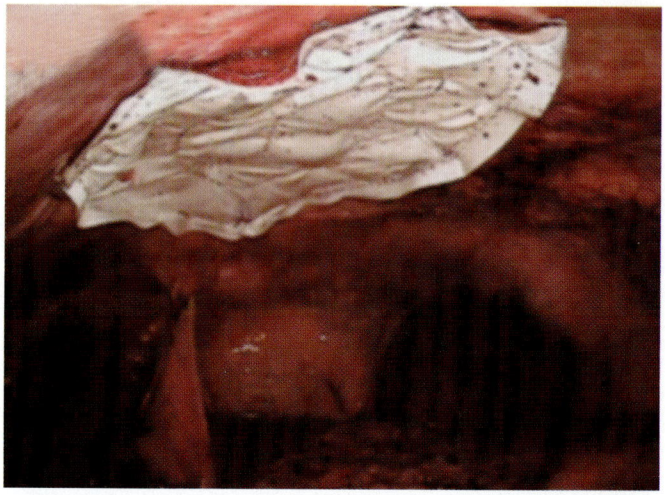

**Fig. 17.21:** Laparoscopic view of the completed procedure

laparoscopic ventral herniorrhaphy, which applies the same concepts of wide coverage and transabdominal suture fixation but uses intraperitoneal mesh. The originally described Stoppa repair positioned the prosthetic mesh in the preperitoneal space between the peritoneum and the transversalis fascia. The modified approach is a retromuscular prefascial prosthetic repair with the mesh placed between the rectus abdominis and the posterior rectus sheath.

*Procedure*: A midline incision is made and the hernia is reduced. The rectus sheath is opened near the linea alba and the retrorectus space is developed to provide 5- to 10-cm overlap of the fascial defect. The perforating vessels that enter the rectus sheath laterally should be preserved. The dissection can be carried inferiorly below the arcuate line between the transversalis fascia and the rectus to allow fixation of the mesh to Cooper's ligament. Similarly, the mesh can be placed between the rectus abdominis and the ribs and internal oblique superiorly for upper abdominal hernias.

If the peritoneum was breached during the course of the dissection, it should be closed or an appropriate mesh safe for intraperitoneal placement should be selected. The overlying muscle provides a rich vascular bed for incorporation of the mesh. Once the mesh is positioned, it is secured in a "clock-face" configuration with transabdominal heavy, monofilament sutures. These are placed via small stab incisions with a Riverdin needle or a suture passer in a mattress fashion and are tied anterior to the rectus sheath. This technique provides wide mesh coverage with secure fixation but without the need to develop subcutaneous flaps. Drains are placed above the mesh or in the subcutaneous space. The fascia is closed or secured to mesh.

## Complications of Ventral Hernia Repair

Many studies that compare laparosopic ventral hernia repair to open techniques show the benefit of the laparoscopic approach in terms of recurrence rates, wound complication rates, and length of hospital stay. The laparoscopic approach, however, lends itself to a variety of potential complications.

### *Bowel Injury*

During abdominal access, lysis of adhesions, and hernia reduction, there is the potential for bowel injury.

### *Bleeding*

Other than the rare trocar injury to a major vessel, the potential for significant bleeding during ventral hernia repair is low because most dissection occurs at the abdominal wall, away from large vascular structures. There are 2 primary causes of bleeding in this procedure. The first potential cause of bleeding is injury to blood vessels during dissection of the adherent abdominal contents. When using scissors or blunt dissection, any significant bleeding should be controlled. Once the bleeding vessel is isolated, it can be ligated with clips or suture, or directly cauterized with cautery or other energy coagulation devices. Uncontrolled bleeding in a laparoscopic operation, although rare, may require conversion to an open approach.

The other main mechanism of bleeding is trauma to the abdominal wall caused by mesh fixation techniques, usually with a suture-passing device. When bleeding is visualized, direct pressure or tying the suture will often stop the bleeding. If bleeding persists, additional sutures may be passed on each side of the site of bleeding through the same skin incision to control the bleeding. Rarely, significant abdominal wall hematomas may occur.

## Postoperative Complications

### Pain

Unlike most laparoscopic procedures, a laparoscopic ventral hernia repair can be very painful, similar to an open operation. Pain is typically due to the fixation of the mesh and is correlated to the size of the mesh placed. Patients with small hernias often are able to go home the day of surgery. Large hernia repairs, however, almost always require a hospital stay for pain management. The pain typically resolves over time and after the initial few days, the pain is usually localized at 1 or 2 of the individual fixation sites. Although this pain usually resolves with conservative management such as rest, heat, and anti-inflammatories, it can persist or recur in some patients.

## Wound Complications/ Fluid Collections

Seroma, a fluid collection in the space where the hernia contents protruded prior to the repair, is a normal occurrence after a laparoscopic ventral hernia repair. The patient should be made aware of this to alleviate the fear that the bulge after the surgery is a recurrent hernia. Seromas typically resolve over time and rarely persist or cause symptoms. If necessary, aspiration should be done using sterile technique to avoid infecting the mesh. Although seromas may be more pronounced after a laparoscopic repair because the stretched overlying skin is not resected as in the open ventral hernia repair, the risk of wound complication is increased in the open repair because of the large incision.

A fluid collection that becomes infected may require mesh removal. There are reports of successful conservative management with antibiotics and drainage guided by computed tomography. For infections with exposed mesh, successful conservative management has included local wound care, wound vacuum-assisted closure, and local debridement, in addition to antibiotics. A wound infection after open ventral hernia repair can lead to the same problems as an infected seroma, including the possibility of mesh removal.

## Recurrence

A ventral hernia repaired without mesh will recur at a higher rate than if mesh is used. Hernia recurrence is minimized if three principles in a mesh repair are followed: (i) clear visualization of the entire abdominal wall, (ii) wide mesh coverage of the defect in all directions, and (iii) secure fixation of the mesh to healthy abdominal wall fascia without tension. Mechanisms of recurrence include missed hernia from lack of visualization of the entire abdominal wall, inadequate mesh coverage leading to protrusion of the mesh into the defect, and inadequate mesh fixation leading to recurrence at the area where the mesh is not adequately fixed to the abdominal wall. The fact that mesh is not inert also allows for recurrence from mesh migration of a portion or all of the mesh and from mesh contraction. Maintaining the principles of clear visualization, wide mesh coverage, and secure fixation, in addition to using mesh that is less likely to contract will minimize recurrence rates for both open and laparoscopic ventral hernia repairs.

# Chapter 18

# Lumbar Hernia (Types of Lumbar Hernia Surgery)

## Hernia of the Superior Lumbar Triangle

Lumbar hernias are rare. DeGarangeot reported the first known case in 1731, the hernia being reduced at autopsy; Petit, in 1783, described a strangulated hernia emerging through the inferior lumbar triangle which now bears his name; and in 1750, Ravaton reported a strangulated lumbar hernia with operation and cure. A century later, Grynfeltt described a hernia through the superior lumbar triangle, distinguishing it from the inferior lumbar triangle. In 1870, Lesshaft independently confirmed the existence of a separate superior lumbar triangle and reported a similar case. By 1890, Macready 25 had collected 25 cases, two of which were through the superior lumbar triangle, which was named the space of Grynfeltt-Lesshaft. In 1925, Virgilio 36 collected 109 cases and found that the Grynfeltt-Lesshaft hernia was more frequent than the Petit's hernia.

### Anatomy (Figs 18.1A and B)

A lumbar hernia may occur anywhere in the lumbar region which is bounded above by the 12th rib, below by the crest of the ilium, in front by a line drawn vertically downward from the anterior extremity of the 12th rib to the crest of the ilium, and behind by the vertebral column and the erector spinae muscles. The two main areas of lumbar hemiation are the superior lumbar triangle (Grynfeltt-Lesshaft) and the inferior lumbar triangle (Petit). If a triangle is present, it is inverted, the base being formed by the lower border of the 12th rib and the portions of the serratus posteroinferior. The anterior border is formed by the internal oblique and the posterior border is the quadratus lumborum; these borders are easily remembered if the area is thought of as the lumbocostoabdominal triangle. The floor of the triangle is the transversalis fascia which is a portion of the fusions of the lumbodorsal fascia which continues anteriorly as the aponeurosis of the transversus abdominis muscle and posteriorly splits into three layers which include the quadratus lumborum and the sacrospinalis. The size and shape of the space depend upon the development of the bordering muscle masses, the length and position of the 12th rib and the position of its muscle attachments, and the position of attachment of the overlying latissimus dorsi. Weak points in the superior lumbar triangle are immediately beneath the 12th rib where the transversalis fascia is not covered by the external oblique and where it is perforated by the 12th dorsal intercostal neurovascular bundle. The inferior lumbar triangle is normally present in adults, occasionally present in children. It is usually triangular shaped with the base being the iliac crest. The posterior border is the free edge of the latissimus dorsi and the anterior border is the external oblique. The musculofascial floor is much stronger than that of the superior lumbar triangle.

### Superior Triangle of Grynfeltt and Lesshaft

It lies above and anterior to triangle of Petit.

#### *Boundaries (Figs 18.2 and 18.3)*

*Above*: 12th rib and lower border of serratus posteroinferior.
*Anteriorly*: Posterior border of internal oblique.
*Posteriorly*: Quadratus lumborum and erector spinae.

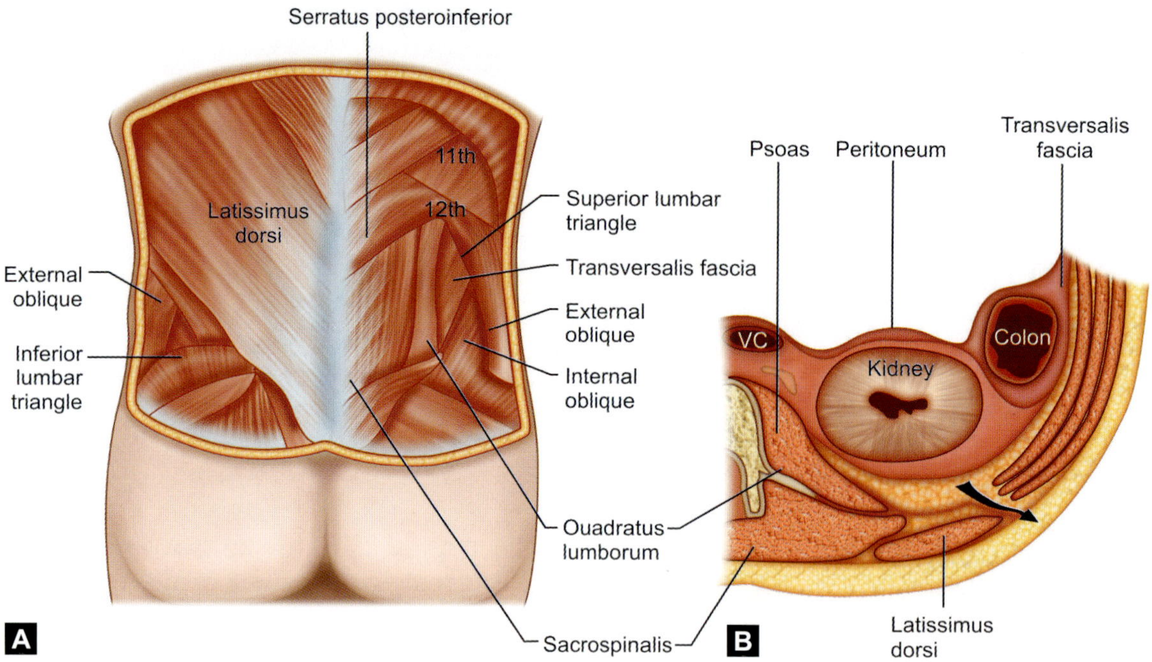


**Figs 18.1A and B:** (A) Anatomical relationships of the inferior and superior triangles. A portion of the latissimus dorsi has been removed to fully expose the deeper superior lumbar triangle; (B) Transverse section through kidney inferior to 12th rib

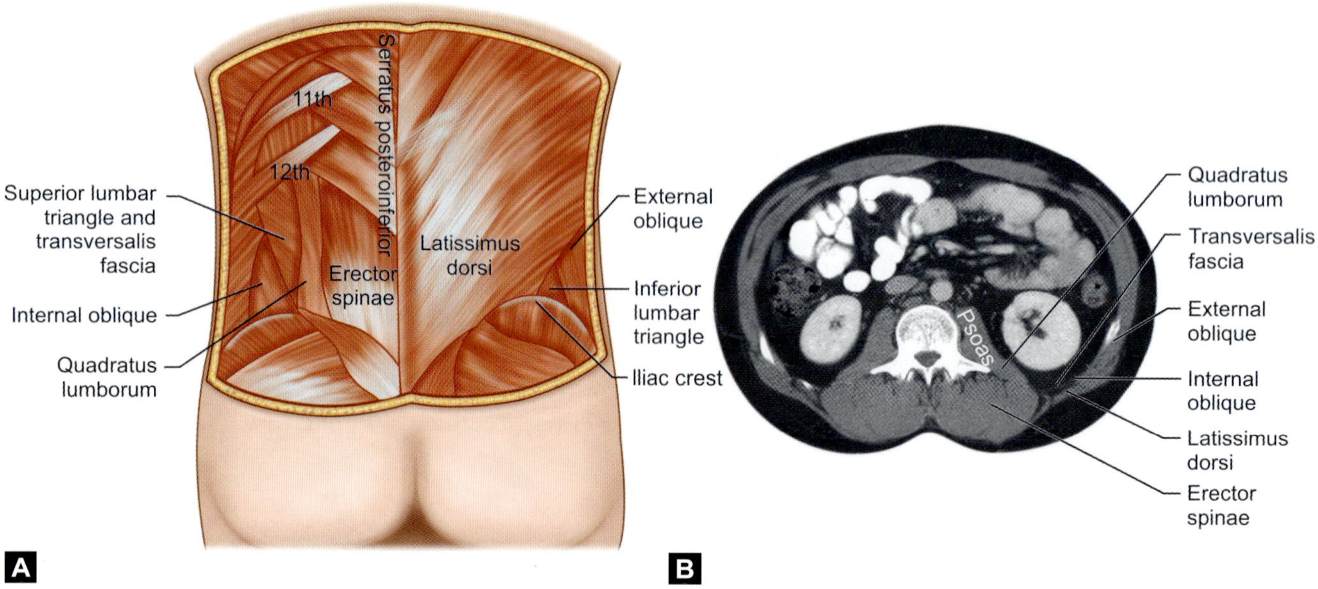


**Figs 18.2A and B:** Posterior abdominal wall—I

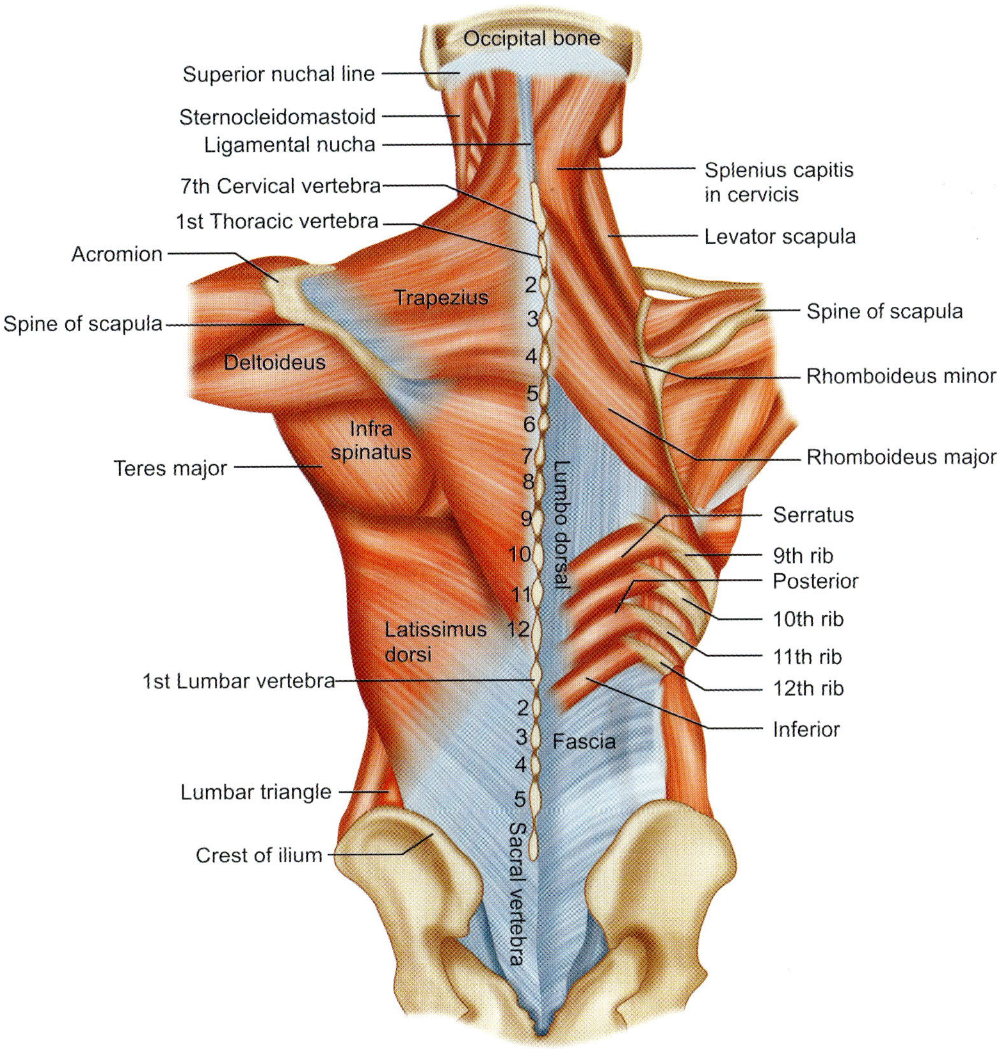


**Fig. 18.3:** Posterior abdominal wall—II

*Floor*: Transversalis fascia.
*Roof*: Latissimus dorsi.

## Etiology

1. *Congenital*: Individually or associated with (a) Other abdominal hernias viz. epigastric, inguinal (b) Lumbocostovertebral syndrome; (c) Neurofibromatosis Type 1.
2. *Acquired*: Trauma, localized muscular paralysis (e.g. polio), postlaparoscopic cholecystectomy.

Lumbar hernia does not include hernia following an operation on kidney which is an incisional hernia (Figs 18.4 and 18.5).

## Presentations

1. Lump
2. Backache with pain radiating to groin due to irritation of lateral cutaneous branch of 10,11,12th intercostal nerves.
3. Obstruction.

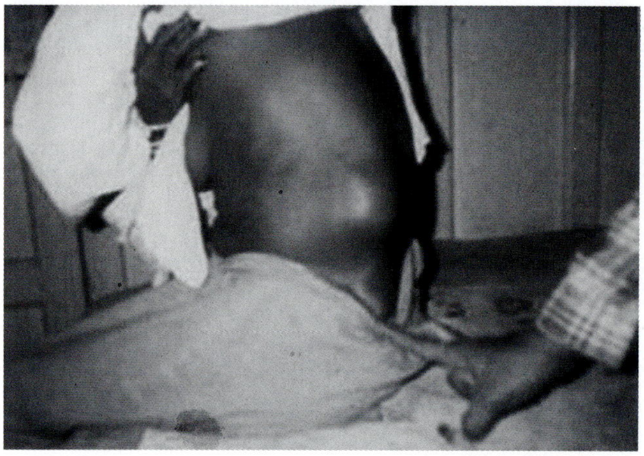

Fig. 18.4: Left lumbar hernia–Anterior view

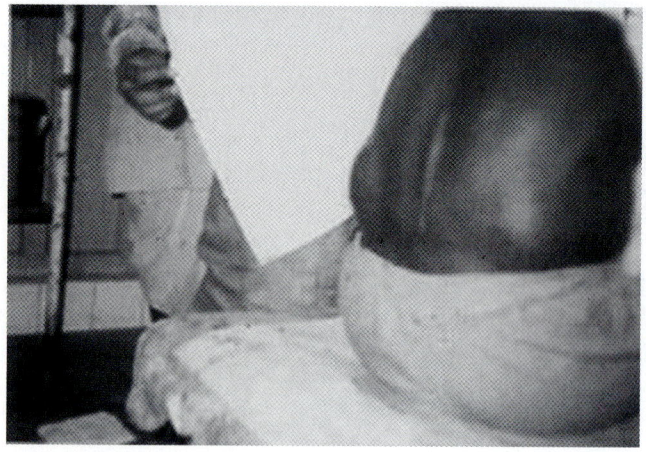

Fig. 18.5: Left lumbar hernia—Lateral view

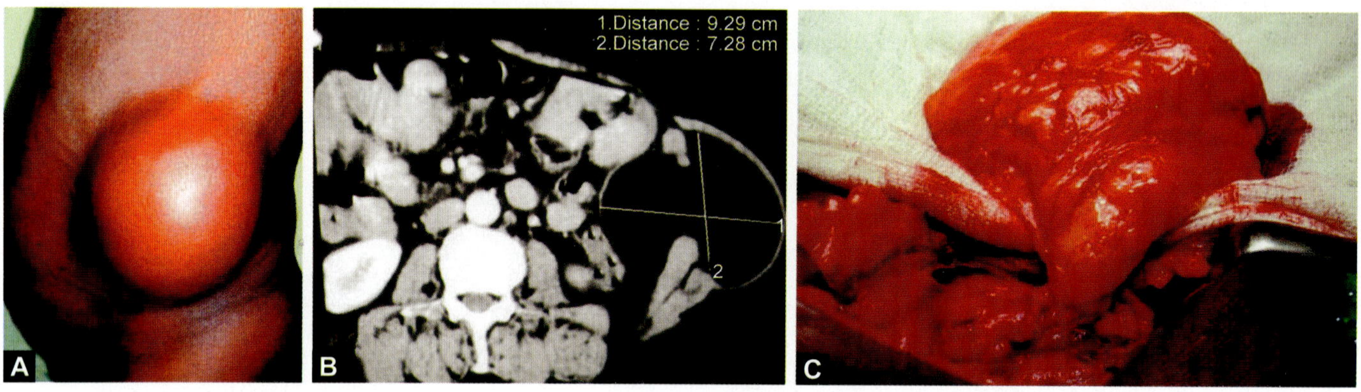


Figs 18.6A to C: Preoperative left lateral view showing lumbar hernia; (B) CT scan of the abdomen shows a left lumbar hernia; (C) Intraoperative view showing herniated fatty mass

### Complications

1. Irreducibility
2. Incarceration
3. Strangulation.

## Lumbar Hernia: Diagnosis by CT

Lumbar hernias occur in the region of the flank bounded by the 12th rib, the iliac crest, and the erector spinae and external oblique muscles. Because CT portrays the anatomic relationships in this region so well. It may be the only radiographic procedure necessary to make the diagnosis of a lumbar hernia. Furthermore, it can be helpful in the assessment of symptomatic patients after flank incision, to differentiate postincisional muscular weakness and intercostal neuralgia from a lumbar hernia.

Lumbar hernias occur in the flank and are most often acquired (spontaneous, post-traumatic, or postoperative) rather than congenital. Symptoms are absent, variable, or confusing because postincisional neuralgia may be indistinguishable from pain caused by a lumbar hernia. A flank bulge may be detectable, but the clinical diagnosis can be very difficult in obese and postoperative patients.

Computed tomography (CT) is able to delineate muscular and fascial layers, a defect in one or more of these layers, and the presence of herniated fat and/ or viscera (Figs 18.6A to C). In all cases of lumbar

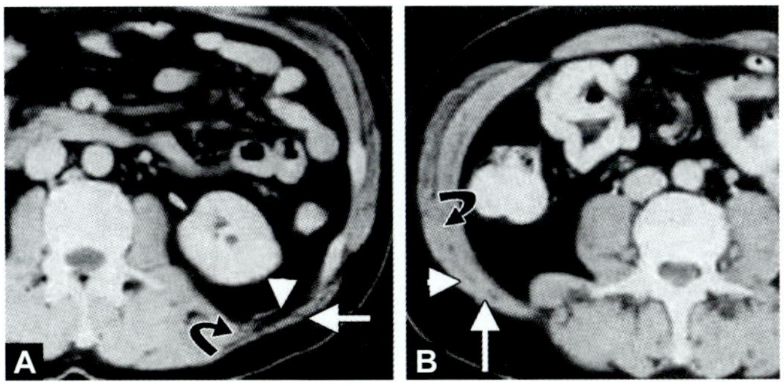


**Figs 18.7A and B:** (A) CT through base of superior lumbar triangle in normal patient showing latissimus dorsi muscle (arrow), serratus posteroinferior muscle (curved arrow), and thoracolumbar fascia (arrowhead); (B) CT through inferior lumbar triangle in normal patient showing inferior triangle region (arrowhead), latissimus dorsi muscle (arrow), and external oblique muscle (curved arrow)

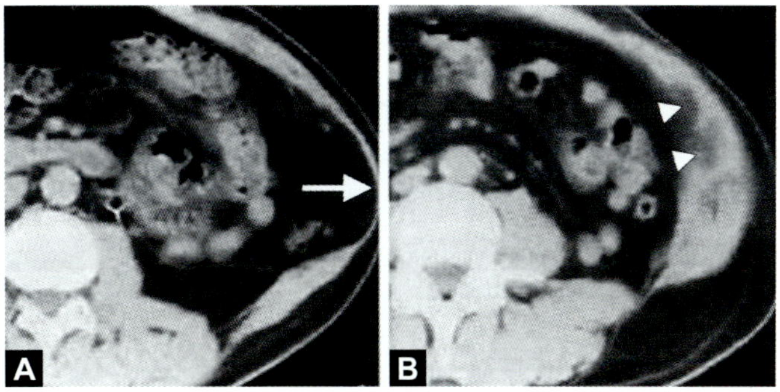


**Figs 18.9A and B:** CT showing postincisional lumbar hernia. (A) External oblique muscle (arrow) is thinned superiorly; (B) Inferior scan shows anterior disruption of transversus abdominis and internal oblique muscles (arrowheads)

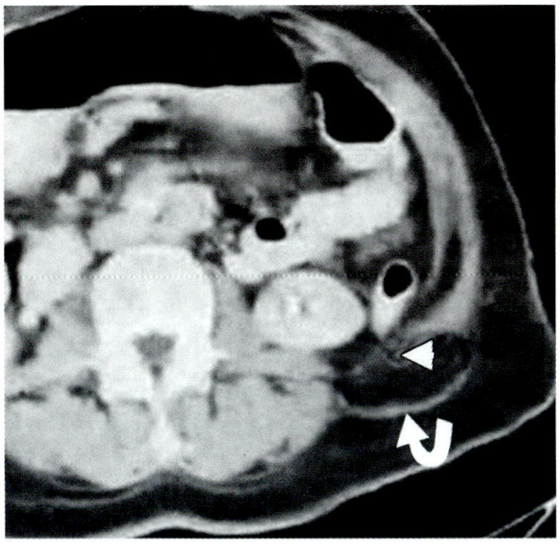

**Fig. 18.8:** CT showing spontaneous lumbar hernia in superior triangle with thinned latissimus dorsi muscle (curved arrow) and disrupted thoracolumbar fascia (arrowhead). Hernia contains extraperitoneal fat

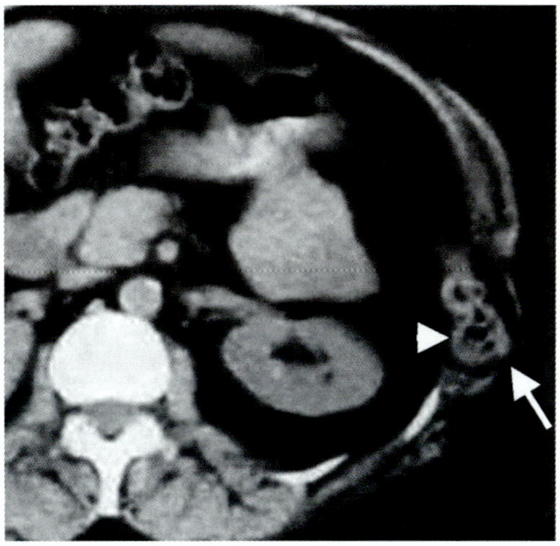

**Fig. 18.10:** CT showing high, postincisional lumbar hernia. Intercostal muscle (arrow) is disrupted. Bowel (arrowhead) is within hernia

hernias, there may be vast differences in the amount of tissue within the hernial sac. They may contain only extrapentoneal fat, extraperitoneal fat plus kidney or colon, as well as intraperitoneal structures (most commonly small bowel). When muscular layers are intact, CT is the only radiographic method necessary for diagnosis. When hernias do exist, CT scan show which fascial or muscular layers are involved and the content of the hernial sac. A normal CT of this region in a symptomatic patient enables the physician to confidently exclude a lumbar hernia and guide therapy away from dealing with a structural abnormality. This is especially important in symptomatic, postincisional patients. When pain is present and no hernia exists, intercostal nerve block often eliminates pain and obviates exploratory surgery to exclude a hernia (Figs 18.7 and 18.8).

Lumbar hernias may manifest as flank ecchymoses and/or hematomas, protruding bulges, localized pain, or referred pain to either the anterior abdominal wall or via sciatic nerve disruption. The classic "seat belt sign" may be present.

Computed tomography has been advocated as the diagnostic study of choice for suspected lumbar hernia in patients whose condition is stable (Figs 18.9 to

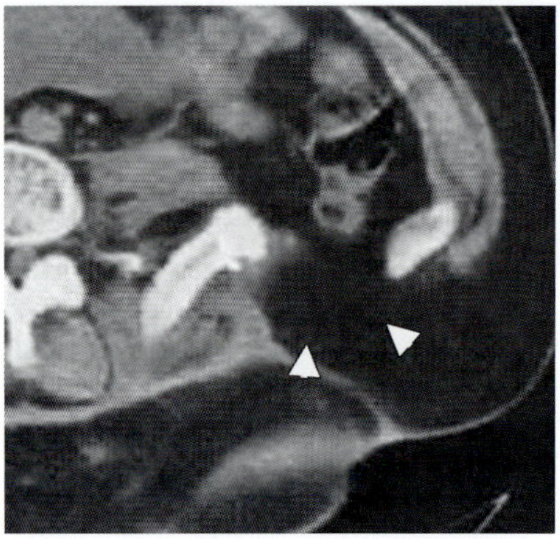

Fig. 18.11: CT shows lumbar hernia that occurred after nonunion of iliac fracture. Thoracolumbar fascia (arrowheads) is thinned and bulging. Hernia contains extraperitoneal fat

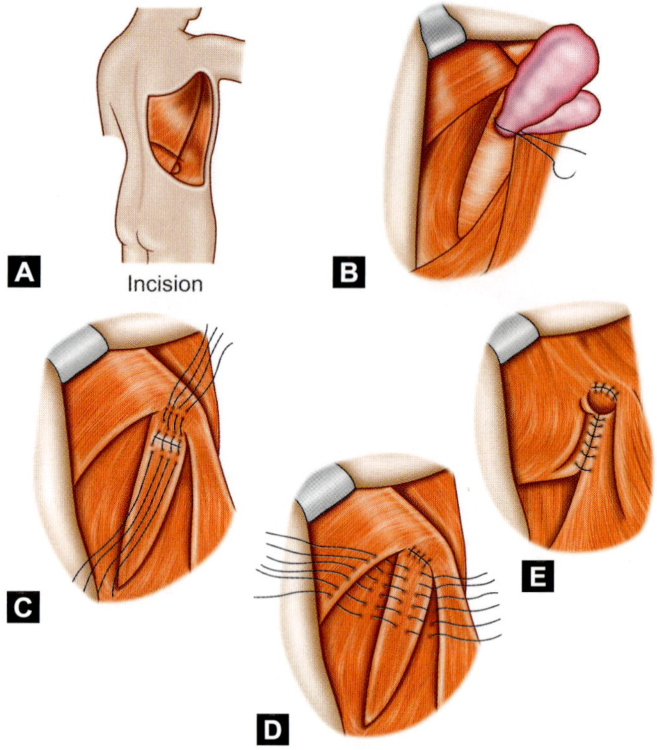


**Figs 18.12A to E:** (A) Incision may be either oblique as shown or vertical for adequate exposure; (B) Identification of defect and ligation of fat-containing sac after inspection of contents; (C) Closure of defect utilizing periosteum of 12th rib; (D and E). Obliteration of triangle with internal oblique, serratus posteroinferior and quadratus lumborum

18.11). Often, CT confirms the diagnosis and may show associated injuries. The anatomy of the adjacent muscle layers and contents of the hernia are usually clearly identified by CT.

## Differential Diagnosis

1. Lipoma
2. Cold abscess.

## Treatment

Before the era of meshplasty, Dowd repair was practized. It involved closure of defect by a pedical flap of tensor fascia lata and gluteus maximus from below the iliac crest with side to side opposition of external oblique and latissimus dorsi for Petit's triangle hernia. For superior triangle flaps from adjacent structures were developed.

Presently if the defect is small and good, strong tissue around, then defect can be closed with continuous polypropylene suture.

For large defect, poor muscular tissue, preperitoneal meshplasty is the preferred treatment. Lately in the laparoscopic era, lumbar hernia are repaired laparoscopically with prosthetic mesh.

### *Surgery for Lumbar Hernia*

*Reported contents of sac*: Contents of the hernias are omentum, small intestine, colon, kidney, stomach, ovary, spleen, and appendix.

A kidney rest is utilized to increase the distance between the 12th rib and iliac crest, and the entire buttock and thigh are prepared to the knee in case a flap of gluteus maximus fascia or fascia lata is required (Figs 18.12A to E). Langan emphasized the helpfulness of marking the hernia with an indelible marker preoperatively.

### *Objectives*

The objectives of operation for hernia are to reduce the hernia, to remove the sac if it is large or simply reduce it within the hernial ring if the sac is small, and to reconstruct the defect. In lumbar hernias, a sac is rarely adherent to the skin, being separated from it by either fat or muscle. The sac should be identified, the neck dissected, and if the content of the sac is properitoneal or peritoneal fat, its pedicle is ligated and the mass excised. Reconstruction of the defect may be accomplished in a variety of ways.

### *Procedure*

The patient is placed in a right lateral position. The swelling is explored through a left flank incision. The retroperitoneal fatty globular mass attached with a tapering pedicle emerging through a narrow constricting ring is discovered to be herniating through the superior lumbar triangle. The constricting ring is released and the pedicle along with the entire herniated mass is excised. A mesh is fashioned as inlay prosthesis and is placed in the extraperitoneal space through the defect in the muscle layer. The defect is repaired with continuous sutures and rest of the wound is closed in layers.

Currently, extraperitoneal mesh repair is considered the optimal treatment for isolated unilateral lumbar hernia. The Rives Stoppa approach, wherein, a large rectangular mesh is fashioned to be placed in the preperitoneal space extending from umbilicus to retropubic space and between the two anterosuperior iliac spines, appear to be the most promising open technique for bilateral lumbar hernia, recurrent hernias or multiple site hernias with comparatively low recurrence rates. Extraperitoneal position of the mesh is advantageous as no bony anchorage is essential. The weight of the intraperitoneal contents is an additional support to maintain the mesh in correct position in the early postoperative period. Laparoscopic transabdominal preperitoneal mesh repair for lumbar hernia confers all the benefits of minimal access surgery to the patient. It is a tensionless repair. It follows the current principle of hernia surgery and is based on the sound physiological principle of diffusing the total intra-abdominal pressure on each square inch of the mesh implanted (Fig. 18.13).

## Treatment

Primary lumbar hernias are rare congenital defects of the abdominal wall. Repair of these rare hernias can be successfully performed via the anterior approach with the use of synthetic mesh—this method of repair is easy, safe, and effective.

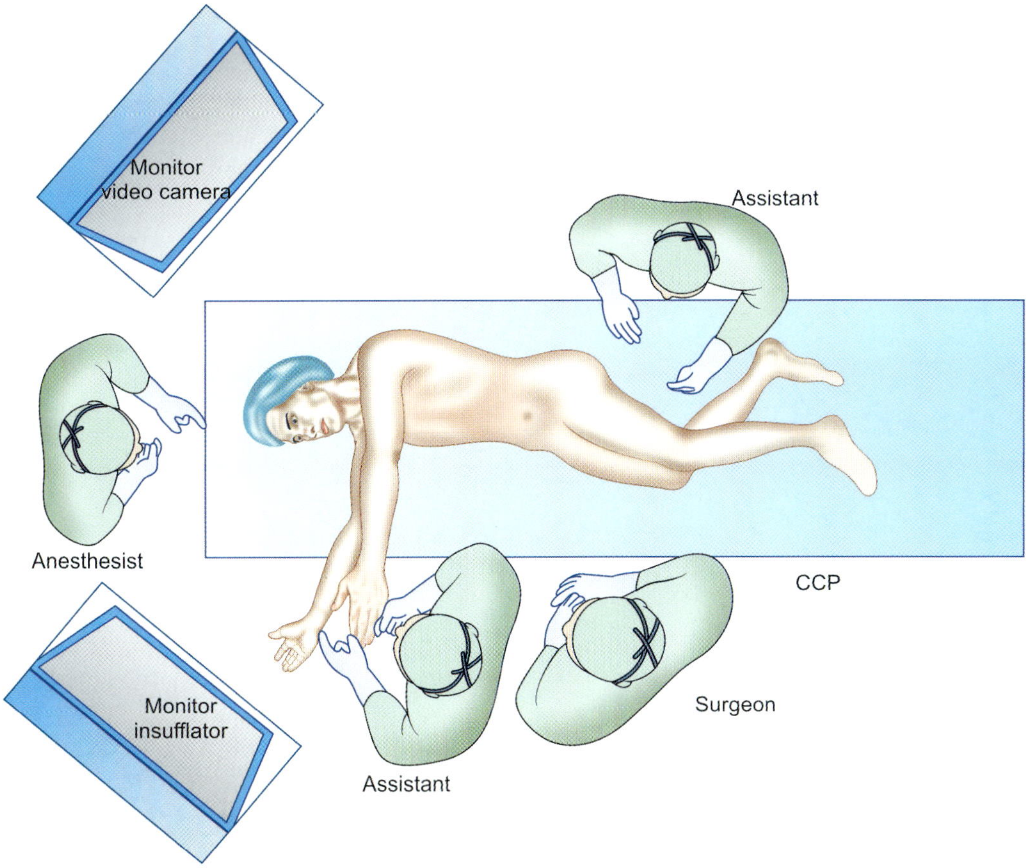


**Fig. 18.13:** Position of patient on operating table with surgery crew

## Laparoscopic Retroperitoneal Repair

Under general anesthesia we performed a retroperitoneoscopic repair of the defect, with a polypropylene prosthesis.

The patient is placed in a semilateral position, on his right side, which optimized exposure and allows the viscera to fall away from the operative field. A small incision is made under the tip of the 12th rib to accommodate a 12 mm distention balloon, placed into the retroperitoneal space. By insufflation, the retroperitoneal space is dissected. The distention balloon is replaced by a 10 mm structural trocar, and with an extra 5 mm trocar near the 11th rib, the retroperitoneal dissection is continued towards the lateral border of the left rectus sheath. A 10 mm trocar is introduced at the umbilicus and a final 5 mm trocar at the left fossa iliaca. The camera is displaced to the 10 mm trocar at the umbilicus. After dissection of the posterior part of the retroperitoneal space, the defect, with a maximal diameter of 5 cm, is visualized. The hernia, containing intraperitoneal fat, is reduced and the borders of the opening are cleared. A 15 _ 15 cm mesh of choice is used to occlude the defect, and it is fixed with the Tacker at the crista iliaca, the musculus quadratus lumborum and the musculus transverses abdominis. A suction drain is placed.

# Chapter 19

# Spigelian Hernia

## Definition

A spigelian hernia is an acquired ventral hernia through the linea semilunaris.

Spigelian hernia (Fig. 19.1) occurs through congenital or acquired defects in the spigelian fascia. This is the area of the transversus abdominis aponeurosis, lateral to the edge of the rectus muscle but medial to the spigelian line, which is the point of transition of the transversus abdominis muscle to its aponeurotic tendon.

Spigelian hernias are an uncommon form of anterior abdominal wall herniation. They constitute less than 2% of a total hernia group composed of femoral. Inguinal. umbilical, and incisional hernias as well as hernias of the linea alba and epigastrium. Because of their relative rarity and sometimes insidious presentation, they often arc not easily discovered clinically and are found at surgery unexpectedly. Furthermore, they are unusual in that they lie in an interstitial position between the external and internal oblique muscles of the anterior abdominal wall. A spigelian hernia most frequently presents as a small intramural mass located along the lateral margin of the rectus sheath halfway between the umbilicus and symphysis pubis and between the internal and external oblique abdominal wall muscles. Obesity, ascites, multiple pregnancies, chronic cough. Blunt abdominal trauma, and rapid weight gain can increase the intra-abdominal pressure and predispose to the formation of a hernia. The hernia derives its name from the anatomist Adriaan van der Spieghel (1578-1625).

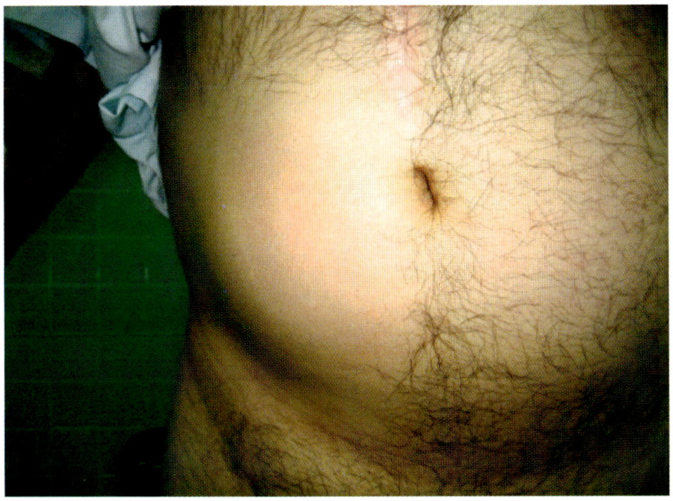

**Fig. 19.1:** Spigelian hernia

### Occurrence

Although cases of spigelian hernia in infants and children have previously been described, these hernias have mainly occurred among adults between 40 and 70 years of age, and generally in obese females who have undergone parturition several times. Many reports on spigelian hernias have emphasized the difficulty in making the diagnosis, for the following reasons: (1) the nonspecific variety of symptoms, (2) their small size, (3) the intramural location of the hernia (usually located between different muscle layers), and (4) the non-diagnostic findings on plain abdominal radiographs (Fig. 19.2). Although uncommon, spigelian hernias account for over 2% of cases undergoing emergency surgery for abdominal wall hernia. A spigelian hernia is an acquired ventral hernia through the linea semilunaris, the line where the sheaths of the lateral abdominal

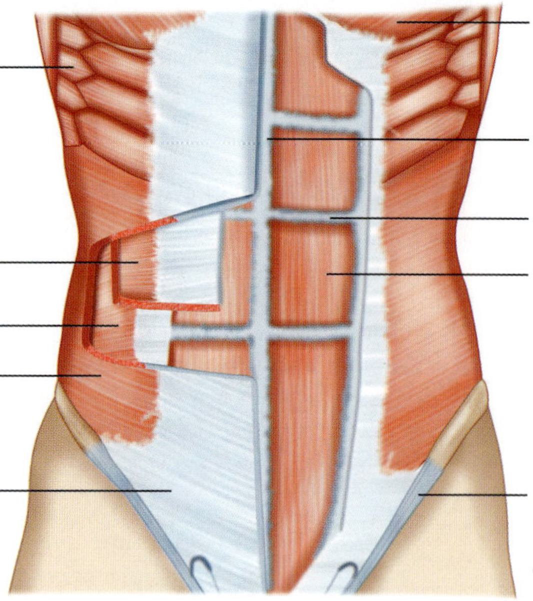


**Fig. 19.2:** Anterior abdominal wall

muscles fuse to form the lateral rectus sheath. Spigelian hernias are nearly always found above the level of the inferior epigastric vessels, and most often occur where the semicircular line—fold of Douglas-cross the linea semilunaris. Fortunately, a spigelian hernia is a relatively rare occurrence. In most instances, the condition does not develop before the age of 40 and is more likely to occur after the age of 50. The hernia is also more likely to develop on the right side of the abdomen rather than the left.

## Symptoms

The patient presents with pain that is localized to the hernial site and is aggravated by any movement that raises intra-abdominal pressure. Later, the pain becomes more dull, constant, and diffuse.

A soft, reducible mass may be present in the lower abdominal area which disappears on pressure. When the mass is reduced, the hernial orifice can usually be palpated. Diagnosis is more difficult when the hernia dissects within the layers of the abdominal wall-internal and external obliques-or may be located at a distance from the linea semilunaris.

The clinical presentation of a spigelian hernia is quite variable but usually insidious. Most frequently only omentum is present within the hernia sac hut all parts of the large and small intestine, the stomach, fat, an endometriosis nodule, ovary, and a Meckel's diverticulum have been reported in a spigelian hernia. Patients frequently are asymptomatic and present with a painless lower abdominal mass which may not be constant. At times the mass may be tender or there may be intermittent abdominal pain without a palpable mass. Symptoms and signs of intestinal obstruction can be superimposed upon these findings.

The entire picture may resemble other conditions.

## Diagnosis

Diagnosis of spigelian hernia is difficult. The absence of typical hernia-type symptoms and the lack of physician experience with such hernias can make early recognition difficult. This is complicated by the fact that the overlying external oblique fascia remains intact, which in effect conceals an underlying fascial defect, making it hard to detect.

Following things may happen to spigelian hernia (Fig. 19.3):

- The sac of spigelian hernia may get diverted due to intact external oblique muscle and aponeurosis and get translocated in interstitial space.
- The sac may get reflected in lateral direction below aponeurosis and present as swelling the either iliac fossa.

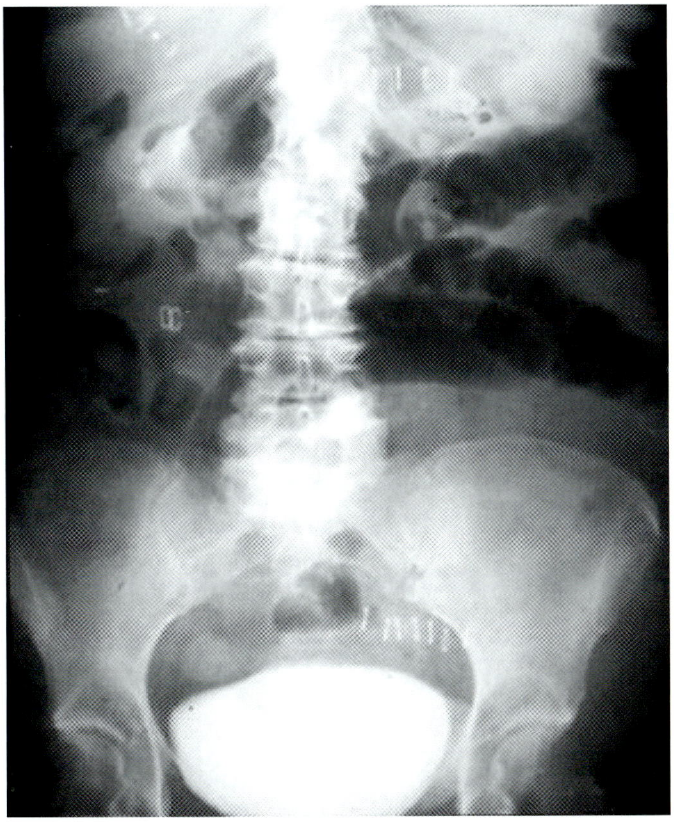

**Fig. 19.3:** A plain abdominal X-ray showing intestinal obstruction in a patient with a spigelian hernia

- The sac may present itself in parallel to rectus abdominis and comes out as a swelling in rectus muscle itself. It looks like it is hematoma of rectus muscle.
- The sac may lie in between the lateral flank muscles.
- The sac may lie in rectus muscle sheaths.

## Clinical Examination

Includes examination of patient with the abdominal muscles relaxed state. Patient should be examined in supine and standing position. There should be thorough examination as the hernia may be reduced at the time of examination. The tenderness at the point of swelling should be noted and taken as high suspicion. If the site is nontender then anterior abdominal muscles may be made taut to exhibit swelling, if any.

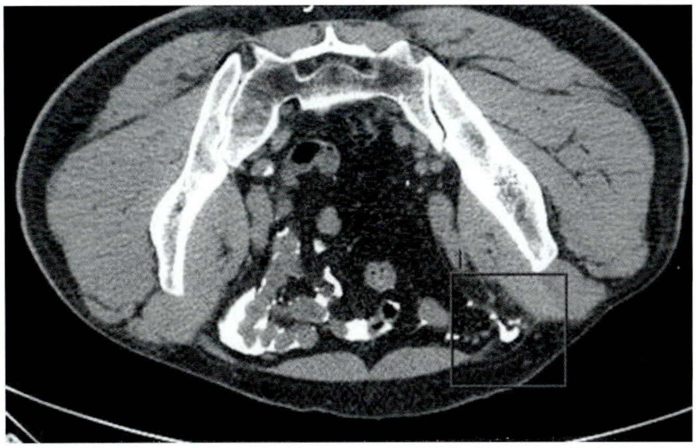

**Fig. 19.4:** Spigelian hernia in CT scan

## Differential Diagnosis

The differential diagnosis includes appendicitis and appendiceal abscess, a tumor of the abdominal wall or a spontaneous hematoma of the rectus sheath or even acute diverticulitis.

## Investigations

The diagnostic procedures are mainly aimed at demonstrating a hernial orifice or sac. Plain abdominal radiographs and gastrointestinal tract studies using barium sulfate are diagnostic only if the bowel has herniated through the defect and appropriate oblique views are obtained.

## Ultrasonography

In today's era sonography is used widely for diagnosis of spigelian hernia. In sonography the study of the semilunar line is done for identifying possible defects. This is the first line of investigation. This is done with the patient in supine and standing positions. The valsalva maneuver is performed to increase the bulge so as to detect it on sonography. The incarcerated spigelian hernia is also well noted sonologically.

## Computed Tomography (Figs 19.4 and 19.5)

Magnetic resonance imaging (MRI scan) is also emerging as the new modality to diagnose difficult to diagnose spigelian hernias.

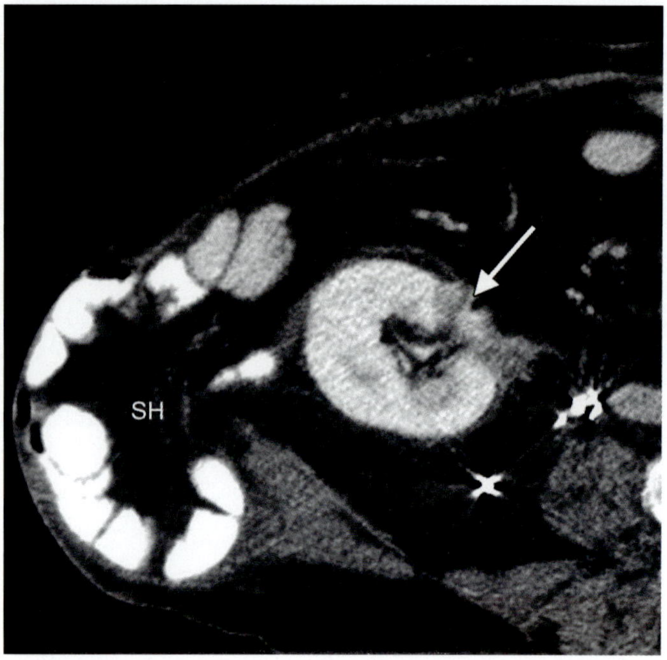


**Fig. 19.5:** Isolated case reports have demonstrated that computed tomography (CT) scanning using closely spaced slices through a limited area may reveal the hernial orifice in the spigelian fascia.This is very reliable imaging technique for spigelian hernia (SH)

### *Treatment*

Spigelian hernias are difficult to treat and they have risk of strangulation; Richter type of hernia has also been reported to occur with spigelian hernia. For this reason, surgery should be advised in all patients. Surgery can be performed either by open technique or by laparoscopically.

### *Preoperative Care*

1. *Anesthesia*: General/Spinal anesthesia is employed for open surgery. General anesthesia is employed for laparoscopic surgery.
2. *Position*: Supine on operating table

### *Conventional Open Surgical Approach*

A transverse incision (Gridiron) is sited over the protrusion. If the hernia is large then elliptical incision is taken to remove excess and redundant skin.If there is doubt or inconsistent diagnosis then paramedian or midline incision is employed.

*Dissection*: External oblique aponeurosis is incised in the direction of its fibers to expose the peritoneal sac. The sac may just lie below aponeurosis or it may be interstitial. In case of gridiron incision the rectus sheath is incised to expose spigelian aponeurosis. Then, the semilunar line is carefully examined along its line to check for multiple defects of spigelian hernia.

*Sac*: The shape of the sac depends upon the hernia size. If the hernia is small then the sac may be of globular or mushroom size shape.The most common sac content is omentum but intestine, appendix, gallbladder, stomach or ovary have been reported.

*Excision of sac*: Excision of the sac can be done in case of large sacs and redundant sac is removed by excision. The remaining part is closed by continuous sutures of absorbable material. Most surgeons simply invert the sac alone; in case of small hernia sac.

*Closure*: The opening in the internal oblique and transverses muscles is closed with polypropylene sutures; in case of repair without prosthetic mesh implant. In case of prosthetic mesh implant the mesh is chosen and fixed preperitoneally or onlay mesh (above the fascia) is fixed. Then, the external oblique aponeurosis is closed with absorbable or nonabsorbable sutures. Subcutaneous fascia may be closed with absorbable sutures.

*Skin closure*: It is done with the suture material of surgeon's choice. The drain is not kept.

## Laparoscopic Surgery for Spigelian Hernia

### Intraperitoneal Onlay Mesh Repair

Intraperitoneal access is performed using Veress needle or open technique. Once abdominal access is obtained, site of hernial orifice is readily identified and ports are placed at least 10 cm away from the hernial defect in the form of an arc of a circle whose center is the hernial defect. Contents are reduced from the sac and adhesiolysis is performed if required to obtain an overlap of 5 cm around the defect for a synthetic mesh. The mesh is fixed using a combination of transabdominal sutures and tacks.

### Transabdominal Preperitoneal Repair (Fig. 19.6)

Once the hernia sac contents are reduced, a peritoneal flap is raised as in transabdominal preperitoneal (TAPP) approach and attempt is made to completely reduce the hernial sac. After dissecting the peritoneal flap for about 5 cm around the hernial defect, Polypropylene mesh is

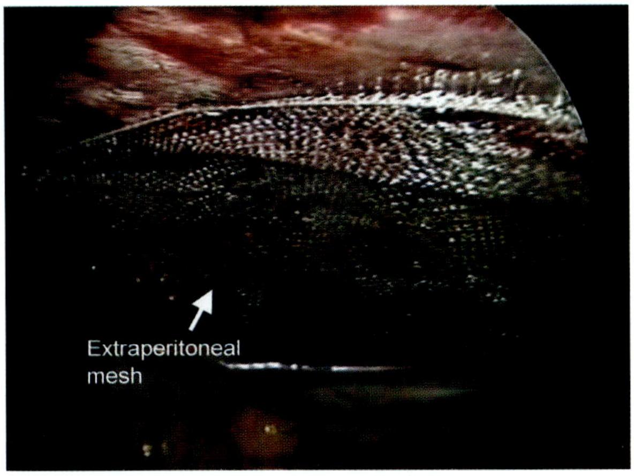


**Fig. 19.6:** TAPP repair for spigelian hernia–after placement of mesh in extraperitoneal space

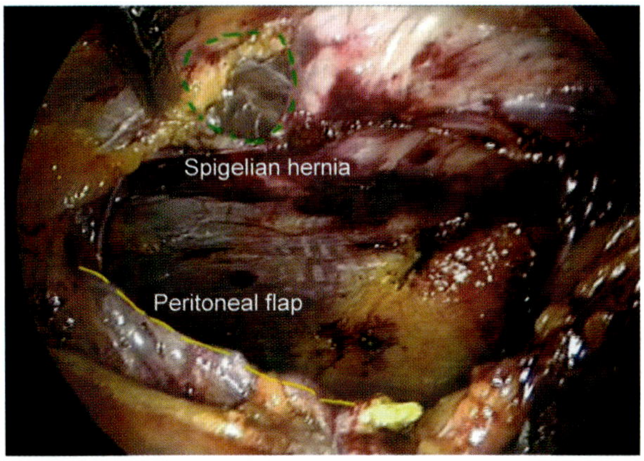


**Fig. 19.7:** TEP repair for spigelian hernia–after reduction of hernia sac

placed in the dissected extraperitoneal space and is fixed using tacks. The peritoneal flap is closed either with tacks or with a continuous suture.

## Total Extraperitoneal Repair (Fig. 19.7)

Endoscopic total extraperitoneal (TEP) repair is performed using 3 midline ports. Extraperitoneal space is created by open access and a balloon. The spigelian hernial sac is identified around arcuate line and reduced completely. The peritoneum is dissected above the arcuate line to have a 5 cm margin around the hernial defect for mesh overlap. A Polypropylene mesh is used to cover the hernial defect. Mesh is fixed to anterior abdominal wall with spiral tacks .

Chapter 20

# Pelvic Hernias

## Obturator Hernia

An obturator hernia is a rare type of abdominal wall hernia (occurrence is 0.073%) in which abdominal content protrudes through the obturator foramen. Because of differences in anatomy, it is much more common in women than in men, especially multiparous and older women who have recently lost a lot of weight. The diagnosis is often made intraoperatively after presenting with bowel obstruction. A gynecologist may come across this type of hernias as a secondary finding during gynecological open surgery or laparoscopy. The Howship-Romberg sign is suggestive of an obturator hernia, exacerbated by thigh extension, medial rotation and adduction. It is characterized by lancilating pain in the medial thigh/obturator distribution, extending to the knee; caused by hernia compression of the obturator nerve. Obturator hernias are rare and a pre-operative diagnosis is exceptional, the vast majority being diagnosed at laparotomy for small bowel obstruction. Obturator hernias represent 0.073% of all. Obturator hernias are a rare cause of small-bowel obstruction, accounting for approximately 0.4% of all cases. Despite advances in modern medicine, the mortality rate of small-bowel obstructions secondary to obturator hernias remains high because of vague presenting symptoms, which make the diagnosis difficult at initial presentation and may delay treatment. Obturator hernias occur predominantly in the seventh and eighth decades of life and are 9 times more frequent in women than men. Large, wide pelvic bones and more horizontally oriented obturator canals, which are prevalent in women, are believed to predispose to the development of obturator hernias. The typical patient with an obturator hernia is a thin, elderly female. Contributing factors are prior pregnancy, chronic illness, malnutrition, and any condition that produces peritoneal weakening. More than 60% of obturator hernias occur on the right side, and about 6 to 15% of cases are bilateral. Obturator hernias have been described: between the pectineus and obturator externus muscles (most common), between the superior and middle fasciculi of the obturator externus muscle, along the course of the inferior branch of the obturator artery and nerve, and between the external and internal obturator membranes (rare).

## Howship-Romberg Sign

One of the most common and distinctive symptoms of an obturator hernia is presentation of the Howship-Romberg sign. This symptom occurs because the obturator hernia causes irritation of the obturator nerve. This symptom is identified by pain that shoots down the thigh to the groin area. This symptom is exhibited in nearly 68% of all patients. First described by Arnaud de Ronsil in 1724.

### Contents of Hernia

- Preperitoneal tissue
- Colon
- Small intestine
- Appendix
- Uterus
- Ovarian tubes
- Ovary

### Anatomy

*The obturator foramen (foramen obturatum; thyroid foramen):* The obturator foramen is a large aperture,

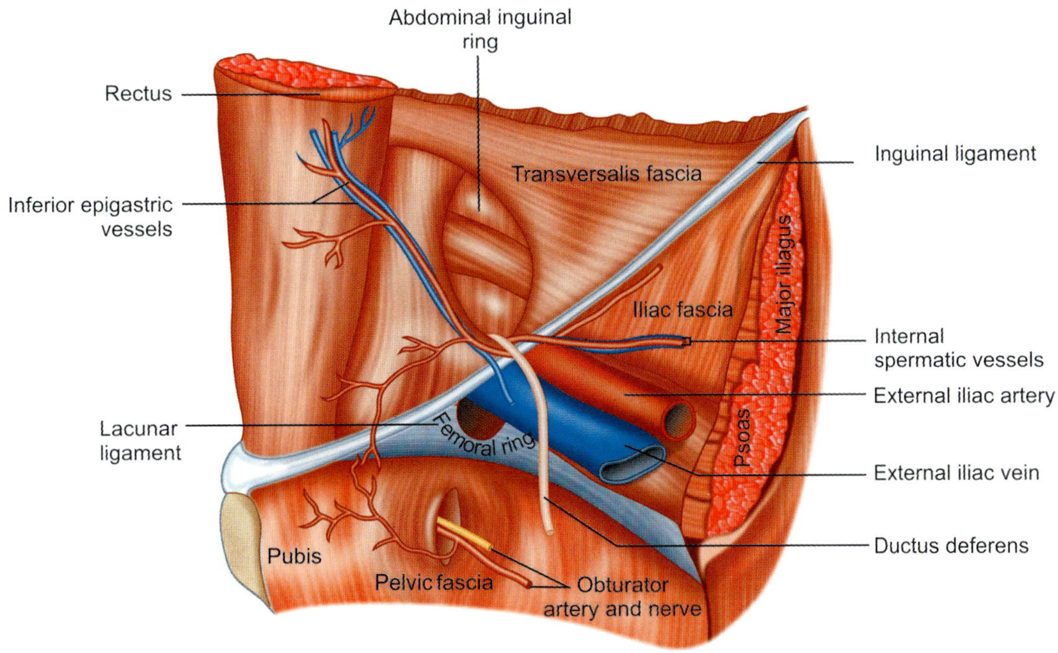


**Fig. 20.1:** Pelvic musculature

situated between the ischium and pubis. In the male it is large and of an oval form, its longest diameter slanting obliquely from before backward; in the female it is smaller, and more triangular. It is bounded by a thin, uneven margin, to which a strong membrane is attached, and presents, superiorly, a deep groove, the obturator groove, which runs from the pelvis obliquely medialward and downward. This groove is converted into a canal by a ligamentous band, a specialized part of the obturator membrane, attached to two tubercles: one, the posterior obturator tubercle, on the medial border of the ischium, just in front of the acetabular notch; the other, the anterior obturator tubercle, on the obturator crest of the superior ramus of the pubis. Through the canal the obturator vessels and nerve pass out of the pelvis (Figs 20.1 to 20.3).

Obturator hernia occurs through the obturator canal, which is 2 to 3 cm long and 1 cm wide, and contains the obturator nerve and vessels. It is bounded superiorly and laterally by the pubic bone and inferiorly by the obturator membrane. Corpus adiposum is a cushion for the obturator nerve. Obturator hernia is nine times more common in females due to their wider pelvis, more triangular obturator canal opening and greater transverse diameter. It occurs most frequently in emaciated patients aged between 70 and 90 years, and hence its nickname, "little old lady's hernia." The loss of protective preperitoneal fat and lymphatic tissue (corpus adiposum) around the obturator vessels and nerves facilitates the formation of hernia.

## Clinical Presentation

The hernia sac may follow the path of the anterior or that of the posterior division of the obturator nerve. Rarely the hernia has been found to descend beneath the superficial part of the obturator membrane. The obturator foramen is occluded by the obturator membrane which is pierced anterosuperiorly by the obturator neurovascular bundle. It is through this deficiency that a hernia occurs. presumably due to the sigmoid, these hernias are more common on the right. The layers the hernial neck passes through include:

- Obturator internus muscle fibers
- Obturator membrane
- Obturator extenus muscle fibers

The hernia will then lie superficial to obturator externis and deep and inferior to pectineus muscle.

The hernia may contain:

- No more than peritoneum filled with fluid, as seen in patients with ascites
- Small bowel (most common)
- Colon
- Appendix
- Omentum
- Meckel diverticulum
- Ovary/fallopian tube
- Uterus.

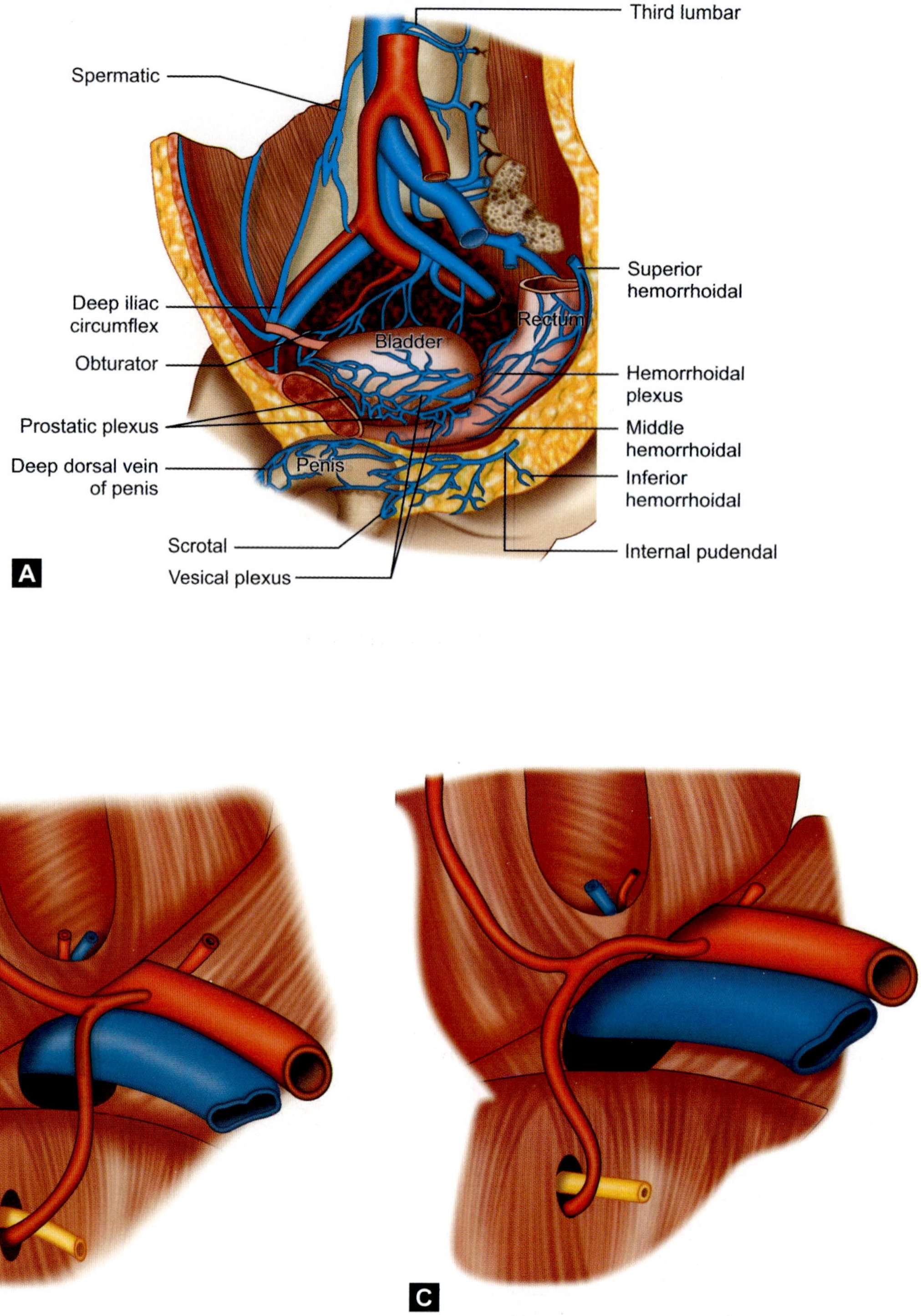


**Figs 20.2A to C:** Pelvic vasculature

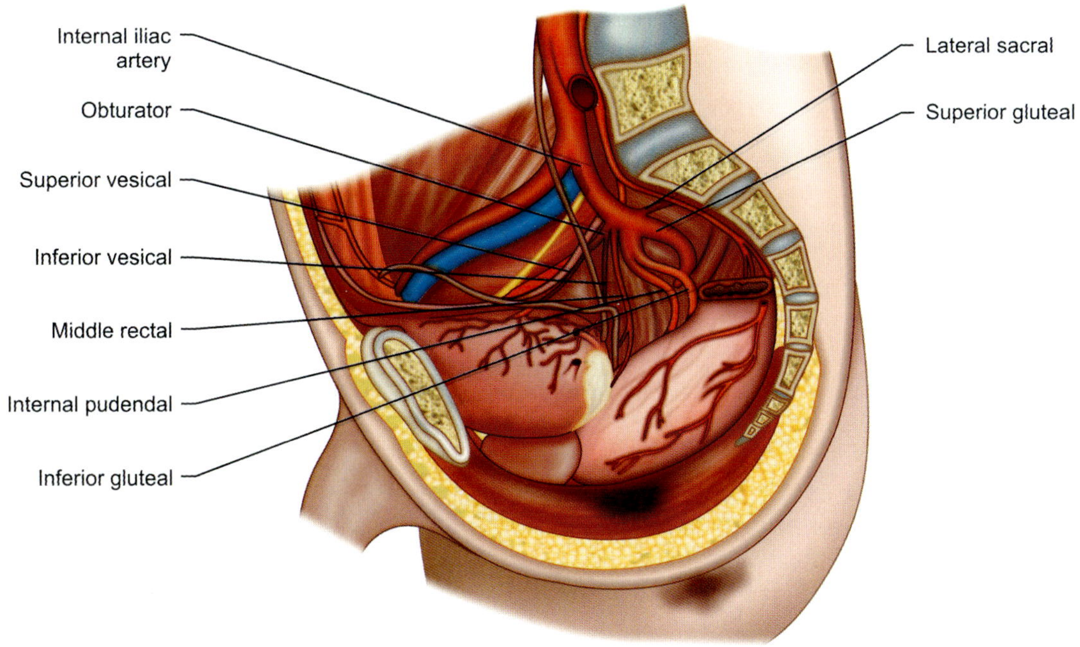


**Fig. 20.3:** Pelvic vasculature-arterial

## Demographics and Clinical Presentation

Typically these hernias occur in elderly women or in other conditions with chronically raised intra-abdominal pressure (e.g. ascites, COPD, chronic cough) and in general are asymptomatic unless they compress the obturator nerve. Howship-Romberg sign (only present in approximately half of cases) contain bowel which incarcerates/obstructs/strangulates.

### Stages of Hernia Formation

Gray et al described three anatomical stages of the formation of obturator hernia. The first stage begins with the entrance of preperitoneal fat into the pelvic orifice of the obturator canal, forming a pilot fat plug. During the second stage, a peritoneal dimple forms and progresses to form a peritoneal sac. During the third stage, symptoms are produced by herniation of the viscera into this sac (Fig. 20.4).

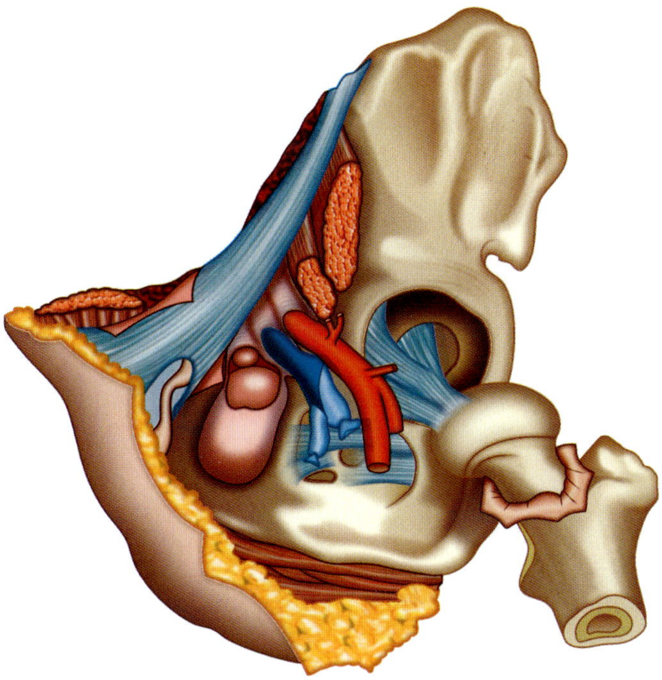

**Fig. 20.4:** Stages of pelvic hernia formation

## Radiographic Features

### Symptoms

- Groin discomfort
- Pain/paresthesia radiating to knee
- Howship-Romberg sign
- Hannington-Kiff sign
- Infarction of bowel
- Tender mass in vaginal examination
- Rheumatoid like pains in groin

### Diagnosis

#### Clinical Tests

*Howship-Romberg sign*: One of the most common and distinctive symptoms of an obturator hernia is presentation of the Howship-Romberg sign. This symptom occurs because the obturator hernia causes irritation of the obturator nerve. This symptom is identified by pain that shoots down the thigh to the groin area. This symptom is exhibited in nearly 68% of all patients. First described by Arnaud de Ronsil in 1724.

*Hannington-Kiff sign*: The Hannington-Kiff sign is a clinical sign in which there is an absent adductor reflex in the thigh in the presence of a positive patellar reflex.

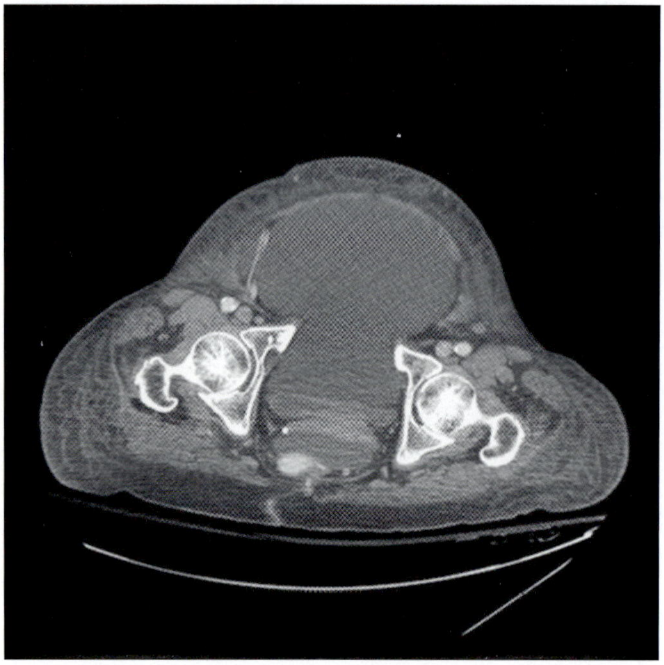

**Fig. 20.5:** CT of pelvic hernia

It occurs in patients with anobturator hernia, due to compression of the obturator nerve. The adductor reflex is elicited by tapping over either the medial epicondyle of the femur or the medial condyle of the tibia, which should cause the adductor muscles of the hip to contract, moving the leg inwards.The sign was described by John G Hannington-Kiff in 1980.

### Radiology

#### Radiographic Features

Several imaging modalities have been described to diagnose obturator hernia including plain radiographs of the abdomen, ultrasonography, and barium enema, but CT of the abdomen and pelvis is most relevant (Fig. 20.5). Recent series have reported that definite and early diagnosis of the obturator hernia can be made in 100% of cases with CT of the abdomen and pelvis (Fig. 20.7). It is minimally invasive, readily available and requires a short time. It is especially useful in the initial period when the patient has non-specific symptoms and vague clinical signs.

However, when there are clinical signs of peritonitis, laparotomy should not be delayed. There is often a delay in the diagnosis and surgical intervention of the obturator hernia because of a hesitation to operate early due to the vague symptoms and history, delayed presentation, advanced age of patients, presence of comorbidities and debilitating conditions.The diagnosis is readily made on cross-sectional imaging, CT/MRI with either fluid or bowel able to be traced along the aforementioned course to lie in the medial upper thigh.

Signs of complication including:
- Bowel obstruction
- Perforation secondary to strangulation.

## Management

Despite its rarity, a variety of operative approaches have been described to repair the obturator hernia. These include the abdominal approach, retropubic approach, obturator approach, inguinal approach and more recently, the laparoscopic approach. The abdominal approach via a low midline incision is most commonly favored, as the advantages of this approach include establishing a diagnosis, avoidance of obturator vessels, better exposure of the obturator ring, and facilitation of bowel resection, if necessary. Many authors prefer a simple closure of the hernial defect with one or more interrupted sutures as it leads to an acceptable recurrence rate of less than 10%.The defect can be closed by synthetic mesh, although a myriad to things have been used in the past, such as costal cartilage, innermost fibers of pectineus muscle, rolled-up tantalum gauze, osteoperiosteal flap from the pubic bone, free omentum and uterine fundus or round ligament.

The laparoscopic approach is an alternative to diagnose, reduce and repair an obturator hernia in selected cases. Both transabdominal and extraperitoneal approaches have been described. This approach is minimally invasive and provides some benefits for these high-risk patients like less postoperative pain, less ileus, fewer pulmonary complications and a shorter hospital stay.

Whatever the approach, the emphasis should be on rapid evaluation, adequate resuscitation and early operative intervention to reduce the morbidity and mortality.

Stepwise approach:

- On presentation; with clinical history and evaluation if the peritoneal signs are present then urgent laparotomy should be done.
- On presentation;with clinical history and evaluation if the peritoneal signs are absent then CT scanning should be done. If obturator hernia is present then urgent laparotomy or laparoscopic repair should be done.

## Surgical Anatomy

The obturator canal is a fiber osseous channel about 3 cm long and just admits the tip of the little finger. The canal lies between the obturator groove on the lower surface of superior pubic ramus and the upper border of the obturator membrane. It is hence understandable that the unyielding nature of the boundaries encourages early strangulation and also makes operative treatment mandatory. The obturator canal is normally occupied by the obturator vessels, nerve and a plug of fat. Loss of this fat in malnourished individuals predisposes to herniation into the empty canal. The obturator nerve lying above the artery is usually on the outerside of the sac. Pressure on the nerve by the contents of hernia is the basis of Howship-Romberg's sign which is pain referred to the knee by acts like straining or coughing. The position of the artery is variable. Classically it lies posterolateral to sac. Normally, there is a small anastomosis between obturator and inferior epigastric arteries. In about 10% of patients the anastomosis is enlarged, in which case the obturator artery arises from the inferior epigastric vessel. The obturator canal is wider in females which partly explains the greater incidence of hernia in females. The content is usually small intestine, rarely cecum, pelvic colon, ovary or Fallopian tube. In 50% of cases, the hernia is of Richter's type. The sac usually stops within the obturator canal but sometimes passes down into the thigh on the deep surface of pectineus, superficial to adductor longus and thus palpable in the thigh. In this situation, it has to be differentiated from femoral hernia. In obturator hernia, the superior pubic ramus can be felt above the lump without discomfort whereas in femoral hernia, the lump will be felt anterior to the superior pubic ramus.

## Surgery

### *Preoperative Hemodynamic Consideration*

If peritoneal signs like obstruction, infarction are present then appropriate fluid and electrolyte replacement is done. Nasogastric tube and urinary catheters are inserted.

## Abdominal Approach

The Trendelenburg position aids dissection. The bowel is inspected and if it dilated to the point of obstruction then retrograde milking of the contents is done.The bowel is packed safely in abdomen from pelvis by warm wet packs. Sac of the hernia is the narrow and small pouch of peritoneum lying in tight obturator canal. Stretching of the obturator canal with a finger is a safe way of releasing the strangulation. If this fails the obturator membrane is divided under vision, the division being in a downward and medial direction. Withdrawal of incarcerated intestine is easier if the hip is flexed and adducted. Rarely, an additional thigh incision medial to the femoral vein is required to push the contents up but in practice is seldom required.

After dealing with the contents, the sac is inverted using artery forceps and then transfixed and excised. But in many cases it is difficult to do this as the peritoneum of the sac is very edematous, friable and tears easily due to the tight constriction, and the delayed diagnosis. In such cases the sac is left *in situ* and the neck closed by non absorbie purse-string sutures. This suffices to prevent recurrence and additional reinforcement is done by suturing the broad ligament or prevesical fascia over the site of the obturator canal.

Approximation of the boundaries of obturator canal inlet by nonabsorbable sutures has been described but, is difficult due to the rigid nature of the boundaries. Even nylon darning to close the canal is suggested.

*Mesh repair*: The defect in the obturator membrane should be repaired using a patch of prosthetic biomaterial placed deep in peritoneum. The hernia sac is inverted and lifted. Then the adjacent peritoneum is freed from the pelvic parietes. The sac is opened and through opening a mesh is placed which should cover the defect up to 3 cm in border.This patch is left in extraperitoneal space.

Other routes of approach to the hernia are obturator and inguinal.

### Obturator Approach

In this approach an incision is made 8 to 10 cm long from a point midway between pubic tubercle and femoral artery, vertically down with the hip slightly flexed and adducted. The Saphenous vein and the external pudenal vessels are divided between ligatures, the fascia lata is incised in the line of the incision, the space between pectineus and adductor longus opened. Pectineus is cut across and dissected up to the neck. The risk to obturator vessels and nerve is high in this approach.

### Inguinal Approach

The approach is extraperitoneal, behind the horizontal ramus of pubis, dividing the external oblique in the line of its fibers. The obturator vessels and nerves can be seen better than in the obturator approach but not as well as in abdominal approach.

## Sciatic Hernia

*Sciatic hernia*: This hernia in the greater sciatic foramen most commonly presents as an uncomfortable mass in the gluteal area. Bowel obstruction may also occur. This type of hernia is only a rare cause of sciatic neuralgia. Sciatic hernias are very rare, and arc reported to be difficult to diagnose by clinical examination.

It is described in both adults and children. In adults, females are more commonly affected. Small bowel, omentum, ureter, ovary, fallopian tube, colon, bladder or Meckel's diverticulum may form the contents of the herniated sac. Various presentations of sciatic hernia could be symptoms of bowel obstruction, ureteric obstruction, pelvic pain, lower back pain or sciatica. Sciatica occurs as a result of compression of the sciatic nerve by the herniated sac (Fig. 20.6). Ureteric obstruction can occur if a ureter is included in the herniated tissue.

Sciatic hernia can also lead to abscess formation in the gluteal region, particularly after perforation of a strangulated bowel.

*Symptoms or history*: Sciatic hernias present with pain originating in the pelvis. Patients may report ipsilateral posterior thigh or buttocks pain or both. Compression of the sciatic nerve may occur, causing pain to radiate down the posterior thigh that is aggravated by dorsiflexion. Owing to a great variety of clinical presentations that depend on hernia content, this uncommon disease is difficult to diagnose. Sciatic hernia of the small bowel may lead to SBO presenting with abdominal pain and intestinal distension, while nausea and vomiting may occur when complicated with incarceration or strangulation. Hernia of the ureter or bladder into the sciatic foramen will manifest as urinary tract symptoms. Other contents like colon, omentum, fallopian tubes, ovary and Meckel diverticulum have also been described.

On rare occasions, sciatic hernias may mimic sciatica, with back pain or leg pain owing to compression of the sciatic nerve.

*Physical examination*: Sciatic hernias pass downward and may present under the lower border of the gluteus maximus muscle in the posterior medial aspect of the thigh. Sciatic hernias, however, are only rarely evident on physical examination. If the ureter herniates into the sciatic foramen it may give rise to a urographic appearance of a redundant, horizontally oriented ureter within a hernia sac that has been called a "curlicue" ureter.

Sciatic hernia is a rare condition that can lead to bowel obstruction, sciatica, pelvic pain, back pain or ureteric obstruction. Clinical diagnosis of this condition is difficult. Ultrasonography and CT are the imaging modalities commonly used to diagnose sciatic hernia, although MRI can be used in cases in which entrapment of the sciatic nerve is suspected. Magnetic resonance neurography (MRN) provides high-resolution images to demonstrate entrapment of the nerve and morphological changes in the nerve. Color Doppler can be useful in surgical planning, as it can provide information regarding bowel viability.

## Treatment

Symptomatic sciatic hernia should be surgically treated as soon as possible, as the risk of strangulation of the bowel

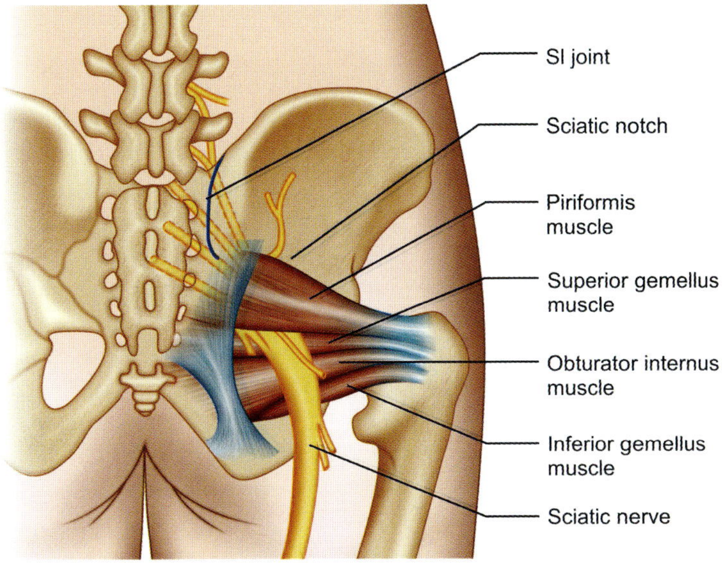


**Fig. 20.6:** Sciatic nerve

is high. A transabdominal or transgluteal approach may be used. A transabdominal approach is recommended in patients who present with bowel obstruction, especially when incarceration or strangulation is suspected; a transgluteal approach may be used when the herniated segments appear viable and reducible.

## Transabdominal Approach

- *Position of patient*: Trendelenberg
- *Incision*: Midline abdominal incision
- *Situation of hernia*: Behind broad ligament in females, anterolateral to rectum in male
- *Dissection*: Contents of the sac are gently drawn out of sac. Gentle traction is given to reduce the contents. If the neck is narrow then it is dilated mainly by fingers. If still unsuccessful , the neck may be incised without injury to nerves. Alternatively or simultaneously, the gentle pressure is given on buttocks to express the contents in abdomen. Then the forceps is inserted and the fundus is catched and invagination of the sac is done. This should be followed by opening of the fundus gaining entry into extraperitoneal space.
- *Prosthetic mesh insertion*: There is large extraperitoneal space created by blunt dissection to expose the wide area of defect. Then prosthetic mesh is pushed into the area covering the defect widely. Mesh is fixed into position by sutures.
- *Closure*: Peritoneum is closed over the mesh. Abdomen is closed in layers.

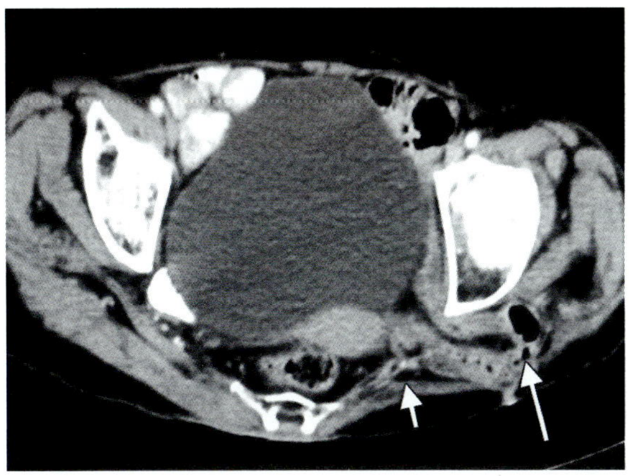

**Fig. 20.7:** CT scan of the pelvis. The long arrow shows herniation of the sigmoid colon through the greater sciatic foramen. The short arrow shows atrophy of the left gluteal muscles

## Laparoscopic Approach

Similar procedure of extraperitoneal repair is done with laparoscopy. The mesh is fixed into extraperitoneal area with tacks. The repair is almost similar to TAPP.

## Perineal Hernias

Perineal hernia is a hernia involving the perineum (pelvic floor) (Fig. 20.11). The hernia may contain fat, any part of the intestine, the rectum, or the bladder; often appears as a sudden swelling to one side (sometimes both sides) of the anus.

A common cause of perineal hernia is surgery involving the perineum. Perineal hernia can be caused also by excessive straining to defecate (tenesmus). Other causes include prostate or urinary disease, constipation, and diarrhea. Atrophy of the levator ani muscle and disease of the pudendal nerve may also contribute to a perineal hernia.

### Perineum

The perineum corresponds to the outlet of the pelvis. Its deep boundaries are—in front, the pubic arch and the arcuate ligament of the pubis; behind, the tip of the coccyx; and on either side the inferior rami of the pubis and ischium, and the sacrotuberous ligament. The space is somewhat lozenge-shaped and is limited on the surface of the body by the scrotum in front, by the buttocks behind, and laterally by the medial side of the thigh. A line drawn transversely across in front of the ischial tuberosities divides the space into two portions. The posterior contains the termination of the anal canal and is known as the anal region; the anterior, which contains the external urogenital organs, is termed the urogenital region (Fig. 20.10).

The muscles of the perineum may therefore be divided into two groups:

1. Those of the anal region.
2. Those of the urogenital region: (A) In the male; (B) In the female (Figs 20.8 and 20.9).

#### *The Muscles of the Anal Region*

| | |
|---|---|
| Corrugator | cutis ani |
| Sphincter ani | externus |
| Sphincter ani | internus |

*The superficial fascia*: The superficial fascia is very thick, areolar in texture, and contains much fat in its meshes. On either side a pad of fatty tissue extends deeply between the Levator ani and obturator internus into a space known as the ischiorectal fossa.

*The deep fascia*: The deep fascia forms the lining of the ischiorectal fossa; it comprises the anal fascia, and the portion of obturator fascia below the origin of Levator ani.

*Ischiorectal fossa (fossa ischiorectalis)*: The fossa is somewhat prismatic in shape, with its base directed to the surface of the perineum, and its apex at the line of meeting of the obturator and anal fasciae. It is bounded medially by the sphincter ani, externus and the anal fascia; laterally, by the tuberosity of the ischium and the obturator fascia; anteriorly, by the fascia of Colles covering the transversus perinei superficialis, and by the inferior fascia of the urogenital diaphragm; posteriorly, by the Gluteus maximus and the sacrotuberous ligament. Crossing the space transversely are the inferior hemorrhoidal vessels and nerves; at the back part are the perineal and perforating cutaneous branches of the pudendal plexus; while from the forepart the posterior scrotal (or labial) vessels and nerves emerge. The internal pudendal vessels and pudendal nerve lie in Alcock's canal on the lateral wall. The fossa is filled with fatty tissue across which numerous fibrous bands extend from side to side.

*The corrugator cutis ani*: Around the anus is a thin stratum of involuntary muscular fiber, which radiates from the orifice. Medially the fibers fade off into the submucous tissue, while laterally they blend with the true skin. By its contraction it raises the skin into ridges around the margin of the anus.

The sphincter ani externus (*external sphincter ani*) is a flat plane of muscular fibers, elliptical in shape and intimately adherent to the integument surrounding the margin of the anus. It measures about 8 to 10 cm. in length, from its anterior to its posterior extremity, and is about 2.5 cm broad opposite the anus. It consists of two strata, superficial and deep. The superficial, constituting the main portion of the muscle, arises from a narrow tendinous band, the anococcygeal raphe, which stretches from the tip of the coccyx to the posterior margin of the anus; it forms two flattened planes of muscular tissue, which encircle the anus and meet in front to be inserted into the central tendinous point of the perineum, joining with the transversus perinei superficialis, the levator ani, and the bulbocavernosus. The deeper portion forms a complete sphincter to the anal canal. Its fibers surround the canal, closely applied to the sphincter ani internus, and in front blend with the other muscles at the central point of the perineum. In a considerable proportion of cases the fibers decussate in front of the anus, and are continuous with the transversus perinei superficialis. Posteriorly, they are not attached to the coccyx, but are continuous with those of the opposite side behind the anal canal. The upper edge of the muscle is ill-defined, since fibers are given off from it to join the levator ani.

*Nerve supply*: A branch from the fourth sacral and twigs from the inferior hemorrhoidal branch of the pudendal supply the muscle.

*Actions*: The action of this muscle is peculiar. (1) It is, like other muscles, always in a state of tonic contraction, and having no antagonistic muscle, it keeps the anal canal and orifice closed. (2) It can be put into a condition of greater contraction under the influence of the will, so as more firmly to occlude the anal aperture, in expiratory efforts unconnected with defecation. (3) Taking its fixed point at the coccyx, it helps to fix the central point of the perineum, so that the bulbocavernosus may act from this fixed point.

The sphincter ani internus (internal sphincter ani) is a muscular ring which surrounds about 2.5 cm of the anal canal; its inferior border is in contact with, but quite separate from, the sphincter ani externus. It is about 5 mm thick, and is formed by an aggregation of the involuntary circular fibers of the intestine. Its lower border is about 6 mm from the orifice of the anus.

*Actions:* Its action is entirely involuntary. It helps the Sphincter ani externus to occlude the anal aperture and aids in the expulsion of the feces.

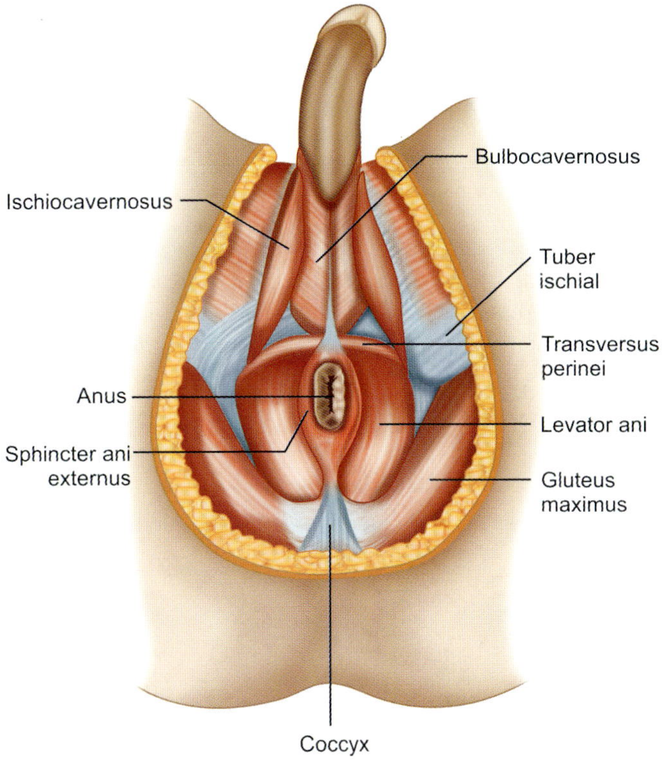


**Fig. 20.8:** Muscles of male perineum

### *The Muscles of the Urogenital Region in the Male (Fig. 20.8)*

- Transversus perinei superficialis
- Ischiocavernosus
- Bulbocavernosus
- Transversus perinei profundus
- Sphincter urethrae membranaceae.

*Superficial fascia*: The superficial fascia of this region consists of two layers, superficial and deep.

The superficial layer is thick, loose, areolar in texture, and contains in its meshes much adipose tissue, the amount of which varies in different subjects. In front, it is continuous with the dartos tunic of the scrotum; behind, with the subcutaneous areolar tissue surrounding the anus; and, on either side, with the same fascia on the inner sides of the thighs. In the middle line, it is adherent to the skin on the raphé and to the deep layer of the superficial fascia.

The deep layer of superficial fascia (fascia of Colles) is thin, aponeurotic in structure, and of considerable strength, serving to bind down the muscles of the root of the penis. It is continuous, in front, with the dartos tunic, the deep fascia of the penis, the fascia of the spermatic cord, and Scarpa's fascia upon the anterior wall of the abdomen; on either side, it is firmly attached to the margins of the rami of the pubis and ischium, lateral to the crus penis and as far back as the tuberosity of the ischium; posteriorly, it curves around the transversus perinei superficialis to join the lower margin of the inferior fascia of the urogenital diaphragm. In the middle line, it is connected with the superficial fascia and with the median septum of the bulbocavernosus. This fascia not only covers the muscles in this region, but at its back part sends upward a vertical septum from its deep surface, which separates the posterior portion of the subjacent space into two.

*The central tendinous point of the perineum*: This is a fibrous point in the middle line of the perineum, between the urethra and anus, and about 1.25 cm in front of the latter. At this point six muscles converge and are attached: viz. the sphincter ani externus, the bulbocavernosus, the two transversus perinei superficialis, and the anterior fibers of the levatores ani.

The Transversus perinei superficialis (Transversus perinei superficial transverse perineal muscle) is

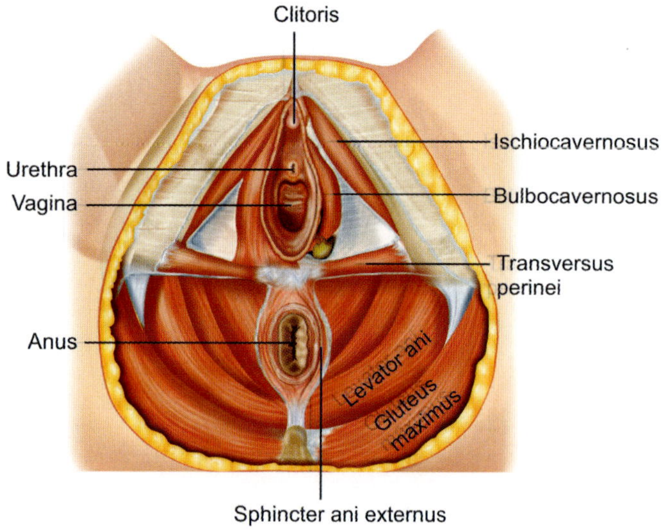


**Fig. 20.9:** Muscles of the female perineum. (Modified from a drawing by Peter Thompson)

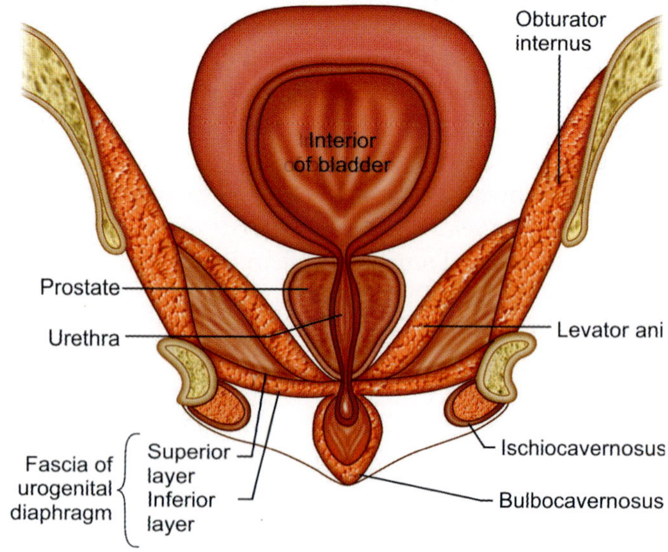


**Fig. 20.10:** Coronal section of anterior part of pelvis, through the pubic arch. Seen from in front. (Diagrammatic)

a narrow muscular slip, which passes more or less transversely across the perineal space in front of the anus. It arises by tendinous fibers from the inner and forepart of the tuberosity of the ischium, and, running medialward, is inserted into the central tendinous point of the perineum, joining in this situation with the muscle of the opposite side, with the sphincter ani externus behind, and with the bulbocavernosus in front. In some cases, the fibers of the deeper layer of the sphincter ani externus decussate in front of the anus and are continued into this muscle. Occasionally it gives off fibers, which join with the bulbocavernosus of the same side.

Variations are numerous. It may be absent or double, or insert into bulbocavernosus or external sphincter.

*Actions*: The simultaneous contraction of the two muscles serves to fix the central tendinous point of the perineum.

The bulbocavernosus (ejaculator urine; accelerator urine) is placed in the middle line of the perineum, in front of the anus. It consists of two symmetrical parts, united along the median line by a tendinous raphé. It arises from the central tendinous point of the perineum and from the median raphé in front. Its fibers diverge like the barbs of a quill-pen; the most posterior form a thin layer, which is lost on the inferior fascia of the urogenital diaphragm; the middle fibers encircle the bulb and adjacent parts, of the corpus cavernosum urethrae, and join with the fibers of the opposite side, on the upper part of the corpus cavernosum urethrae, in a strong aponeurosis; the anterior fibers, spread out over the side of the corpus cavernosum penis, to be inserted partly into that body, anterior to the ischiocavernosus, occasionally extending to the pubis, and partly ending in a tendinous expansion which covers the dorsal vessels of the penis. The latter fibers are best seen by dividing the muscle longitudinally, and reflecting it from the surface of the corpus cavernosum urethrae.

*Actions*: This muscle serves to empty the canal of the urethra, after the bladder has expelled its contents; during the greater part of the act of micturition its fibers are relaxed, and it only comes into action at the end of the process. The middle fibers are supposed by Krause to assist in the erection of the corpus cavernosum urethrae, by compressing the erectile tissue of the bulb. The anterior fibers, according to Tyrrel, also contribute to the erection of the penis by compressing the deep dorsal vein of the penis as they are inserted into, and continuous with, the fascia of the penis.

The ischiocavernosus (*erector penis*) covers the crus penis. It is an elongated muscle, broader in the middle than at either end, and situated on the lateral boundary of the perineum. It arises by tendinous and fleshy fibers from the inner surface of the tuberosity of the ischium, behind the crus penis; and from the rami of the pubis and ischium on either side of the crus. From these points fleshy fibers succeed, and end in an aponeurosis which is inserted into the sides and under surface of the crus penis.

*Action*: The ischiocavernosus compresses the crus penis, and retards the return of the blood through the veins, and thus serves to maintain the organ erect.

Between the muscles just examined a triangular space exists, bounded medially by the bulbocavernosus, laterally by the ischiocavernosus, and behind by the transversus perinei superficialis; the floor is formed by the inferior fascia of the urogenital diaphragm. Running from behind forward in the space are the posterior scrotal vessels and nerves, and the perineal branch of the posterior femoral cutaneous nerve; the transverse perineal artery courses along its posterior boundary on the transversus perinei superficialis.

*The deep fascia*: The deep fascia of the urogenital region forms an investment for the transversus perinei profundus and the sphincter urethrae membranaceae, but within it lie also the deep vessels and nerves of this part, the whole forming a transverse septum which is known as the urogenital diaphragm. From its shape it is usually termed the triangular ligament, and is stretched almost horizontally across the pubic arch, so as to close in the front part of the outlet of the pelvis. It consists of two dense membranous laminae, which are united along their posterior borders, but are separated in front by intervening structures. The superficial of these two layers, the inferior fascia of the urogenital diaphragm, is triangular in shape, and about 4 cm in depth. Its apex is directed forward, and is separated from the arcuate pubic ligament by an oval opening for the transmission of the deep dorsal vein of the penis. Its lateral margins are attached on either side to the inferior rami of the pubis and ischium, above the crus penis. Its base is directed toward the rectum, and connected to the central tendinous point of the perineum. It is continuous with the deep layer of the superficial fascia behind the transversus perinei superficialis, and with the inferior layer of the diaphragmatic part of the pelvic fascia. It is perforated, about 2.5 cm below the symphysis pubis, by the urethra, the aperture for which is circular and about 6 mm in diameter by the arteries to the bulb and the ducts of the bulbourethral glands close to the urethral orifice; by the deep arteries of the penis, one on either side close to the pubic arch and about halfway along the attached margin of the fascia; by the dorsal arteries and nerves of the penis near the apex of the fascia. Its base is also perforated by the perineal vessels and nerves, while between its apex and the arcuate pubic ligament the deep dorsal vein of the penis passes upward into the pelvis.

If the inferior fascia of the urogenital diaphragm be detached on either side, the following structures will be seen between it and the superior fascia: the deep dorsal vein of the penis; the membranous portion of the urethra; the transversus perinei profundus and sphincter urethrae membranaceae muscles; the bulbourethral glands and their ducts; the pudendal vessels and dorsal nerves of the penis; the arteries and nerves of the urethral bulb, and a plexus of veins.

The superior fascia of the urogenital diaphragm is continuous with the obturator fascia and stretches across the pubic arch. If the obturator fascia be traced medially after leaving the obturator internus muscle, it will be found attached by some of its deeper or anterior fibers to the inner margin of the pubic arch, while its superficial or posterior fibers pass over this attachment to become continuous with the superior fascia of the urogenital diaphragm. Behind, this layer of the fascia is continuous with the inferior fascia and with the fascia of Colles; in front, it is continuous with the fascial sheath of the prostate, and is fused with the inferior fascia to form the transverse ligament of the pelvis.

The transversus perinei profundus arises from the inferior rami of the ischium and runs to the median line, where it interlaces in a tendinous raphé with its fellow of the opposite side. It lies in the same plane as the sphincter urethrae membranaceae; formerly the two muscles were described together as the constrictor urethrae.

The sphincter urethrae membranaceae surrounds the whole length of the membranous portion of the urethra, and is enclosed in the fasciae of the urogenital diaphragm. Its external fibers arise from the junction of the inferior rami of the pubis and ischium to the extent of 1.25 to 2 cm and from the neighboring fasciae. They arch across the front of the urethra and bulbourethral glands, pass around the urethra, and behind it unite with the muscle of the opposite side, by means of a tendinous raphé. Its innermost fibers form a continuous circular investment for the membranous urethra.

*Nerve supply*: The perineal branch of the pudendal nerve supplies this group of muscles.

*Actions*: The muscles of both sides act together as a sphincter, compressing the membranous portion of the urethra. During the transmission of fluids, they like the bulbocavernosus, are relaxed, and only come into action at the end of the process to eject the last drops of the fluid.

### *The Muscles of the Urogenital Region in the Female (See Fig. 20.9)*

- Transversus perinei superficialis.
- Ischiocavernosus.
- Bulbocavernosus.
- Transversus perinei profundus.
- Sphincter urethrae membranaceae.

The transversus perinei superficialis (transversus perinei; superficial transverse perineal muscle) in the female is a narrow muscular slip, which arises by a small tendon from the inner and forepart of the tuberosity of the ischium, and is inserted into the central tendinous point of the perineum, joining in this situation with the muscle of the opposite side, the sphincter ani externus behind, and the bulbocavernosus in front.

*Action*: The simultaneous contraction of the two muscles serves to fix the central tendinous point of the perineum.

The bulbocavernosus (sphincter vagina) surrounds the orifice of the vagina. It covers the lateral parts of the vestibular bulbs, and is attached posteriorly to the central tendinous point of the perineum, where it blends with the sphincter ani externus. Its fibers pass forward on either side of the vagina to be inserted into the corpora cavernosa clitoridis, a fasciculus crossing over the body of the organ so as to compress the deep dorsal vein.

*Actions*: The bulbocavernosus diminishes the orifice of the vagina. The anterior fibers contribute to the erection of the clitoris, as they are inserted into and are continuous with the fascia of the clitoris, compressing the deep dorsal vein during the contraction of the muscle.

The ischiocavernosus (erector clitoridis) is smaller than the corresponding muscle in the male. It covers the unattached surface of the crus clitoridis. It is an elongated muscle, broader at the middle than at either end, and situated on the side of the lateral boundary of the perineum. It arises by tendinous and fleshy fibers from the inner surface of the tuberosity of the ischium, behind the crus clitoridis; from the surface of the crus; and from the adjacent portion of the ramus of the ischium. From these points fleshy fibers succeed, and end in an aponeurosis, which is inserted into the sides and under surface of the crus clitoridis.

*Actions*: The ischiocavernosus compresses, the crus clitoridis and retards the return of blood through the veins, and thus serves to maintain the organ erect.

The fascia of the urogenital diaphragm in the female is not so strong as in the male. It is attached to the public arch, its apex being connected with the arcuate pubic ligament. It is divided in the middle line by the aperture of the vagina, with the external coat of which it becomes blended, and in front of this is perforated by the urethra. Its posterior border is continuous, as in the male, with the deep layer of the superficial fascia around the transversus perinei superficialis.

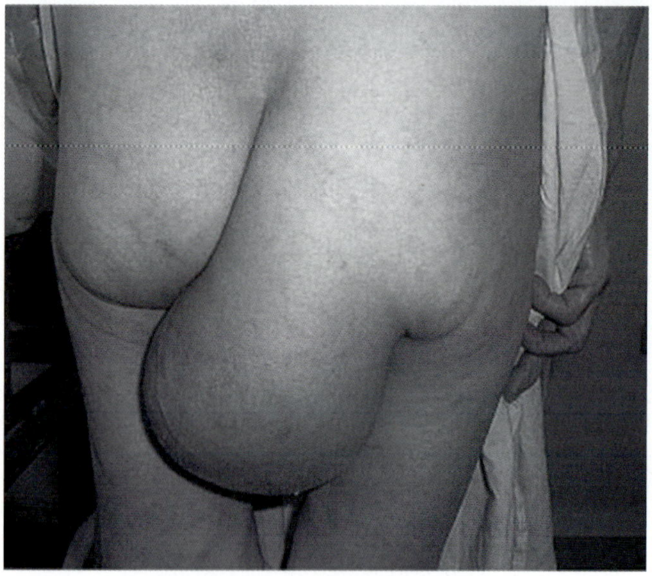

**Fig. 20.11:** Perineal hernias

Like the corresponding fascia in the male, it consists of two layers, between which are to be found the following structures: the deep dorsal vein of the clitoris, a portion of the urethra and the constrictor urethra muscle, the larger vestibular glands and their ducts; the internal pudendal vessels and the dorsal nerves of the clitoris; the arteries and nerves of the bulbi vestibuli, and a plexus of veins.

The transversus perinei profundus arises from the inferior rami of the ischium and runs across to the side of the vagina. The sphincter urethrae membranaceae (constrictor urethrae), like the corresponding muscle on the male, consists of external and internal fibers. The external fibers arise on either side from the margin of the inferior ramus of the pubis. They are directed across the pubic arch in front of the urethra, and pass around it to blend with the muscular fibers of the opposite side, between the urethra and vagina. The innermost fibers encircle the lower end of the urethra.

*Nerve supply*: The muscles of this group are supplied by the perineal branch of the pudendal.

Spontaneous development of perineal hernias is a very rare condition and many techniques have been described for repairing the pelvic floor defect.

*Occurrence*: Posterior primary perineal hernias are very unusual findings and they may be congenital or acquired. They occur most commonly between the ages of 40 and 60 years and are five times more common in females than in males, due to the broader female pelvis and attenuation of the pelvic floor during pregnancy.

## Clinical Investigations

Signs and symptoms are confined to complaints of a mass in the perineum or buttock, which may cause some discomfort when sitting. The classic signs of hernia, such as perineal bulging, size that varies when abdominal pressure is applied, tympanites and peristalsis, allow diagnosis to be made. However, perineal hernias may be mistaken for other diseases of the perineum and adjacent organs, such as lipomas, fibromas, rectocele, cystocele and prolapse of the rectum. One particular condition from which perineal hernias must be distinguished is sciatic hernia. However, when a perineal hernia is reduced, the direction of reduction together with the palpable defect in the pelvic floor identifies the hernia as perineal rather than sciatic.

*Investigations*: Radiographic demonstration of such hernias via plain film or barium had already been reported before the advent of CT/MRI scanning (Figs 20.12 and 20.13). They can show that the herniation of the sigmoid colon is adjacent to the distal rectum and going into the buttock. In the normal pelvis, CT scans are adequate to display the muscle anatomy of the pelvic floor, thereby allowing the identification of any muscle perineal defect.

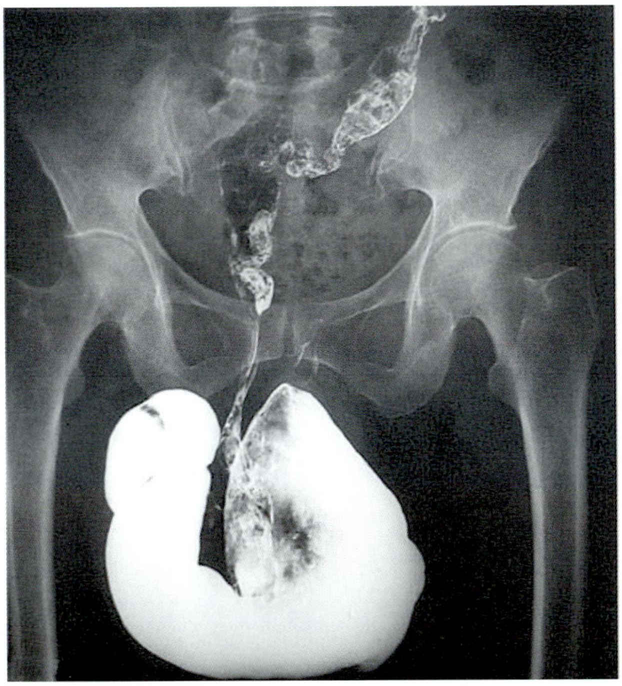

**Fig. 20.12:** Barium enema shows a perineal hernia with loop of sigmoid colon in sac

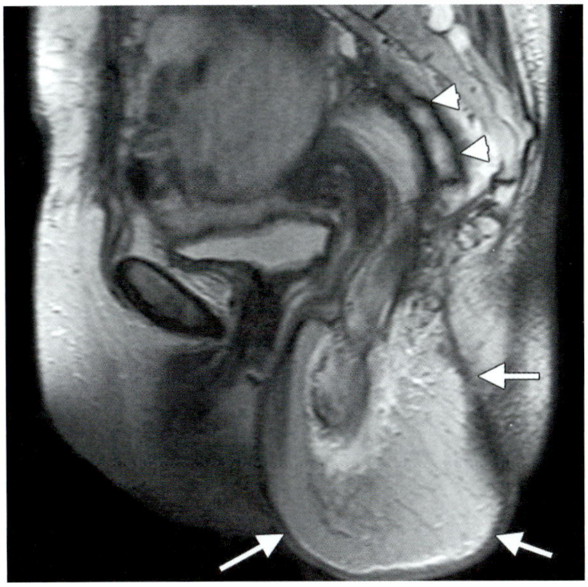

**Fig. 20.13:** MRI perineal hernias

## Treatment

Simple closure of the pelvic defect by bringing together the levator ani muscles along the midline is occasionally feasible, the pelvic floor is usually deficient and requires support using autogenous or prosthetic materials.

The perineal approach is usually difficult in the repair of perineal hernias, unless these are accompanied by an abdominal access.

A new laparoscopic approach for repairing postoperative perineal hernias, involving the use of synthetic mesh, has recently been reported and regarded as safe and effective.

Surgical repair can be done either through a transabdominal approach or transperineally.

# INDEX

**Page numbers followed by *f* refer to figure and *t* refer to table**